THE

CHOLESTEROL

HOAX

Sherry A. Rogers, M.D.

Sand Key Company, Inc.
PO Box 19252
Sarasota, FL 34276

Handwritten annotations:

↑ Cholesterol is merely ↑ of toxicity. We should

er—

cholesterol is responsible for 21

cholesterol drugs — accelerate aging & usher in disease.
- you must check. Liver enzymes, "Danger anyone"
- 1leads to intestinal inflamation + poor absorption of nutrients
- it works by poisoning a Liver enzyme that makes Cholesterol & CoQ10 — CHF. MI, exhaustion, HTN, CA

We need chol for our brain + sex hormones & libido

We need chol in the cell membrane to properly release cytokines, to kill CA cells.

↑ CA rates, as chol depletes CoQ10, Vit E + Betacarotene, all help reverse CA

& chol., damages brain receptors where happy hormones fit to make us feel terrific.

The Cholesterol Hoax

Sherry A Rogers, M.D.

Copyright © 2008 by Sand Key Company, Inc.

Sand Key Company, Inc.
PO Box 19252
Sarasota, FL 34276

1-800-846-6687
www.prestigepublishing.com

Library of Congress Control Number: 2007942760

ISBN: 978-1-887202-06-0

Printed in the United States of America

Table of Contents

Chapter III
Fracturing the Myths About Cholesterol 91

Chapter V
You Can Catch a Heart Attack: The Infection Connection 210

Chapter VI
The Nutrient Connection 240

Chapter VII
The Toxic Connection   **294**

Chapter VIII
Creating Your Cholesterol Reversing Plan and More   347

Chapter IX
Resources   381

Index   407

Dedication

We have slept in our Caribbean tree house
And the cornfield by the pond,
In the milk house at the barn
And in French castles, of which we're fond.

From the office fold-out couch,
To the romantic bungalow on the Key,
On the sailboat in New England,
I have slept embraced by *Thee*.

From Rome to that floor in Shanghai,
Sometimes we didn't have a bed.
From Melbourne to the Yangtze,
Each place I've laid my head.

Each night has become my favorite night,
With which no other could compare.
The reason is plain and simple:
It's because you, *my Precious,* were always there.

I dedicate not only this book, but also my whole life to God's most precious earthly gift to me, *Luscious*, who has grown more luscious every day for over 38 phenomenally blessed years.

i

About the author: Sherry A. Rogers, M.D., is board certified by the American Board of Family Practice, board certified by the American Board of Environmental Medicine, a Fellow of the American College of Allergy, Asthma and Immunology and a Fellow of the American College of Nutrition. She has been in solo private practice in environmental medicine for over 38 years in Syracuse, NY where she sees patients form all over the world. She has lectured at Oxford and in 6 countries where she has taught well over 100 physician courses, has published over a dozen books including the landmark book *Detoxify or Die* (prestigepublishing.com), 20 scientific papers, textbook chapters, was environmental medicine editor for *Internal Medicine World Report*, received the American Academy of Environmental Medicine Rinkle Teaching Award for Teaching Excellence, has a referenced newsletter for 19 years, a non–patient consulting service, a lay and professional lecture service, is the guest on over 100 radio shows a year, and more.

Foreword

I had to chuckle when I recently discovered a website created by AstraZeneca Pharmaceutical, the manufacturer of Crestor. This widely touted statin has been hailed as a wonder drug that dramatically decreased cholesterol levels. Yet their very own website offers the following caveat: "Crestor has not been determined to prevent heart disease, heart attack, or strokes." Well there you have it. Kudos to AstraZeneca for being so honest, at least about that part of it!

As Dr. Rogers so thoroughly shows, cholesterol never was a deficiency of statin drugs. Their hidden dangers are exposed, and then the reader is instructed in the much more healthful non-prescription alternatives. Next she explores scores of myths about cholesterol, complete with the scientific evidence. The next five chapters are devoted to showing how to identify much more serious risks of heart death than cholesterol and how to correct them. There is nothing else like it. How it would change the face of medicine, law and insurance coverage if read by every physician and layperson. But more important is the impact on the individual's health and longevity.

I have to admit that as a Harvard-trained physician, I was at first filled with incredulity. But once I settled into the book, and dispensed with my ill-founded prejudices, I came to appreciate that *The Cholesterol Hoax* is groundbreaking, full of well-kept medical secrets and clinical wisdom to empower the reader as never before, regardless of their cholesterol level. Bravo to Dr. Rogers for being so passionate in her quest for true healing, not merely bludgeoning a symptom with the latest side effect-ridden drug, and then providing the instruction the health-conscious consumer needs in order to make a life-saving difference. It is bound to become a classic and deserves to be read and reread, by physician and lay alike.

Martha Stark, M.D.
Boston MA, 2008
Clinical Instructor in Psychiatry, Harvard Medical School
Faculty, The Center for Psychoanalytic Studies, Massachusetts General Hospital, Harvard Medical School
Faculty, Continuing Education Program, Department of Psychiatry, Beth Israel Deaconess Medical Center, Harvard Medical School
Faculty, Massachusetts Institute for Psychoanalysis
Author of *Working With Resistance, Primer on Working with Resistance*, and *Modes of Therapeutic Action*

iii

Introduction

This book may herald one of the most important steps you've ever taken toward your health, **even if you don't have high cholesterol**. Folks who know me know that I never write a book just limited to the disease on the cover. I always write with **the plan to empower everyone toward better health,** and regardless of which end of the spectrum they are on. So whether your cholesterol is sky high or your Ultrafast Heart Scan calcium score is in the dangerous level or you are healthy or do not even have high cholesterol, this book is loaded with information you need to make yourself healthier and stay that way. Whether you are on death's doorstep or are exceedingly healthy or just want to have that athlete's edge, there is enormous empowerment in store for you.

And of course, if you've been told you have high cholesterol, you'll find the answers you've been looking for (and many you didn't even know existed) in here, complete with the scientific backup, so that you can feel comfortable sharing it with your physician. I'll begin by showing you . . .

1. The hidden dangers of high cholesterol prescription medications which go far beyond depression, heart disease, cancer, impotency, brain loss, nerve damage, kidney and liver death, amnesia, Alzheimer's, suicide or painful death by rhabdomyolysis. For starters, they deplete your body of vitamins and minerals and fatty acids needed to slow aging and stave off cancer and heart disease.

2. How drugs guarantee you will develop other illnesses quicker, which magically require even more drugs. For once you step onto that medication merry-go-round and take even one drug, it guarantees you'll tumble into an avalanche of drugs.

3. But don't worry, because I'll give you many alternatives for lowering your cholesterol that are safer, cheaper, oftentimes more effective, and non-prescription to choose from.

4. Then we will crack the many myths that cholesterol propaganda has generated and give you the real scoop. For starters,

- Cholesterol is not the cause of arteriosclerosis and is not dangerous until it is oxidized, and that's easily prevented, without drugs.
- Cholesterol is absolutely essential in the body for preventing the brain loss of Alzheimer's.
- Cholesterol is crucial in fighting off cancer, building our stress and sex hormones, making bile for digestion and detoxification, and protecting the body against aging and depression, as just a few examples.

Together we will crack many more myths about cholesterol. For example:

- Cholesterol is not the main cause of heart attacks.
- In fact, half the people who have a heart attack never had high cholesterol.
- But they did have a normal or low "good cholesterol" or HDL. It needs to be much higher than you have been told.
- Furthermore, there are many other parameters such as elevated hsCRP, fibrinogen, homocysteine and more that are much more dangerous risk factors than cholesterol. But because one brand of cholesterol drug alone brings in over $10 billion a year (more than five times the FDA annual budget), cholesterol is stressed.
- And you'll learn why you should ignore that advice that cholesterol-lowering drugs should be taken even if you don't have high cholesterol to protect against heart disease.

5. The good news is that most of these more dangerous parameters are easily cured with non-prescription, inexpensive nutrients and phytonutrients.

6. And you will be happy to learn that you don't need to torture yourself with a low cholesterol diet; the body desperately needs cholesterol. Besides that, **the liver makes 80% of the cholesterol, regardless of your diet.** But there is one food additive hidden in most processed and fast foods that should be eliminated because it is a major cause of high cholesterol. Harvard researchers have shown for decades it makes the body go berserk in revving up its cholesterol production. But the FDA for some reason has allowed food manufacturers to say there is none on the label when the food contains a damaging 500 mg of trans fats per miniscule half cup serving!

7. Then for the fun part. I want to help you find the real underlying causes of your high cholesterol so that you can actually cure it. You do not need to take anything "forever". Sometimes the cause is a hidden tooth infection that dentists are unable to find on x-ray, or an asymptomatic very common stomach bug that migrates through the blood to drill holes in the coronaries. This causes the body to respond by making cholesterol to patch up the damage.

I'll also show you how everyday, unavoidably ubiquitous pollutants in our air, food, and water damage the ability of the body to properly metabolize cholesterol. For example, plasticizers or phthalates from water and other beverage bottles leach out plastics that then sit in your cells to damage their ability to properly metabolize cholesterol. Lots of other everyday pollutants that are commonly found in all human bodies, like Teflon from your frying pan or mercury from fish and dental fillings can also damage your cholesterol chemistry. And I'll give you the entire scientific backup for everything I say because I want you to be armed with the truth. For **high cholesterol is merely the smoke detector. It is a messenger warning of raging toxicity. We should not shoot the messenger when we can fix and correct what it is warning us about.**

The great news is that by correcting the damage caused by these pollutants and getting them out of the body, we simultaneously turn back the hands of time. It's a win-win situation, because as you learn to correct your cholesterol once and for all, you simultaneously will slow down aging and most likely cure a lot of other conditions that you thought you just had to learn to live with. In other words, **having high cholesterol is a blessing because you never would have found this book and begun to learn how to not only normalize your cholesterol, but also improve your health in a multitude of even more important ways.**

Admittedly there is more in here than the average person needs. But since your biochemistry and your medical history are unique, no one knows just how much you will need to do in order to become well. And bear in mind that **no one thing is appropriate for everyone.** On the flip side, there is something for everyone. You will also find some things repeated. That is not because I forgot or think you did, but because that is one way we learned in medical school. Former facts were brought to a different light as we learned new things and it helped to collate them for an even deeper understanding. Also I am an admitted reference junkie. Because I teach physician courses I want the scientific back up for everything. But if I provided a reference after each sentence, it would not only make reading sheer drudgery, but the vastly increased weight of the book would discourage many from ever picking it up. I have put author names of scientific papers in parentheses for papers that are particularly important or that I have not referenced elsewhere. But there is not a name after each sentence. Never the less, the references are either in this book or in our other books or in our referenced monthly newsletters of 18 years.

Even if you're marvelously healthy, this book will empower you to stay that way and even reach improved levels of wellness. The fact is you will be brought to new levels of knowledge that exceed what 90% of physicians know. And you must know this in order to heal yourself, since **no one can heal you except you.**

So do I think that I'm smarter than 90% of physicians? Absolutely not. As the oldest of eight children, I knew there was no money for college, much less medical school (much less for a female in the 60's). Consequently, I studied to win scholarships and worked through high school, college and medical school. Even though I was never at the head of my class, having had over 20 incurable diagnoses was an absolute blessing. It showed me that the years of medical school training were useless if I was going to actually cure any disease. Drugs are great for emergencies or acute situations, but for chronic ongoing medical problems they are dangerous, for they guarantee **the sick will get sicker quicker** and "need' exponentially more drugs.

Then why are prescription drugs the mainstay of medical practice? Why does every disease become an automatic deficiency of the latest medication? Why does every symptom dictate a lifetime sentencing to drug dependency? Power and money. For example, the famed *New England Journal of Medicine* shows us that over 87% of the physicians who create the rules or recipes for all physicians to follow, called practice guidelines, are on the payroll of or have received money from the pharmaceutical industry. There's big money in a lifetime of drugs, while there's no money in health.

We have a spectrum of readers using this book. If you are completely new to empowerment medicine, where you actually learn to find causes and cures of your symptoms so that they do not become a lifetime sentencing to some overpriced and side effect-ridden drug, **welcome to the first day of the rest of your life.** Some of you readers are admittedly at much higher levels of comprehension, because you have followed our monthly newsletter for years and read several of the books. I refuse to "dumb it down", but insist on continually bringing you to higher levels of health control. So for newcomers, if parts overwhelm you, just keep plowing through because you'll surprise yourself at how much you learn. I want you to see how having **high cholesterol was a blessing in disguise**, leading you now to an understanding of how to heal diseased and aging blood vessels and the organs that depend upon them, and how to bring your body to new levels of wellness. After 38 years in medicine, I still find that empowering folks from all walks of life to learn how to heal their bodies without drugs is most fascinating.

You will learn how common non-prescription medicines can triple your heart attack risk. And you'll learn how several easy tests (that are rarely checked) actually predict who will have a heart attack in the next 5 years. But you can become an expert in learning how to harness and even reverse the damage.

Most people spend more time choosing a car or knowing the scores of their favorite teams than they invest in learning how to control their health. We only have one body, so we need to become experts in its repair so that it performs beyond our wildest expectations for a lifetime.

I can't wait to empower you! So let's get started.

Chapter I

Cholesterol-Lowering Drugs Can Kill You

Introduction

So you've been told that you have high cholesterol and need to take a cholesterol-lowering medication for the rest of your life. If you don't, cholesterol will glue itself to the lining of your heart blood vessels and plug them up. You'll die of a sudden heart attack or stroke.

But this is wrong. Cholesterol by itself, naked, is not the villain and does not cause heart attacks. Furthermore, controlling your cholesterol does not guarantee you won't have a deadly heart attack. But taking cholesterol-lowering medications does guarantee you will have an avalanche of new symptoms, which can include fatal heart disease. And did you know that half the folks who have a heart attack never even had high cholesterol? As we move along I'll give you the scientific proof for every statement, all from leading conventional medical journals. For I want you to know more about heart health than most physicians you will ever see. After all, it is your heart, and you have total responsibility for its well-being. The encouraging part is you have more control over your heart health and longevity than any physician. **Health cannot be bought, but luckily, it can be taught.**

Certainly heart attacks are epidemic. **Every half minute a person dies of a heart attack in United States, making heart attack the number one cause of death for adults in the U.S.** (*National Heart, Lung and Blood Institute Fact Book: Fiscal Year 1995.* Bethesda Maryland, US Department of Health and Human Services, March 1996: 30-52. Monograph). Most women over 50 years of age think heart disease doesn't affect them, and that their biggest health threat is breast cancer. But a woman's chances of dying of breast cancer are 2.8% versus the staggering 31% probability of dying of heart disease. **The chance of a woman over 50 having a heart attack is more than ten times higher than getting a breast cancer** (Tecee). Heart disease kills three out of every five people. **But only half the people who have a heart attack had high cholesterol** (Rubins). And for those taking cholesterol-lowering medications, these drugs can actually hurry their demise and definitely usher in new and seemingly unrelated diseases. Let's look at the side effects of the cholesterol-lowering drugs.

The Major Cholesterol-Lowering Drugs, Statins

Cholesterol-lowering drugs invite accelerated aging and disease. Once I show you what they do, I doubt you'll ever take another one again. And as I'll show you, there are many healthier alternatives. Or you may choose to just plain learn how to get rid of your high cholesterol, as I'll show you in subsequent chapters, so you will not have to take any remedy forever.

When you look at the number of adults who are taking the statin cholesterol-lowering drugs, clearly we will never run out of uninformed people who are looking for an easy way out. Although over 15 million people already take the cholesterol-lowering drugs in the United States, many policymakers want to extend that to 36 million more adults, including those who don't even have high cholesterol. They want folks to use them prophylactically, and currently children are the next market target, but more on all of this later.

Let's look at Lipitor, the number one prescribed cholesterol-lowering drug. It is so profitable that **Lipitor brings in well over $10 billion a year, which is over five times the annual budget of the entire FDA.** In fact Lipitor is the best selling drug in the history of the world to date, with annual sales increasing 23% in some fiscal periods, causing Pfizer's net income to quadruple (Hensley). Following are some of the common generic names as well as the brand names of cholesterol-lowering statin drugs and of course, there are new ones continually emerging as the patents run out on the old ones. I'll be telling you more about their details and dangers.

Statin Drugs

Brand name	Generic name
Lipitor	atorvastatin
Mevacor	lovastatin
Pravochol	pravastatin
Zocor	simvastatin
Lescol	fluvastatin
Crestor	rosuastatin
Altocor	lovastatin extended release
Pravigard	pravastatin with buffered aspirin
Advicor	lovastatin plus extended release niacin
Baycol	(withdrawn, too dangerous) cerivastatin

Right now, Lipitor, Zocor, Lescol, Pravachol, Advicor, Mevacor, and the generic lovastatin are the main statin cholesterol-lowering prescription drugs. They average well over $100 a month (some more than quadruple that) and are loaded with side effects, many of which people have died from. In fact the last statin drug to be pulled off the market (Baycol) had over 8,400 law suits against it and now they're not sure if the German company Bayer AG has enough money to cover all of these legal cases. Over 100 people died and many more got serious muscle disease with extreme pain and weakness (called rhabdomyolysis).

When you are on any statin drug, it is recommended that you check your liver enzymes monthly, which further adds to the expense and alerts you that this is dangerous medicine. And you can add to the list of side effects many other symptoms like seemingly harmless bloating, diarrhea, and constipation, which invariably lead to intestinal inflammation and poor absorption of nutrients, which in turn leads to an avalanche of diseases, and all for a bargain of over $1200 a year! But you will learn here that statin dangers don't stop there. They trigger Alzheimer's and cancer. So let's make sure you know about the major problems with the cholesterol-lowering statin drugs.

The Lowdown on Cholesterol-Lowering Drugs

(1) **Statin drugs work by poisoning a liver enzyme that makes cholesterol.** When the body makes cholesterol, it uses many pathways but one major bottleneck is a rate-limiting enzyme in the liver called **HMG COA reductase (3-hydroxyl-3-methylglutaryl-coenzyme A reductase)**. The *statin category of cholesterol-lowering prescription medications all work by turning off or poisoning this main enzyme that the liver uses to make cholesterol.* It sounds pretty good, doesn't it? But I guess prescribing physicians forgot their physiology and biochemistry, because **we need cholesterol to keep the brain from aging**. Clearly this drug class will bring on a lot more Alzheimer's and senility, which are already soaring to unprecedented levels. More on the amnesia, depression, nerve, heart and muscle damage and suicide that statins bring on later.

(2) Furthermore, **turning off cholesterol production fuels the Viagra epidemic, because you need cholesterol to make your sex hormones** like testosterone, estrogen and progesterone. Without cholesterol you also get impotency and rock bottom libido. So no wonder poor libido is a side effect of statin drugs. You also need cholesterol for other hormones, like the stress hormones of the adrenal gland, so there will be more fatigue or downright exhaustion, irritability, road rage, and hostile aggression. Another adrenal hormone also needed for healthy libido, DHEA, is made from cholesterol (for folks wanting to cure libido problems, refer to *The High Blood Pressure Hoax*). The body also uses cholesterol to make another hormone that is inappropriately called vitamin D, not only necessary for strong bones but also for the prevention of

osteoporosis, diabetes, multiple sclerosis, depression, cancer, psoriasis, and arteriosclerosis.

(3) And **we need cholesterol in the cell membranes** so that they can properly release **cytokines,** like tumor necrosis factor. Only healthy cell membranes with sufficient cholesterol can release chemicals that we make inside of our cells **to kill cancer cells.** In addition, you need cholesterol for every cell membrane receptor site. These docking sites or "knobs" allow hormones to actually turn on the cells' functions. Without sufficient cholesterol in the cell membranes, you can pour on hormones, even prescription substitutes, but they won't work, because their docking sites are deformed. For example, the vitamin D receptor has to be healthy enough to accept vitamin D and allow it to turn on redifferentiation, a process that makes cancer cells go back to being normal cells. No wonder studies show that there's a **higher cancer rate among people taking cholesterol-lowering drugs** (Newman).

(4) If these side effects were not enough, the same enzyme that statin drugs inhibit or poison, HMG COA reductase, is used by the body to make the fat-soluble vitamin, coenzyme Q10. This vitamin-like substance is crucial for life! By poisoning the body's production of CoQ10, **statin drugs actually create a life-threatening coenzyme Q10 deficiency**. In people uninformed enough to take the statin drugs (rather than find what's broken and fix it, as you will learn), they slowly avalanche into a host of diseases caused by a silent deficiency of this important vitamin-like nutrient, CoQ10. With low CoQ10 from the statin drugs, you can usher in congestive heart failure, which kills more people each year than cancer and kills more quickly than cancer does. The average survival when you get cancer is 6 years, while the average survival when you get diagnosed with congestive heart failure is 5 years. But CoQ10 deficiency doesn't stop there.

To prescribe a statin drug without boosting your CoQ10 should be illegal. For **CoQ10 deficiency often causes fatal cardiomyopa-**

thy, heart attack, congestive heart failure, exhaustion, cancer, myopathy (muscle diseases), fibromyalgia, depression resistant to anti-depressants, high blood pressure, gum disease and tooth loss, hair loss, liver disease, sudden complete memory loss or amnesia, cataracts, angina, folic acid deficiency, damaged cell membranes, fatigue, accelerated aging and much more (Bliznakov, Rao, Folkers, Thompson, Hebert, Newman, Westphal).

In fact, CoQ10 deficiency not only accelerates getting a variety of diseases, but a **low CoQ10 level predicts that you can die within 6 months** (Jameson). A physician who would merely prescribe a statin drug and turn you lose without even measuring your CoQ10, much less supplementing it, is dangerously irresponsible and shows lack of scientific knowledge of the mechanism of action of the very drug he is authorized to prescribe. But the physician is not alone in his ignorance, for the authoritative specialists who dictate the practice guidelines or rules of medicine for doctors don't recommend CoQ10 either. Could that have anything to do with the fact that was published in *The New England Journal of Medicine* in 2002 (Choudhry) showing that over 87% of these "experts' who dictate the rules of medical practice are financially linked to the pharmaceutical industry? For when you finally get one or more of the diseases from your statin drug killing off your CoQ10, you will invariably have to buy more drugs for your new symptoms. And this is just a glimpse: the power of the pharmaceutical industry over medical practice is staggering, as physicians, prestigious medical journal editors and congressmen have documented (Cauchon, Cohen, Haley, Angell, Rogers).

Why is CoQ10 so important? For starters, CoQ10 has proven necessary to stop some of the dangerous side effects of chemotherapy in cancer patients and has even *caused cancer progression to come to a screeching halt, even reversing or causing a melting away of tumors* (Lockwood). Of course, that means it was the last part of an enormous total load, or the proverbial last straw to unload from

6

the camels back so the patient could now stand on all fours again. *I never want you to come away with the idea that any nutrient is a solo act by itself.* They all work in concert. It is only when they are the last straw that they become the dramatic cases you hear about. Clearly, if CoQ10 has reversed some end-stage cancers, and being deficient is like fertilizer for cancer, **you definitely do not want to be on a statin drug if you have (or ever had) cancer**.

Meanwhile, if you're already on one of the statin drugs, **start CoQ10 today** and keep it up until you read further to identify the cause and cure of your high cholesterol. For **without enough CoQ10, you are a sitting duck for everything from heart attacks to cancer.** And even if you have nothing wrong with you and feel fine, a trial of one bottle may leave you thinking more clearly or with energy you didn't even know you were missing.

(5) **Cholesterol drugs axe nutrients and invite cancer!** Not only do the statin drugs lower the CoQ10, they deplete your vitamin E (alpha-tocopherol) and vitamin A precursor, beta-carotene, by as much as 22%. These three vitamins are necessary to not only prevent heart attacks, but cancer. That is one of many reasons why **statin drug-takers also have a higher rate of cancer** (Newman). Furthermore, beta-carotene is also crucial in reversing cancers once they have started. As Harvard researchers have shown, high doses of beta-carotene make the cancer gene go back to normal and make cancer cells commit suicide! No drug has this type of power. That is one reason the cancer program (using all non-prescription items) spelled out in *Wellness Against All Odds* is so healing (prestigepublishing.com or 1-800-846-6687).

No wonder studies show that there's a **higher cancer rate among people taking cholesterol-lowering drugs, for they deplete not only CoQ10, but also vitamin E and beta-carotene.** In one study, the common cholesterol lowering-drug simvastatin (Zocor) lowered vitamin E (alpha-tocopherol) 16.2%, beta-carotene 19.5%

and CoQ10 (ubiquinol-10) by 22%. If that were not enough, it also lowered the insulin levels 13.2 % (Jula). These deficiencies not only contribute to cancer but heart death, Alzheimer's, diabetes, and accelerated degeneration. Not a good choice when there are so many other ways to safely normalize cholesterol, as you will learn.

(6) Statin drugs damage the good effect of vitamin E. Many docs are prescribing cholesterol-lowering drugs like Lipitor for people who do not even have high cholesterol. They do it for the antioxidant effect. But ironically, **Lipitor decreases vitamin E levels. This vitamin E axing by statin drugs makes it easier for cholesterol to stick to blood vessel walls causing coronary artery disease, heart attack, and death.** In fact, **Lipitor reduced vitamin E levels a walloping 18% in another study, forcing cholesterol to plaster itself onto arterial walls** (by increasing the LDL oxidation as you'll learn) by 18%. Meanwhile taking Lipitor and vitamin E supplements (750 I.U. a day of the natural form) increased vitamin E levels 62% (Manuel-y-Keenoy). Statin drugs clearly interfere with your antioxidant status by dropping your level of vitamin E. And by the way, regarding those highly publicized studies that showed vitamin E was of no use? They were fraught with bad science to make unknowledgeable folks shun vitamins. Many of the studies, for example, used inferior synthetic vitamin E, which in fact is only one of the 8 parts of real natural vitamin E. So, yes, they were right, but for the wrong conclusion. Synthetic vitamin E made in a lab that is only one of 8 essential parts of the vitamin is not good for you. In fact, synthetic vitamin E counters the benefits of good vitamin E you get from food and natural supplements. But more on that later.

In one study they showed that after you come home from a late-night out with a heavy high-fat meal, you are much more prone to having a heart attack before morning. But a mere 500 mg of vitamin C and 800 IU of vitamin E can counteract the damage and protect you (Plotnick). Funny they didn't publicize that study on TV.

8

So as well as requiring coenzyme Q10 supplementation, you should also use vitamin E supplements if you're on statin drugs. And in case your doctor wonders if the vitamin E will affect the cholesterol-lowering effect of statin medications, it does not. It only improves your status. The best form of vitamin E actually contains all eight natural components of vitamin E, not just alpha tocopherol, like cheap grocery store vitamins. Use **E-Gems Elite** (Carlson), two a day.

(7) As well, **statin cholesterol-lowering drugs decrease the ability of insulin to metabolize sugars**. When insulin loses its power to lower sugar, the body makes more insulin. But high insulin promotes arteriosclerosis by many mechanisms. Damaging the action of insulin also promotes diabetes (which is already escalating at breakneck speeds) and accelerates aging. Another heart-damaging mechanism of high insulin is that it ushers in the metabolic syndrome (also called Syndrome X), which consists of any or all of the following: high cholesterol or high triglycerides, high blood pressure, overweight with inability to reduce the weight and much more. Fortunately it is totally curable with nutrients, as you will learn. Any one of these high insulin consequences alone shortens your life dramatically (Jula).

(8) But the harm of statin drugs doesn't end here. When you take statin drugs there is a **14-fold increased risk of developing polyneuropathy** (Gaist). This nerve damage can cause a wide range of symptoms from numbness and tingling to impotency or paralysis. But when you seek a neurological consult and get your $1000 MRI, physicians often see these baffling symptoms as a deficiency of yet another drug, sometimes even as a deficiency of the antidepressant Prozac.

(9) **Statins have caused serious amnesia within minutes.** To give you an idea of how serious and hidden the side effects of cholesterol-lowering statin drugs are, "One day former astronaut, Duane Graveline, came back from a walk and failed to recognize

his wife" (Westphal). Investigations proved the cause of this serious and sudden amnesia was the statin drug Lipitor that he had begun several weeks before. I'm wondering how many pilots of commercial airlines are on this stuff!!! Duke University physicians and scientists have reported over 60 cases of statin-induced serious amnesia. It goes away if you are smart enough to stop the drug, and recurs if you are dumb enough to ever take it again (Wagstaff). More details on this later.

(10) **Cholesterol drugs cause miserable people.** Studies show that folks taking statin cholesterol-lowering statin drugs are not happy (Morales). One out of three has low energy, does not feel content, is no longer happy, and has other subtle and affective (mood) changes. And of course, if you look at how they work in the body, they should make someone depressed and have mood swings. In poisoning the enzyme that the body uses to make cholesterol, you poison the ability of the body to make coenzyme Q10, which you need in the brain to be happy. Also by poisoning the ability of the body to make enough cholesterol, you damage the brain receptors or docking sites where the "happy hormones" fit or plug in like pieces of a puzzle to make us feel terrific. The cell membrane receptors for our "happy hormones" are malformed when they don't have enough cholesterol and other nutrients. So regardless of how much of the neurotransmitter poisons for happiness (like Prozac) that you may take, they can't work because the receptor sites in the cell membrane are broken. Medications become powerless to turn on the mood of happiness.

(11) **Cholesterol drugs guarantee an avalanche of new symptoms, especially cancer and more serious heart disease**. There is so much more that the cholesterol-lowering drugs do that I'll just show you a smattering. As an example, when you don't have enough cholesterol, it damages the receptors on the surface of every cell that transport crucial vitamins to the inside of the cell. Folic acid is a pivotal B vitamin, because it protects our genetics from damage by environmental chemicals. When there is not

enough folic acid, genetic damage results in cancers, birth deformities, mental illness, arteriosclerosis, accelerated aging, heart disease, colitis, cervical dysplasia (suspicious PAP smears), depression, Parkinson's disease, Alzheimer's, and multiple other medical problems. Many researchers have shown that **low cholesterol** (as you have with cholesterol-lowering drugs) **damages the folic acid receptors** (Chang, Rothberg). That is another mechanism by which they can usher in cancer. Furthermore, **statins work by actually poisoning the gene** that controls the enzyme the liver uses to make cholesterol (Parker). Who knows what the long-term effects of poisoning our genes will be, but certainly this could have an effect on the increased rate of cancer that was reported in the *Journal of the American Medical Association* among folks using cholesterol-lowering drugs (Newman).

Let's look at just another example of how far-reaching a low-cholesterol can be and how it triggers an avalanche of seemingly unrelated symptoms. In the cell membrane there are electrically charged channels or pores that pump calcium in and out of the cell. When there is insufficient cholesterol, the **calcium pumps no longer work** (Fujimoto). This back-up of calcium stuck inside the cell causes irregular heartbeat (cardiac arrhythmias like atrial fibrillation), chest pain (angina), high blood pressure (hypertension), and shortness of breath and ankle swelling (congestive heart failure). These are the leading causes of eventual heart death that cardiologists treat.

Unfortunately the main categories of drugs cardiologists prescribe to compensate for damaged membrane calcium pumps are called **calcium channel blockers.** At the outset it sounds pretty logical that if the calcium pumps don't work, we should poison them so that too much calcium does not get inside the cell to cause all those nasty symptoms. But that allows the doctor to ignore finding the underlying cause of the symptoms and correcting it, as you will learn how to do later on. A major problem is that these calcium channel blocker drugs (the number one category of prescribed drugs by cardiologists, and usually prescribed for life) have been proven to slowly deteriorate and **shrink the brain and deteriorate the intellect** within less than five years (Norvasc, Procardia, Calan, Dilacor, etc., and other calcium channel blocker drugs are in *Detoxify or Die*, page 172). Rather than merely block the damaged calcium channels, *Detoxify or Die* shows you how to repair them. Then you can avoid a lifetime of these drugs that shrink the brain within 5 years. Because if you don't, when these drugs eventually fail to work, the resulting heart failure and arrhythmias are treated with ablation. Translation: Rather than understand how to fix the problem, when medicines fail to work, doctors actually burn out part of the heart with lasers inserted into blood vessels (cheaper and easier than surgery)!

Statins Rot the Brain

Before we go further, I want to be sure you appreciate how dangerous statins are for the brain. **Cholesterol-lowering drugs cause memory loss, amnesia, Alzheimer's, and mimic strokes.** While doing one of my favorite radio shows, *The Power Hour* (powerhour.com), I learned of a medical doctor, NASA research scientist, and astronaut, all rolled into one, who had been on the show before me talking about his experiences with sudden amnesia from Lipitor. During one of his annual flight physicals his cholesterol was found to be a tad elevated so he was put on Lipitor. Within a month, upon returning from his morning walk, he didn't recognize his wife, his house, didn't know he was a doctor, and in fact he didn't remember much of anything. The medical workup resulted in the diagnosis of TIA (transient ischemic attack, which means a mini-stroke from which folks always recover). When he asked his doctors whether Lipitor might be the cause, they laughed.

The next year during his physical they also prescribed Lipitor again and the same thing happened. Even though he was a doctor with superlative credentials as well as a real life rocket scientist, once he had stepped over that line where he appeared to cast doubt upon the wonders of drugs, he became a *persona non grata*. For over 38 years in medicine I have seen this happen to anyone regardless of their credentials from the twice Nobel Prize winner Linus Pauling right on down to psychiatrists, surgeons, internists and anyone else who dares to question drugs (or develop symptoms of multiple chemical sensitivity, as another example). They either get maligned, ignored and otherwise discredited or distracted with trumped up investigations.

Since all of his medical colleagues totally denied that Lipitor could cause amnesia, he created a web site to see if others had had these problems, opening up to a world of people with even scarier symptoms than his. For one company CEO, his wife asked him to pick up some grocery items as long as he was going out to the hardware store. Hours later when he opened his trunk at the hardware store to put his packages inside, he was startled to find the grocery items and the same hardware items, with their receipts confirming he had already purchased them all that day. But where had those stolen hours gone? Too bad he hadn't forgot to take his Lipitor!

The bottom line is that there are airline pilots, airline traffic regulators, drivers on our high-speed highways including those carrying tons of dangerously toxic materials who are already balancing coffee, sandwiches and cell phones while on these drugs as they tool along at 75 mph. In fact everywhere folks on these drugs surround us, as over 50 million Americans take them. **We are in a sea of dangerous minds that have had cholesterol stolen from their brains.** When the critical period strikes for each mind when it suddenly cuts out and stops functioning is a total crapshoot.

Furthermore, robbing the body of cholesterol synthesis also (1) deprives the brain of dolichols, messengers or neurotransmitters, (2) damages our NF-kB production that then ushers in cancers, and causes (3) **unusual ligament and tendon rupture** (like we saw with some antibiotics), (4) heart failure, and (5) fatal muscle/joint weakness and pain and (6) finally death via rhabdomyolysis. And this just scratches the surface of statin side effects.

Just recall Cox-2 inhibitors like Vioxx, the female hormone Premarin made from a carcinogenic horse urine estrogen (that was forced on women for decades before they proved it quadrupled their cancer rate), or the many other FDA drug withdrawals that were proven to accelerate disease and death. The message is clear for anyone who has even a remote knowledge about the body. **You cannot poison enzymes in God's miraculous molecular biochemistry and expect to get away with it, especially when you are poisoning the synthesis of a major constituent of every cell in the body.**

Folks, this is serious, because **over 150,000 people are estimated to have this statin-induced amnesia at some point.** Will he be on the highway in front of you and your precious family, or will he be the surgeon operating on you, or will he be the pilot of your plane? Or will it just be a worker at a nuclear facility or the fellow who somehow put PCB-containing fire retardant into cattle feed, raising the cancer incidence enormously throughout the US Midwest, or the guy who put melamine into pet food?

Appreciating the gravity of this hidden and ignored epidemic of mind rot, Dr. Graveline subsequently wrote two great, easy to read books that you may want to get from "The Power Hour", *Lipitor, Thief of Memory* and *Statin Drugs, Side Effects, and the Misguided War on Cholesterol* (thepowerhour.com or 1-877-817-9829).

Meanwhile, researchers have shown that **statins actually cause an increase in the death rate** of 1% per year (Jackson). More importantly, other researchers are showing that anywhere from one week to over 10 years later people can have serious memory loss from the statin drugs (Wagstaff). Furthermore, there's lots of medical proof of how statin drugs not only damage brain chemistry, but are probably going to usher in an unprecedented epidemic of Alzheimer's (Meske). Can you really afford to purposely damage your brain and shorten its productive lifespan?

Statins Silently Create a Selenium Deficiency

We could fill a whole book, just on the side effects of statin drugs. There are many other little-known side effects that have serious ramifications. One study came from the prestigious journal, *Lancet*; showing **statin drugs create a selenium deficiency** (Moosmann). Yet I have never heard of any cardiologists who measure selenium on their patients for whom they have prescribed a life sentence on statins. Selenium is important in not only detoxification of daily chemicals as well as medications, but for processing of thyroid hormones (for cholesterol control, weight control, energy, depression, constipation). As well, selenium is crucial for protecting against cancer, maintenance of muscle strength, control of gene function and mitochondrial function where energy is created inside of our cells. So you can see how **other diseases can silently emerge.** Yet when your physician is not checking intracellular selenium, he will never know what has happened to you.

Cholesterol Drugs Cause Miserable People

I often am asked, "My husband isn't the same since he started on his cholesterol medicine. Could there be a connection? His doctor says 'No'."

Studies show that folks taking statin cholesterol-lowering drugs (Lipitor, Crestor, Mevacor, Zocor, etc.) are not happy. One out of three has low energy, does not feel content, is no longer happy, and has other subtle and affective (mood) changes (Morales). In another study, folks with low cholesterol naturally (on no medications) also had more major depression and suicide (Partonen).

And of course if you look at how cholesterol-lowering drugs work in the body, it should make someone depressed and have mood swings. They work by poisoning the enzyme the body uses to make cholesterol with. By doing this you poison the ability of the body to make coenzyme Q10 which you need in the brain to be happy. Also by poisoning the ability of the body to make enough cholesterol, you damage the brain receptors where the "happy hormones" fit or plug in like pieces of a puzzle to make us feel terrific. When the receptors are malformed because they don't have enough cholesterol and other nutrients, no matter how much Prozac that you may take for happiness, it can't work. It doesn't have a receptor site in the cell membrane that is working properly, so it cannot turn on the mood of happiness. Likewise if folks have low cholesterol from other reasons (environmental chemicals can do it), the same abnormal brain membrane chemistry applies. One man's misery can infect the family.

Watch Out for Combination Cholesterol-Lowering Drugs

If the statin drugs were not cause enough for worry by themselves, the FDA is now allowing pharmaceutical companies to make combinations of statin drugs with a second health-robbing drug. Unfortunately, sometimes the danger of two drugs is not cumulative, but synergistic. In other words, one plus one does not equal two, but more like five in terms of dangerous side effects when two drugs are combined. Let's look at some of the examples that you want to avoid. **Caduet not only contains a statin to poison the HMG-CoA reductase enzyme in the liver that makes cholesterol, but it contains a calcium channel blocker.** You just learned that this category of drug is proven by MRI to shrink the brain and rot intellect within 5 years.

Colestid's second drug is a bile acid sequestrant, meaning it sops up your cholesterol like a sponge, so you cannot absorb cholesterol. It sounds like a good thing, doesn't it? But in the process of being a sponge for cholesterol, it also sops up your **precious bile.** But you **need bile to detoxify everyday chemicals,** many of which you'll learn later actually caused your high cholesterol in the first place. If that were not dangerous enough, **you need bile for the absorption of fat soluble vitamins, like A, D, E, and K that you need to prevent cancer, heart diseases, and every other disease**. And don't overlook the fact that **beta-carotene, lipoic acid and CoQ10** are fat-soluble vitamins. As I've referenced in previous *TW* (*Total Wellness*, the monthly referenced 8-page newsletter for 18 years, prestigepublishing.com or 1-800-846-6687) issues, many of these fat-soluble vitamins can make cancer cells revert back to normal cells, *after* every thing that medicine has to offer has failed (called re-differentiation). No drug does that. No, this is not a drug we want hidden in your cholesterol drug.

Likewise, **Vytorin is another combination drug that contains an inhibitor of cholesterol absorption,** stopping your absorption of life-saving fat-soluble nutrients. **Zetia** is just the same cholesterol sponge in a solo act, as it has no statin added**.**

Non-Statin Type Cholesterol-Lowering Drugs

Other classes of cholesterol-lowering medications include gemfibrizol, known by its brand name, Lopid. As with the statins, this category can also cause myopathy, the mysterious condition of profound muscle aches, pain and weakness (Margarian). One diagnostic clue is an elevated CK (creatinine kinase) blood level that is a tip-off proving deterioration of muscle. This drug class can also deteriorate the kidneys as well as the heart muscle (called rhabdomyolysis), both of which can be lethal.

Other dangerous classes of cholesterol-lowering drugs include those that tie up bile acids in the gut, like Colestid and Questran. These are particularly nasty because once more in sopping up bile, you inhibit absorption of heart-protecting fat-soluble vitamins, A, D, E, and K, beta-carotene, lipoic acid and coenzyme Q10, plus life-saving fatty acids. This provides a fast ticket to any disease including cancer. In fact, even the *Journal of the American Medical Association* showed over 23 years ago that these drugs increased gallbladder disease, and create beta-carotene deficiencies (Lipid Research Clinics Program).

But by far the worst cholesterol-lowering drug was Atromid (clofibrate). Did you know that when we need experimental animals in the laboratory with cancer one of the quickest ways to get it is by giving them clofibrate? It causes cancer by damaging the genes, which can be measured as a simple blood test called 8-OHdG (8-hydroxy-2'-deoxyguanosine), as it tells if you are on your way to cancer or metastases (Qu). This cholesterol drug also damages the mitochondrial genes (responsible for energy synthesis), leading to accelerated aging, chronic fatigue, and more. It is off the market now, without fanfare, after decades of use.

So from this section, you can add the following list of cholesterol-lowering drugs to the solo statin drugs that you learned about earlier.

Other Cholesterol-Lowering Drugs

> Caduet (a statin and a calcium channel blocker)
> Colestid (a statin and a bile acid sponge)
> Vytorin (a statin with a cholesterol sponge)
> Zetia (just the cholesterol sponge)
> Questran (a bile acid sponge)
> Welchol (a bile acid sponge, colesevalam)
> Lofibra (fenofibrate)
> Tricor (fenofibrate
> Lopid (gemfibrizol)
> Atromid (phased out, but 3 above are related, clofibrate)

Do they think we have enough drugs to poison cholesterol synthesis and absorption? And don't forget that the really scary part is that these "sponges" are not only sopping up your crucial fat-soluble vitamins, but crucially important fatty acids and phosphatidyl choline that you need to prevent all sorts of diseases, especially cancer which rivals arteriosclerosis for the number of people it kills every year. To prescribe these drugs is totally unconscionable in my book without (1) making sure folks are on supplemental nutrients, and then (2) measuring their levels to be sure you've given enough to compensate for the nasty effects of the drug. But I'll make you an expert in that later.

Let's Save You Some Money

Meanwhile when you read further, in the next chapter you will learn about safer and more natural alternatives to prescription statin cholesterol-lowering drugs. And in subsequent chapters you'll actually learn how to cure your high cholesterol so that you will need nothing at all. In the meantime however, let's save you some money, especially since over 40% of the US population doesn't have insurance. Zocor, for example, averages $405 for ninety 20 mg tablets. But the generic equivalent simvastatin costs $249. However, through **Life Extension Pharmacy** this generic costs $20. Likewise, Pravachol 40 mg (90 tablets) averages around $435, generic pravastatin $203, and **Life Extension Pharmacy** generic $37 (available at 1-877-877-9700 or lifeextensionrx.com). Quite an enormous savings.

Watch Out for Dangerous Docs Who Prescribe Cholesterol-Lowering Drugs to Lower Your CRP

CRP, C-reactive protein, is a simple blood test that any doctor can (and should) do routinely. Why? Because **CRP is a stronger predictor of an early heart attack or stroke than is a high cholesterol level** (Ridker 2002, Krumholz, Rifai). Furthermore, a high CRP blood test is an indicator of increased risk of depression (Ford). Unfortunately, *The New England Journal of Medicine* published studies showing statin drugs cut the risk of heart attack by lowering CRP by 21% (Nissen, Ridker 2005). So docs jumped on the bandwagon and began prescribing statins for folks who didn't have high cholesterol, but who had high CRP. However researchers used very high doses of cholesterol-lowering drugs to accomplish this 21% reduction in CRP. These higher doses are more likely to give a greater suppression of coenzyme Q10, plus more side effects like fatal rhabdomyolysis. There are better, safer, and cheaper ways to lower CRP. But they don't support the drug industry coffers.

What you shouldn't expect to see in medical journals dedicated to drug-oriented medicine is that one part of natural **vitamin E** (actually, one of its 8 parts, alpha-tocopherol) **can lower the CRP not 21% like statins, but by 52%,** more than double of what the dangerous statin drugs can do. But hang on. Another **part of vitamin E, gamma tocopherol safely lowers CRP by 61%, almost triple the improvement of statin drugs and at 1/5th the cost of statin drugs, and with none of the deadly side effects** (Himmelfarb, Jiang).

But don't expect to ever see anything this inexpensive, harmless, non-prescription and superior to drugs in pharmaceutical-sponsored medical journals (Angell). You see, real vitamin E is not one thing but actually is 8 entities, four tocopherols and four tocotrienols. But the junk vitamins that merely state "vitamin E" (as in cheap grocery store vitamins) are usually just the synthetic alpha-tocopherol made in a laboratory. It does not contain all of the eight parts. Now you can begin to understand why vitamin E had such bad press a few years ago (Devaraj, Miller). In "shifty science" researchers did not use the whole vitamin E in their studies that showed it was useless. They only used part of vitamin E (and often synthetic), not the whole thing the way God designed it. So of course, vitamin E came out looking bad, like it didn't work. It shouldn't have! Then the equally unknowledgeable media picked up on it and authoritatively unannounced to innocent audiences that vitamin E was powerless.

Meanwhile, when information-challenged cardiologists read the article about using statin drugs to lower CRP, they thought it sounded so good that they even started pushing statin drugs on people who did not have high cholesterol, in the misguided attempt to stave off arteriosclerosis, especially coronary artery disease. They had no idea that **gamma tocopherol** was infinitely safer, cheaper, more physiologic, and **gave triple benefit in lowering the dangerous CRP compared with statins**. You can add **Gamma E-Gems**, 1-2 a day to your 1-2 **E-Gems Elite** to begin to lower your CRP, but more on this later.

Watch Out for Too Low a Cholesterol

When it comes to prescribing cholesterol-lowering drugs for people who do not even have high cholesterol, beware: **too low a cholesterol is just as dangerous as too high.** As you've already learned, cholesterol is essential for all membrane structure and function, hormones, hormone receptors, cytokine release for fighting infection, cancers and autoimmune disease. In essence, folks with a **cholesterol under 160 mg/dL have double the risk of brain hemorrhage and increase their risk of cancers of the liver, lung, pancreas, and leukemia, plus cirrhosis and suicide** (Neaton). In another study, having a low cholesterol made sure folks had more than double their death rate from non-cardiac conditions (Behar). **A low cholesterol, besides doubling the chance of death, dramatically damages mental-health leading to depression, suicide, mania**, and more (Cassidy, Boston, Engleberg).

Remember, too low a cholesterol triggers an avalanche of seemingly unrelated symptoms. In the cell membrane that has enough cholesterol, electrically charged channels pump calcium in and out of the cell. **When there is insufficient cholesterol, the calcium pumps no longer work (Fujimoto). This causes irregular heartbeat (cardiac arrhythmias like atrial fibrillation), chest pain (angina), high blood pressure (hypertension), and shortness of breath and ankle swelling (congestive heart failure).**

Too low a cholesterol is associated with increased risk of heart disease, cancer, suicide, depression, Alzheimer's, neurologic disease, violence and accidents, as it should be (Meilahan, Kritchevsky, Hiatt, Muldoon).

The Politics of Medicine

Other drugs kill the heart, too. I keep hearing folks ask how the FDA can let dangerous drugs on the market. But this reflects a naïve understanding of the power of the pharmaceutical industry. Remember you learned earlier that in one year, one of all the cholesterol-lowering drugs brings in more than five times the entire annual budget for the FDA. And you need only cursorily read *The Wall Street Journal* to learn how frequently drugs are withdrawn after having been granted FDA approval. Let me give you a little more information about a recent drug withdrawal, as one example, so that you understand the process better.

In August 2001 the *Journal of the American Medical Association* published an article showing that Vioxx, the popular prescription arthritis medicine, increased the rate of heart attack. But it wasn't withdrawn until four years later, staying on the market to reap enormous profits. *The Wall Street Journal* (Burton) even reported on a Harvard study confirming that **Vioxx increased the heart attack risk 39% within just the first one to three months of use**. But that didn't change a thing. Nor did scientific reports in leading medical journals and newspapers (Fitzgerald, Topal, Whalen). Does that give you an idea of the power of the pharmaceutical industry?

Other researchers at Vanderbilt University who studied over 24,000 patients came to the same conclusion and published their work in the British medical journal, *Lancet*. Needless to say, although this information was over two years old, kept resurfacing, and had been published in the most prestigious journals in studies involving nearly 100,000 patients, it was conveniently ignored until the lawsuits emerged. And remember millions of people are still taking drugs that work on the same chemistry. They are just not smart enough to realize that if one NSAID can damage the heart, then the others with similar chemistry have that potential as well. And as I showed in *Pain Free In 6 Weeks*, the NSAID (non-steroidal anti-inflammatory drugs, like ibuprofen, Motrin, etc.) for pain relief cause over 100,000 cases of congestive heart failure a year, as an example of just one of the many ways they damage the heart. Remember, congestive heart failure kills more people each year and faster than cancer does. And NSAIDs create high blood pressure and damage cartilage chemistry, nearly guaranteeing the eventual need for a joint replacement (which is epidemic).

Contrast that with tryptophan which is an essential amino acid, meaning the body needs it every day. It has been a safe supplement for decades. Then a shoddy manufacturing error arose when a Japanese company making tryptophan tried to skimp on one of the steps in their genetic engineering process. This resulted in a very toxic tryptophan, which caused over at 30 deaths by eosinophilic myalgia syndrome (*TW*). Quickly, the FDA raided every health food store in the country and tryptophan was off the shelves within days. And even more odd is the fact that it has never returned. We never see this type of speed with prescription drugs.

And if that were not bad enough, all sorts of other **commonly prescribed drugs can actually cause high cholesterol**. For example, chlorthalidone for blood pressure (Ames) and **beta-blockers** like propranolol also create high cholesterol in some folks (Tanaka, Waal-Manning). Hundreds of other drugs work by poisoning pathways so that your symptom goes away and you think the prescriber is a miracle worker. Meanwhile **all drugs deplete nutrients** (Pelton) that can then lead to the inability of the body to properly metabolize cholesterol. When high cholesterol is seen, immediately a statin drug is prescribed. And you now know the devastating roller coaster ride you can take once you begin that class of drugs.

Prescription Drugs,
The Number One Cause of Death in the U.S.

With so many safer, more effective and cheaper substitutes available for lowering your cholesterol that you will learn about in the next chapter, why have you and your doctor not heard of them? The reason is not so pure, but very simple: money.

What is the number one cause of death in the United States? It's not high cholesterol or accidents by cars, planes, or trains. It's not wars. It's not drug addiction, and it's not even disease, so that lets out heart disease, cancer, strokes, diabetes and more. In Third World countries, infections and malnutrition are major causes of loss of life. But **in United States the number one cause of death** is not any of those things. **It is prescription drugs** (Null, *TW*).

As Jay Cohen, M.D., professor of medicine at the University of California, San Diego has provided the sterling and startling evidence for the doubting Thomas. He meticulously documented how the drug industry surreptitiously hires physicians as consultants who just coincidentally happen to be on the very FDA committees that are responsible for approval of their drugs. As well, they hire expensive lobbyists who encourage FDA physicians to speed the approval process. And they hire scientists and physicians to do the research on the drugs, but reserve the right to throw out any research that casts a negative light on their products. In fact the drug companies forbid hired researchers to talk about or publish discoveries about adverse reactions. And they hire ghostwriters who have never had anything to do with the drug experiments to write the convincing research papers for publication in the leading medical journals (Cauchon, Cohen, Haley, Angell).

The situation gets much stickier once the drug has been approved, because there is even sloppier handling of adverse reactions. First of all, officials state that only 1-5% of adverse reactions to drugs get reported. Dr. Cohen does an unprecedented and highly commendable job of detailing over the last decade how, even though the FDA had the evidence that hundreds of people were dying from specific drugs, it took over a year before many drugs were withdrawn from the market. The reason? These drugs were bringing in billions (not mere millions) of dollars a year, making a few hundred lawsuits from folks who died a spit in the ocean comparatively. Besides that, recognition that the drug was responsible and then proving it against a dozen slick attorneys hired by the drug companies would be beyond the average person's means.

There are many other great books on the market also complementing this enormous amount of evidence for collusion between the drug industry and the FDA: Dr. Ralph Moss's *Questioning Chemotherapy*, former New York State assemblymen Daniel Haley's *Politics of Healing*, esteemed University of Chicago professor Dr. Sam Epstein's *The Politics of Cancer Revisited,* George Washington University Medical School professor Thomas Moore's *Prescription for Disaster* and *Deadly Medicine*, Harvard and Johns Hopkins associated Peter Breggin's *Toxic Psychiatry*, and Harvard psychiatrist Joseph Glenmullen's *Prozac Backlash*, Breggin's *Talking Back to Ritalin,* etc. And did you ever wonder how the ridiculous notion that high cholesterol should be treated as a statin drug deficiency has so fiercely controlled medicine? Just recall that the *Journal of the American Medical Association* showed that over 87% of physicians on boards that dictate how medicine is practiced are financially connected to the drug industry (Choudry).

Of all these great works, I think the job that Dr. Jay Cohen has done with *Overdose (*1-800-669-CALM*)* is the most casily readable and convincing. And I haven't even begun to touch on one of the most important points that he reveals. That is that most people can get away with far lower doses than the doses they have been prescribed, thereby sparing them from becoming a statistic for the number one cause of death in the United States.

25

Who's Side is the FDA On?

Meanwhile, you might wonder how medications like a Vioxx stayed on the market so long when they more than quadrupled the rate of heart attack. That's because 93% of the votes cast to keep COX-2 meds on the market in 2005 were made by those receiving consulting fees from the drug industry. And this article came right out of the *Journal of the American Medical Association* where reference was made regarding **FDA Drug Advisory Committee meetings between 1998 and 2000, where 92% had at least one voting member on the pharmaceutical payrolls creating a voting member with a serious conflict of interest.** In fact, exclusion of members with serious conflicts would have resulted in recommendations to remove two out of three of these drugs from the market. Look at the lives that could have been saved (Lurie).

Just in case you are not thoroughly convinced that you have to take control because no one else will be looking out for you, then let me give you just one more tiny example. The FDA in 2007 approved its first over-the-counter (nonprescription) diet pill (Matthews). It actually is the same exact chemical as the prescription pill (Xenical) made by the same factory only in a smaller dose (duh.... like the average person couldn't figure out to increase the dose). You might think that this sounds good, but to take it for only six months costs over $360 for a total weight loss of only 5 pounds! For those who did not take the drug but did everything else the same, they lost half as much (but didn't have to spend $360).

The biggest problem was that this diet pill works as a gastric and pancreatic lipase inhibitor. In other words, you don't absorb your fat because it poisons the body's enzyme needed to help absorb fats. This might sound good until you remember that you are already too smart to be fooled, for you know it also will inhibit the absorption of your fat soluble vitamins, A, D, E and K plus CoQ10, beta-carotene and lipoic acid, plus fatty acids and phosphatidyl choline. This is a fast ticket to accelerated aging and every disease from heart disease to cancer. Interestingly there were no vitamin absorption studies required for this drug to pass into non-prescription status (nor prescription status). Comparing the people who took the prescription drug versus those who did not take it revealed more abdominal pain, nausea, diarrhea, tooth and gum problems, respiratory infections, fatigue, dry skin, sleep disorders, irregular menstrual periods, anxiety and psychiatric problems including depression and ankle swelling (*PDR*). And why shouldn't it since it's inhibiting the absorption of so many nutrients. Plus 7% of folks taking this diet pill got diabetes. Is someone looking out for what's best for you? Just look at the facts and decide.

And in terms of statin drugs, allow me to give you just one more example and then we can move on. A widely publicized study in the *New England Journal of Medicine* (Amarenco) using Lipitor concluded that all people who have had a stroke should be on Lipitor. But every one of the 11 authors was either a Pfizer employee or a Pfizer consultant. Now since 5.4 million Americans and 55 million people worldwide have had a stroke, this would be a staggering monetary boon (Cohen). But the saddest part was that the results of the study didn't even warrant the conclusion that it' s beneficial. In fact, **the chance off a second hemorrhagic stroke increased 67% in folks using Lipitor versus those using nothing.** But unfortunately even the author of an authoritative accompanying editorial called for widespread use of Lipitor. And wouldn't you know, he was also a consultant for Pfizer (Cohen). Do we have a crooked system or what? Oh, by the way, that authoritative paper also recommended that all people with TIA (transient ischemic attack) be on Lipitor. Ironically, remember that's one of the many dangerous side effects of Lipitor.

If you still have even the slightest doubt about the unprecedented power of the pharmaceutical industry, I urge you to get the *60 Minutes* archived transcript for the TV program aired July 29, 2007. They carefully documented one congressional event, pas-

27

sage of the Medicare prescription bill. With over a thousand Pharma lobbyists, the congressmen reported how they were stalked and cajoled into wee hours of the morning on Capitol Hill, while the unprecedented extension of voting time went from minutes to hours. Attached to the bill was the inability of the United States government to negotiate with pharmaceutical companies for the most favorable price for Medicare prescription drugs. As a result, compared with the VA hospital system which does negotiate for the best price, **Medicare pays well over $800 a year for Lipitor per patient, while the VA pays less than half of that, around $300.** And Zocor was even worse at over $1000 being paid by the government for Medicare recipients versus over 10 times less for VA persons. And then at the end of the show they showed how over 15 congressman and other government employees went on to be lobbyists and related employees of the pharmaceutical industry. One congressman's beginning salary with a pharmaceutical company within weeks of passage of the bill was $2 million a year for starters. As one of the congressmen intimated, Pharma owns the government.

I really did not want to bog you down with the politics of medicine, but folks are often so incredulous that they are not being protected, that they find it hard to not put their total trust in the drug world. Many are dead now because of their trust. If you are still in doubt, take a stroll through the references I've provided at the end of this chapter, bearing in mind this is just a smattering of the proof, since it is not the focus of this book. The **focus is to empower you beyond your wildest dreams**.

The CoQ10 Quagmire

You recall statins turn off CoQ10 production in the body (Ghirlanda, Folkers, Willis, Mortensen). And with depleted CoQ10, the LDL cholesterol becomes a bad guy when it is oxidized for lack of CoQ10 (Thomas). For **without sufficient CoQ10 to protect the LDL** cholesterol from free radicals stealing electrons from it, it now becomes a wildly ravenous molecule that steals back electrons from the artery wall and glues itself onto the wall in the process. This **is a major reason why taking statin drugs is no guarantee you will not die of a heart attack. In fact, they promote heart disease** as well as a stable full of other nasty symptoms. I shudder when I rarely hear of a cardiologist who covers a statin prescription with CoQ10 even though it is incontrovertibly proven to be of benefit (Bargossi, Langsjoen).

Prescription of a statin drug without boosting your CoQ10 should be illegal. For CoQ10 deficiency can cause fatal cardiomyopathy, heart attack, congestive heart failure (which usually carries a death sentence of 5 years), exhaustion, cancer, myopathy, depression resistant to anti-depressants, high blood pressure, gum disease and tooth loss, hair loss, liver disease, sudden complete memory loss or amnesia, cataracts, angina, cancer, folic acid deficiency, damaged cell membranes, and much more (Bliznakov, Rao, Thompson, Hebert, Newman, Westphal). In fact, it not only accelerates getting a variety of diseases, but aging and **low CoQ10 levels predict that you can die within 6 months** (Jameson). **A physician who would only prescribe a statin and turn you lose without even measuring your CoQ10 much less covering it, is dangerously irresponsible and shows lack of scientific knowledge of the very drug he is authorized to prescribe.**

One of my favorite CoQ10 sources is sublingual so it spares you one more capsule to ingest and get rid of. **Q-ODT** (oral dissolving tablet) is 80 mg easily absorbed under the tongue. Use 1-3 under the tongue 2-3 times a day. You can not only actually measure your coenzyme Q10 level on the **Cardio/ION Panel** as I will show you later, but it also contains an even better organic acid assay (hydroxymethylglutarate) which will show you if a particular dose is high enough for your body individuality. For we all have individual biochemical needs. That is the beauty of organic acids; they demonstrate your individual dose requirements, regardless of how you measure up against the "average person".

Many other drugs also deplete CoQ10 by a variety of other mechanisms. These include the blood thinner warfarin (coumadin), the chemotherapy drug adriamycin (doxorubicin), the blood pressure and heart drugs called beta-blockers like Inderal, Atenolol, some diabetes, epilepsy, and colitis drugs, and the food additive in "fat-free" or "guilt-free" foods: olestra "fights fat" by actually stopping CoQ10 absorption (as well as the absorption of fat soluble vitamins like A, D, E, K, lipoic acid and beta carotene) (Bliznakov, Fuke, *TW*).

The Bare Minimum Nutrients if You're on Statins

Clearly it should be illegal to prescribe a statin drug without also prescribing coenzyme Q10 (Langsjoen, Thomas, Mabuchi, Lamperti, Cohen). So until you and your doctor are able to get rid of your cholesterol drug, at least take some rudimentary nutrients to counter the nasty effects. One start is by taking extra coenzyme Q10 in the form of Q- ODT. Since **Q-ODT** is 80 mg of coenzyme Q10 in an oral dissolving tablet (ODT), there is no capsule for your body to detoxify. You merely put the tiny tablets under your tongue twice a day and let them dissolve and get absorbed just like nitroglycerin would. Second would be vitamin E with all 8 of its natural components, as in **E Gems Elite.** At least take the following to begin to repair your deficits and damage:

E Gems Elite	1-2/day
Gamma E Gems	1-2/day
Cod Liver Oil	1-3 tsp/day
Super 2 Daily	2/day
Phos Chol	1-3tsp/day
Liquid Multiple Minerals	1-2/day
Q-ODT	1-3 under the tongue, 1-3 times/day

Busy Executive Summary

If you feel great and don't have anything else wrong with you except for high cholesterol, don't worry, you shortly will. For it is against nature to poison one of the primary cholesterol synthesizing enzymes in the human liver with a nasty chemical. Statin cholesterol-lowering drugs can cause serious amnesia within minutes, guarantee an avalanche of new symptoms including cancer, while the other symptoms become mysteriously undiagnosable and untreatable. The next prescribed drug can further kill the heart. Worst of all cholesterol-lowering drugs create new heart disease. Killing cholesterol does not save lives. Prescription drugs are the number one cause of death in the U.S.

Until you are able to read further and get off your drugs, at least take two of the chief nutrients that cholesterol drugs destroy, coenzyme Q10 and vitamin E that has all 8 components. High cholesterol is not a deficiency of some statin drug. If God wanted you dependent upon the pharmaceutical companies for the rest of your life, He would have figured out a much better system. And as you read on, you'll see that indeed He has.

Sources for this Chapter's Recommendations

- Q-ODT, intensivenutrition.com, 1-800-333-7414
- Gamma E Gems, E-Gems Elite, Cod Liver Oil, Super 2 Daily, Liquid Multiple Minerals, carlsonlabs.com, 1-800-323-4141
- PhosChol, nutrasal.com, 1-800-777-1886
- *Statin Drugs, Side Effects, and the Misguided War on Cholesterol,* and *Lipitor, Thief of Memory,* thepowerhour.com, 1-877-817-9829
- *Overdose,* painstresscenter.com, 1-800-669-CALM
- Generic Statins, lifeextensionrx.com, 1-877-877-9700

References:

Steinberg D, Parthasarathy S, Khoo JC, Witztum JL, et al, Beyond cholesterol: modification to low-density lipoprotein that increase its atherogenesis, *New Engl J Med*, 320: 9 15-24, 1989

Thomas S. R., Neuzil J., Stocker R, Inhibition of LDL oxidation by ubiquinol-10. A protective mechanism of coenzyme Q in atherogenesis? *Mol Asp Med,* 18 (suppl.): s 85-103, 1997

Amarenco P, et al, High-does atorvastatin after stroke or transient ischemic attack, *New Engl J Med*, 35; 6:349-59, Aug 10, 2006

Rubins HB, et al, Distribution of lipids and 8500 men with coronary artery disease, *Am J Cardiol* ,75:1196-1201, June 15, 1995

Manuel-y-Keenoy B, Vinckx M, Vertommen, et al, Impact of vitamin E supplementation on lipoprotein peroxidation and composition in type 1 diabetic patients treated with Atorvastin, *Atherosclerosis*, 175: 369-76, 2004

Jula A, Marniemi J, Ronnemas T, et al, Effects of diet and simvastatin on serum lipids, insulin, and antioxidants in hypercholesterolemic men: a randomized controlled trial, *J Am Med Assoc*, 287; 5:598-605, 2002

Hensley S, Pfizer's net income quadruples on Lipitor sales, fewer charges, *Wall Street J*, B2, Jan 20, 2005

Lurie P, et al, Financial conflict of interest disclosure and voting patterns and Food and Drug Administration Drug Advisory Committee meetings, *J Am Med Assoc*, 295; 16:1921-28, Apr 26, 2006

Morales K, et al, Simvastatin causes changes in an affective processes in elderly volunteers, *J Am Geriatr Soc*, 54:7-76, Jan 2006

Newman TB, Hulley SS, Carcinogenicity of lipid-lowering drugs, *J Amer Med Assoc*, 275;1:55-60, 1996

Nissen SE, Tuzcu EM, Schoenhagen P, et al, Statin therapy, LDL cholesterol, C-reactive protein, and coronary artery disease, *New Engl J Med*, 351; 1:29-38, Jan 6, 2005

Ridker PM, Cannon CP, Morrow D, et al, C-reactive protein levels and outcomes after statin therapy, *New Engl J Med*, 352: 1:20-28, Jan 6, 2005

Ridker PM, Rifai N, Cook NR, et al, Comparison C-reactive protein and low-density lipoprotein cholesterol levels in the prediction of first cardiovascular events, *New Engl J Med*, 347; 20:1557-65, Nov 14, 2002

Krumholz HM, Seeman TE, Merrill SS, et al, Lack of association between cholesterol and coronary heart disease mortality and morbidity and all-cause mortality in persons older than 70 years, 272; 17:1335-40, Nov 2, 1994

Rifai N, Ridker PM, Proposed cardiovascular risk assessment algorithm using high sensitivity C-reactive protein and lipid screening, *Clin Chem*, 47; 1:28-30, Jan 2001

Wang XL, Rainwater DL, Mahaney MC, Stocker R, Co-supplementation with vitamin E and coenzyme Q10 reduces circulating markers of inflammation in baboons, *Am J Clin Nutr*, 80; 3:649-55, Sep 2004

Himmelfarb J, Kane J, McMonagle E, et al, Alpha and Gamma tocopherol metabolism in healthy subjects and patients with end-stage renal disease, *Kidney Internat*, 64; 3:978-91, Sep 2003

Jiang Q, Ames BN, Gamma tocopherol, but not alpha-tocopherol, decreases proinflammatory eicosanoids and inflammation damage in rats, *FASEB J*, 17; 8:816-22, May 2003

Devaraj S, Jialal I, Alpha-tocopherol supplementation decreases serum C-reactive protein and monocyte interleukin-6 levels in normal volunteers and type 2 diabetic patients, *Free Rad Biol Med*, 29; 8:790-92, Oct 15, 2000

Neaton JD, Blackburn H, Jacobs D, et al, Serum cholesterol level and mortality findings for men screened in the Multiple Risk Factor Intervention Trial. Multiple Risk Factor Intervention Trial Research Group, *Arch Intern Med*, 152; 7:1490-1500, July 1992

Behar S, Graff E, Reicher-Reiss H, et al, Low total cholesterol is associated with high total mortality in patients with coronary heart disease. The Bezafibrate Infarction Prevention (BIP) Study Group, *Heart J*, 18; 1:52-9, Jan 1997

Cassidy AT, Carroll BJ, Hypocholesterolemia during mixed manic episodes, European Archives, *Psych Clin Neurosci*, 2002 June, 252; 3:110-14

Boston PF, Dursun SM, Reveley MA, Cholesterol and mental disorder, *Brit J Psychiat*, Dec 1996, 169; 6:682-9

Engleberg H, Low serum cholesterol and suicide, *Lancet*, March 21,1992 339; 8795:727-79

Ford DE, Erlinger TP, Depression and C-reactive protein in US adults: data from Third National Health and Nutrition Examination Survey, *Arch Intern Med*, 2004 May 10, 164; 9:1010-14

Steinberg K, Arthasarathy S, Witztum JL, et al, Beyond cholesterol: Modification of low-density lipoprotein that increase its atherogenicity, *N Eng. J Med*, 320:915-24, 1989

Cox DA, Cophen ML, Effects of oxidized low-density lipoprotein on vascular contraction and re-laxation: Clinical and pharmacological implications in atherosclerosis, *Pharmacol Rev*, 48:3-19, 1996

Meyer M, Is this the drug for you? Doctors say millions more should take cholesterol drugs -- but are there risks?, *AARP Bulletin*, 20-21, Nov. 2002

Chang WJ, Rothberg KG, Kaman BA, Anderson RGW, Lowering cholesterol content of MA104 cells inhibit receptor-mediated transport of folate, *J Cell Biol*, 118: 63-69, 1992

Illingworth DR, et al, Comparative effects of lovastatin and niacin in primary hypercholesterolemia, *Arch Intern Med*, 154:1586-95, 1994

Rothberg KG, Yingon YS, Kaman BA, Anderson RGW, Cholesterol controls the clustering of gly-cophospholipid-anchored membrane receptor for 5-methyltetrahydrofolate, *J Cell Biol*, 111:2931-38, 1990

Fujimoto T, Calcium pump of the plasma membrane is localized in caveolae, *J Cell Biol*, 120:1147-57, 1993

Mochizuki H, Oda H, Yokkogoshi H, Amplified effect of taurine on PCB-induced hypercholes-terolemia in rats, *Adv Exp Med Biol*, 442:285-290, 1998

Wiseman H, Halliwell B, Damage to DNA by reactive oxygen and nitrogen species: role in inflam-matory disease and progression to cancer, *Biochem J*, 313:17-29, 1996

Graham R, Bayer's insurance not enough for Baycol suits, *Wall Street Journal*, B5, Mar. 14 2003

Magarian GJ, Lucas LM, Colley C, Gemfibizil-induced myopathy, *Arch Intern Med*, 151:1873-74, Sept 1991

Qu B, Li QT, Halliwell B, et al, Mitochondrial damage by the "pro-oxidant" peroxisomal proliferator clofibrate, *Free Rad Biol Med*, 27; 9/10:1095-1102, 1999

Wiseman H, Halliwell B, Damage to DNA by reactive oxygen and nitrogen species: role in inflammatory disease and progression to cancer, *Biochem J*, 313: 17-29, 1996

Gaist D, et al, *Neurology*, 58: 1333-1337, 2002).

Delany RM, Identifying hidden risk: specific assessment and therapy of lipid subclasses, in *The Heart On Fire: Modifiable Risk Factors Beyond Cholesterol*, 10th International Symposium on Functional Medicine, I. F. M., Gig Harbor WA (1-800-228-0622)

Burton TM, Callahan P, Vioxx study sees heart-attack risk, *The Wall Street Journal*, B2 Oct. 30th, 2003

Atkins D, Psaty BM, Koepsell TD, Longstreth WT, Larson EB, Cholesterol reduction and the risk of stroke in men. A meta-analysis of randomized, controlled trials, *Ann Intern Med*, 119: 136-45, 1993

Hebert PR, Gaziano JM, Hennekens CH, An overview of trials of cholesterol-lowering and risk of stroke, *Arch Intern Med*, 155: 50-55, 1995.

Suurbula M, Agewall S, Fagerberg B, Swendehag I, Wikstrand J, on behalf of the Risk Intervention Study (RIS) Group. Multiple risk intervention in high-risk hypertensive patients, *Arterioscler Thromb Vasc Biol*, 16: 462-70, 1996

Johansson J, Olsosn A, Bergstrand L, Elinder LS, Nilsson S, Erik U, Molgaard J, Holme I, Waldius G, Lowering of HDL-2b by probucol partly explains the failure of the drugs to affect femoral arteriosclerosis in subjects with hypercholesterolemia, *Arterioscler Thromb Vasc Biol*, 15: 1049-10 56, 1995

Ridker PM, Rifai N, Clearfield M, et al, Measurement of C-reactive protein for the targeting of statin therapy in the primary prevention of acute coronary events, *New Engl J Med*, 344: 1959-65, 2001

Pearson TA, Commentary: lipid-lowering therapy in low-risk patients, *J Am Med Assoc*, 279: 1659-61, 1998

Perrault S, Hamilton VH, Grover S, et al, Treating hyperlipidemia for the primary prevention of coronary disease: are higher doses of lovastatin cost-effective?, *Arch Intern Med*, 158: 3 75-81, 1998

Tecee MA, Dasgupta I, Doherty JU, Heart disease in older women, *Geriatrics*, 58; 12:333-39, 20

Cohen JS, Do you really need maximum-does Lipitor?, *Life Extension*, Fort Lauderdale, 49-58, Aug 2007

Parker RA, Pearce BC, Clark RW, Gordon DA, Wright JJ, Tocotrienols regulate cholesterol production in mammalian cells by post-transcriptional suppression of 3-hydroxy-3-methylglutaryl-coenzyme A reductase, *J Biol Chem*, 268 (15) 11230-8, May 25, 1993

Plotnick GD, et al, Effect the antioxidant vitamins on the transient impairment of endothelium-dependent brachial artery vasoactivity following a single high-fat meal, *J Am Med Assoc*, 278;20:682-86, Nov 26, 1997

Matthews AW, Glaxo weight-loss drug. Alli wins and nonprescription usage, *Wall Street Journal*, D3, Feb 8, 2007

Jackson PR, et al, Statins for primary prevention: at what coronary risk is safety assured?, *Brit J Clin Pharmacol*, 52: 439-446, 2001

Wagstaff LR, et al., Statin-associated memory loss: analysis of 60 case reports and review of the literature, *Pharmacotherapy*, 23; 7:871-880, 2003

Meske V, et al, Blockade of HMG-CoA reductase activity causes changes in micro-tubule-stabilizing protein tau via suppression of geranylgeranylpyrophosphate formation: implications for Alzheimer's disease, *Europ J Neurosci*, 17:93- 02, 2003

Graham R, Bayer's insurance not enough for Baycol suits, *Wall Street Journal*, B5, Mar. 14 2003

Fitzgerald GA, Coxibs and cardiovascular disease, *New Engl J Med*, 351: 1709-11, Oct. 21, 2004

Topal EJ, Failing the public health – Rofecoxib, Merck, and the FDA, *New Engl J Med*, 351: 1707-9, Oct. 21, 2004

Whalen J, Study by Vioxx critic links drug to extra coronary cases, *Wall St. J*, D3, Jan 25, 2005

Coenzyme Q10 References:
Bargossi AM, Battino M, Gaddi A, et al. Exogenous CoQ10 preserves plasma ubiquinol levels in patients treated with 3-hydroxy-3-methylglutaryl coenzyme A reductase inhibitors, *Internat J Clin Lab Res*, 24: 171-6, 1994

Fuke C, Krikorian, SA, Couris RR, Coenzyme CoQ10: A review of essential Functions and clinical trials, *Pharmacist*, 28-41, Oct 2000

Langsjoen PH, Langsjoen AM, Coenzyme Q10 in cardiovascular disease with emphasis on heart failure and myocardial ischaemia, *Asia Pacific Heart J* ,7; 3: 160-168, 1998

Langsjoen PH, et al, Treatment of statin adverse effects with supplemental coenzyme Q10 and statin drug discontinuation, *BioFactors*, 25 (1-4): 147-52, 2005

Langsjoen PH, et al, The clinical use of HMG CoA-reductase inhibitors and the associated depletion of coenzyme Q10. A review of animal and human publications, *BioFactors*, 18 (1-4): 101-11, 2003

Mabuchi H, et al, Reduction of serum ubiquinol-10 and a ubiquinone-10 levels by atorvastatin in hypercholesterolemia, patients, *J Atheroscler Thromb*, 12; 2:111-19, 2005

Lamperti C, Muscle, coenzyme Q10 level in statin-related myopathy, *Arch Neurol*, 62; 11: 1109-12, Nov 2005

Mortensen AS, et al, Coenzyme Q10: clinical benefits with biochemical correlates suggesting a scientific breakthrough in the management of chronic heart failure, *Int J Tissue React*, 12; 3: 155-62, 1990

Folkers K, Langsjoen P, Tamagawa H, Lovastatin decreases coenzyme levels in humans, *Proc Natl Acad Sci USA*, 1990; 87:8931-34

Bliznakov EG, Wilkins DJ, biochemical and clinical consequences of inhibiting Coenzyme Q10 biosynthesis by lipid-lowering HMG-CoA reductase inhibitors (statins): A critical overview, *Advances in Therapy*, 1998; 15; 4:218-28.

Lockwood K, Moesgaard S, Folkers K, et al, Progress on therapy of breast cancer with vitamin Q10 and the regression of metastases, *Biochem Biophys Res Commun*, 1995; 212:172-177

Gaby AR, The role of coenzyme Q10 in clinical medicine: Cardiovascular disease, hypertension, diabetes mellitus and infertility, *Alt Med Rev*, 1996; 1(3): 168-175

Langsjoen PH, Folkers K, Long-term efficacy and safety of coenzyme Q10 therapy for idiopathic dilated cardiomyopathy, *Amer J Cardiol*, 1990:65; 521-3

Baggio E, Gandini R, Plancher AC, Passeri M, Carmosino G, et al, Italian multicenter; study on the safety and efficacy of coenzyme Q10 as adjunctive therapy in heart failure, *Clin Invest*, 1993; 71:S145-9

Politics of Medicine References:

Cohen JS, *Overdose.The case against the drug companies: prescription drugs, side effects, and your health*, Tarcher/Putnam/Penguin Books, New York, 2001, available from 1-800-669-CALM.

Cauchon D, FDA advisers tied to industry: Approval process riddled with conflicts of interest, *U.S.A. Today*, Sept. 25, 2000

George CF, Adverse drug reactions and secrecy, *British Medical Journal* , 304; 23: 1328, 1992

Angell, M, Is academic medicine for sale?, *New England Journal of Medicine*, 342: 1516-18, May 18, 2000

Angell, M, *The Truth About the Drug Companies*, Random House, NY, 2004

Lazarou J, Pomeranz BH, Corey PN, Incidence of adverse drug reactions in hospitalized patients: a meta-analysis of perspective studies, *Journal American Medical Association*, 279; 15: 1200-1205, April 15, 1998

Stelfox HT, Chua G, Detsky AS, Conflict of interest in the debate over calcium-channel and agonists, *New England Journal of Medicine*, 338; 2:101-6, Jan. 8, 1998

Haley D, *Politics of Healing*, Random House, NY, 2004

Other Disease-Producing Side Effects of Statin Drugs:

Pelton R, LaValle JB, Hawkins EB, Krinsky DL, *Drug-Induced Nutrient Depletion Handbook*, 2nd Edition, 1-800-837-5394

Newman TB, Hulley SB, Carcinogenicity of lipid-lowering drugs, *J Am Med Assoc*, 55-60, 1993

Mortensen SA, Leth A, Rohde M, Dose-related decrease of serum coenzyme Q10 during treatment with HMG-COA reductase inhibitors, *Mol Asp Med*, 18 (suppl): S137-44, 1997

Palomaki A, et al, Enhanced oxidizability of ubiquinol and alpha-tocopherol during lovastatin treatment, *FEBS Letter*, 410: 254-8, 1997

Bliznakov EG, Wilkins DJ, Biochemical and clinical consequences of inhibiting coenzyme Q10 biosynthesis by lipid-lowering HMG COA reductase inhibitors (statins): a critical overview, *Advances in Therapy*, 15; 4:219-28, Jul/Aug 1998

Ghirlanda G, Oradei A, Manto A, et al, Evidence of plasma CoQ10-lowering effect of HMG-CoA reductase inhibitors: a double-blind, placebo-controlled study, *J Clin Pharmacol*, 33: 226-29, 1993

Willis RA, Folkers K, Tucker JL, Tamagawa H., et al., Lovastatin decreases coenzyme Q levels in rats, *Proc Nat Acad Sci USA*, 87: 8928-30, 1990

Folkers K, Langsjoen P, et al, Lovastatin decreases coenzyme Q10 levels in humans, *Proc Nat Acad Sci USA*, 87:8931-4, 1990

Pelton R, LaValle JB, Hawkins EB, Krinsky DL, *Drug-Induced Nutrient Depletion Handbook,* 2nd Edition, 1-800-837-5394

Bliznakov EG, Lipid-lowering to drugs (statins), cholesterol, and coenzyme Q10. The Baycol case--a modern Pandora's box, *Biomed Pharmacother*, 56:56-9, 2002

Jameson S, Statistical data support prediction of death within six months on low levels of coenzyme Q10 and other entities, *Clin Invest*, 71 (suppl):137-39, 1993

Thompson PD, Zmuda JM, Guyton JR, et al, Lovastatin increases exercise-induced skeletal muscle injury, *Metabolism* 46:1206-10, 1997

Herbert PR, Gaziano JM, Chan KS, Hennekens CH, Cholesterol-lowering with statin drugs, risk of stroke and total mortality: an overview of randomized trial, *J Am Med Assoc,* 278:313-21, 1997

Westphal SP, You're my wife?, *New Scientist*, p14, Dec. 6, 2003

Ames RP, Hill P, Increase in serum lipids during treatment of hypertension with chlorthalidone, *Lancet*, i: 721-3, 1976

Tanaka N, Sakaguchi S, Oshige K, Nimura T, Kanehisa T, Effect of chronic administration of propanolol on lipoprotein composition, *Metabolism,* 25: 1071-5, 1976

Waal-Manning HJ, Simpson FO, Beta-blockers and lipid metabolism, *Brit Med Jl*, ii: 705,1977

Meilahan EN, Ferrell RE, Naturally occurring low blood cholesterol and excessive mortality, *Coron Artery Dis*, 4:843-53, 1993

Kritchevsky SB, Kritchevsky D, Serum cholesterol and cancer risk: an epidemiologic perspective, *Annal Rev Nutr*, 12: 391-416, 1992

Hiatt RA, Fireman BH, Serum cholesterol in the incidence of cancer in a large cohort, *J Chron Dis*, 39: 8 61-70, 1986

Muldoon MS, Manuck SM, Matthews KM, Lowering cholesterol concentrations and mortality: a quantitative review of primary prevention trials, *Brit Med J,* 301: 309-14, 1990).

Morales K, et al, Simvastatin causes changes in an affective processes in elderly volunteers, *J Am Geriatr Soc,* 54:7-76, Jan 2006

Partonen, Association of low serum total cholesterol with major depression and suicide, *Br J Psychiatry*, 175; 259-262, 1999

Moosmann B, Behl C, Solano protein synthesis and side effects of statins, *Lancet*, 363: 892-94, 2004

Lipid Research Clinics Program, The Lipid Research Clinics Coronary Primary Prevention Trial results, *J Am Med Assoc*, 251:351-64, 1984

Chapter II

Quick Fixes for Lowering Cholesterol the Smart Way

The good news is there are oodles of safer, cheaper, and better non-prescription alternatives to lower your cholesterol. This chapter will show you some of the simplest, safest, least expensive, non-prescription and most effective ways of normalizing your cholesterol without dangerous drugs. You've just learned that drugs all have side effects that put you on a fast track for other diseases. For the folks who have had a heart attack but do not have high cholesterol, the good news is that you will learn in this chapter some of the many ways to guard against sudden cardiac death. For remember, **half the folks who die of a sudden heart attack never had high cholesterol**. As well, **half the folks who get a sudden heart attack,** irrespective of whether they had high cholesterol, **don't live**. So it behooves us all to learn everything presented here.

Furthermore, once anything invasive has been done to coronary vessels, such as angioplasty, bypass graphs, or stents, the tissues are even more reactive. **Half the folks are already clotting off their "new "vessels within 6 months of the procedure.** And if you have cholesterol plaques or calcifications in your coronaries already or other risk factors for early cardiac death, you can learn some of the ways to reverse them, in subsequent chapters. Last, but never least, for those who think they are well, have no high cholesterol problem, and have not had a heart attack or heart surgery yet, read on. You may be in silent deep trouble and not even know it, as half the sudden deaths have been at surprisingly younger ages, many in thin, active folks. But buck up. You, too, can empower yourselves to stave off these events.

To B or Not to B

Vitamin B3, also called niacin, is a wonderfully natural way to lower cholesterol, and in fact is one of the oldest, safest, and best researched. It is even available as a prescription drug Niaspan®, but that has the side effects of liver toxicity. Fortunately, there is a form of niacin that is far superior to the prescription Niaspan, called **Niacin-Time**. What are Niacin-time's advantages?

- It is formulated with a sustained release form wax matrix that allows slow release over 5-7 hours. You want to be treating your high cholesterol for as long as possible throughout the day with sustained corrective levels.
- The natural beeswax matrix is safer than the synthetic petro-chemical concoctions for coating pills for sustained release used by pharmaceutical companies.
- The wax matrix makes Niacin-Time less likely to cause the flushing, tingling or the transient hot flash that is associated with niacin.
- Medical studies have proven Niacin-Time is better than the prescription form, with better absorption and fewer side effects
- It is non-prescription, so you have control.

After reviewing the data, the odds, and seeing the effects in folks first-hand, **Niacin-Time** is a great place to start to lower your cholesterol. Take 500 mg of Niacin-Time, one or two twice daily. Depending on your body burden of factors causing your high cholesterol, it may be all you need. For others they may need to combine other cholesterol-lowering agents with it. And for others, as you will learn in subsequent chapters, these treatments will not be enough, for they need to get to the root cause. But take heart, I'll guide you through it all.

Meanwhile, if your doctor insists on using the prescription form of Niaspan (because it is controlled by him and is in the *PDR (Physician's Desk Reference* book of drugs), remind him that studies comparing Niaspan (or Advicor which is lovastatin plus extended release niacin) versus the special wax matrix of Niacin-Time, showed superior bioavailability (gets into the blood stream better) for Niacin-Time (Figge). And then you may hear that niacin has been associated with abnormal liver enzymes, for example, elevated alkaline phosphatase. It is always a good idea to check the levels of liver enzymes, but bear in mind that a high percentage of people who are on placebo also have elevated liver enzymes and that the very abnormality that caused the high cholesterol may indeed be the culprit for the liver enzyme elevations (Keenan).

More importantly, as you will learn here, vitamin B3 works in harmony with other nutrients. Only pharmaceutical companies try to use nutrients as though they were solo drugs. But nutrients are not solo acts; they simply were not designed to work that way. So when you bombard someone with Niaspan, the prescription form of niacin, of course there is more chance of liver toxicity since you are using unphysiologically high doses. Contrast this with the lower doses needed for Niacin-time because (1) you will learn how to combine it with complimentary nutrients that allow a lower dosage, and (2) its superior bioavailability confirmed in medical tests also allows a lower, safer dose, translating into less chance of liver problem (which I have never seen with Niacin-Time).

But Niacin-time's benefits don't end here. As you will learn, there are many other indicators of early heart attack, many of which are much more serious, much more deadly, and faster acting than having a high cholesterol. Some of these dangerous factors include:

(1)   **A high fibrinogen**, a protein that indicates there is nasty inflammation going on somewhere which is making the blood eager to throw clots.
(2)   **A low HDL**, for remember many folks who had serious heart attacks or sudden death never had high cholesterol, but many had a low or low normal (below 60) "good" HDL cholesterol.
(3)   **Elevated lipoprotein A, called Lp(a).**

The good news is **Niacin not only safely decreases cholesterol synthesis, but also works better than the statins at lowering fibrinogen, raising HDL, and lowering Lp(a)** (Illingworth, Shepherd, Jin). Niacin fixes all these, and it is a natural vitamin that the body needs anyway. In one study in the *Journal of the American Medical Association*, **niacin raised the good cholesterol or HDL 29% and lowered triglycerides 28%, while the statin drug failed to do this** (Elam). In fact niacin works so well that it has even reversed cholesterol transport (Jin), which translates into **reversing coronary artery disease** (Brown). But I'll tell you more about this later. Meanwhile, **there isn't a more logical first choice than Niacin-Time**.

The Least Expensive Cholesterol Treatment
Also Helps Other Abnormalities

This is so important, let's review: Niacin or vitamin B3 has been known for over 50 years to be good for lowering cholesterol (Altschul), so good in fact that it is one of the few vitamins that has become a prescription drug. Niaspan® is a prescription capsule that is a time released form of niacin or nicotinic acid, vitamin B3, to give steadier levels in the body. But studies have shown that **Niacin-Time** (Carlson) is superior to Niaspan®, as well as being, much cheaper, non-prescription, and with a natural beeswax-matrix that makes it sustained-release, for a continuous release over 5-7 hours (Aronov) as opposed to the plasticizers used by the pharmaceutical industry for sustained release.

If that were not good enough news, Niacin-Time does more than just lower cholesterol by about 16%. It also **lowers the bad cholesterol LDL-C** (which plasters cholesterol onto the arterial wall) by 21%. But it does more. It also **raises the good cholesterol HDL** (that carries cholesterol off the arterial wall and dumps it into the gut) **by 29%** (Alderman, Elam). Remember that having a low HDL is one of the only risk factors that many people with serious heart disease had. They never had high cholesterol. But Niacin-

Time does even more. Having elevated lipoprotein(a) is another far more dangerous risk factor than having a high cholesterol or even a high oxidized LDL cholesterol. **None of the statins help to lower the Lp(a), but niacin is one of the few treatments for lowering lipoprotein(a) or Lp(a)** (Aronov, Carlson), in addition to actually **reversing coronary vascular lesions** (Brown). If that were not enough, Niacin-Time also lowers triglycerides. What drug can compete with nature's niacin? What pharmaceutical drug made in a lab can compete with what God has designed to:

(1)   Lower cholesterol 16%,
(2)   Lower LDL-C 21%,
(3)   Lower Lp (a)
(4)   Raise HDL 29%
(5)   Lower triglycerides 26%

If you're already on a statin drug for your cholesterol, adding Niacin-Time has enabled many to lower their doses of statin drugs, thereby decreasing the outrageous costs (over $4 a capsule now) and decreasing the chances of the serious side effects of statin drugs which include the fatal rotting away of the heart and other muscles, rhabdomyolysis (Gardner). And for folks who need higher doses but get flushing and tingling, you can use a half or whole aspirin to cut the reactions until you learn how to get yourself healthier and not need it (Whelan).

Doses of niacin over 2000 milligrams can cause an elevated homocysteine. Since higher doses are the ones associated with flushing, I would recommend finding the additional factors that are needed to bring your cholesterol to normal, rather than beating it to death with just vitamin B3 by using the vitamin like a solo drug. Remember, nutrients work in synergy in the body. **The body is a magnificent orchestration of chemical interactions.** As you'll learn, there is more than one way to lower cholesterol; in fact most people use several complementary modalities, since most folks are complexly deficient. So **when one modality doesn't work, don't push it to the limit, see what else is missing.**

The drawbacks? Whenever you use excessively high levels of a nutrient, especially when it is unbalanced with other nutrients, as most of the medical studies are, you can expect adverse effects. Elevated liver enzymes and increased blood sugar were the main problems, plus a small percentage of people had the classic flushing that made B3 intolerable to them (Aronov, Elam). But I have observed that **once folks have their nutrient levels measured and corrected, as you will learn to do, they can use much lower doses of nutrients to achieve the same cholesterol-lowering effect, and thereby avoid unwanted side effects.** And remember vitamin B3 is not just for lowering high cholesterol and raising the HDL but, depending on an individual's deficiencies, it works for depression, leg pains, angina, memory loss, schizophrenia, energy, peripheral vascular disease, and much more. On the flipside, statin drugs don't have a litany of other beneficial effects and the body does not require them.

The great news is that studies prove the special beeswax matrix coating of Carlson's Niacin-Time make it better absorbed, more effective, safer and it's infinitely cheaper than the **Niaspan** prescribed by physicians. In fact it had **double the absorption**, which translates into better bioavailability, hence a lower dose can be used, making it **less likely to create flushing or liver problems**. As proof of this, compared to the Rx, **the dropout rate from Niacin-Time flushing was reduced from 25% to 3%.**

When you factor in that Niacin-Time is cheaper as well as safer, plus doubles your levels allowing you to use half as much, there's no contest (Aronov, Keenan). And contrary to other forms of niacin, it is **safe for diabetics** while it has the added benefit of not only **raising the HDL cholesterol but also lowering triglycerides** (Elam). Non-prescription Niacin-Time is beyond a doubt the best-proven form of B3, and far superior to the commonly prescribed

B3 form. The dose to start with is one **Niacin-Time** 500 mg two or three times a day and move it to four times a day if needed. To be or not 2B, but definitely B3 in the form of Niacin-Time (Carlson, 1-800-323-4141 or carlsonlabs.com).

The Yeast Solution

Do you want something else to start to lower your cholesterol naturally or to add to an existing treatment? How about the tongue-twister red yeast rice? It turns out that over a thousand years ago in China, folks started adding purple-colored yeast, *Monascus purpureus* to steamed rice and then fermenting the mixture. The result was red-colored rice; it was used as a food-coloring agent as well as for improving digestion and blood circulation (Ma). The amazing fact is that somehow it was discovered that red yeast rice contains statins, the most prevalent one being lovastatin, the very statin that was the first prescription cholesterol-lowering drug Mevacor®. But in contrast to the prescription, I'll show you why red yeast rice has virtually no side effects (Wang, Li, Heber).

I know it sounds a bit odd that a particular fungus strain, *Monascus purpureus,* used for centuries as a natural food additive to color foods could lower cholesterol. But when rice is fermented with this fungus it creates a pallet of chemicals that target the cholesterol-making enzyme in the liver, HMG CoA reductase. Remember this is the same liver enzyme that statins poison. But instead of using nature's full pallet of chemicals, **drug manufacturers have stripped statins down to one part of this pallet and modified them with chemical attachments** so they could become a new patentable drug for lowering cholesterol. **They stole the chemistry from nature, and then dangerously modified it** so it could be a unique thus patentable drug. In doing so they have stripped it of its natural harmonizing properties and created something that is potentially toxic. **In their attempt to "one-up" nature, they invariably create a laundry list of side effects.**

In fact, the majority of pharmaceutical drugs are copied from nature and derived from fungal chemistry. As usual though, pharmaceutical companies do not use the whole natural product produced by the yeast (nature), but only part of it. **By artificially fractionating a natural product, you lose the harmony of the other components.** This is why drugs have so many side effects and natural agents do not. The harmony of the other components is necessary to maximize the good effects without creating harmful ones. Pharmaceutical chemists always seem to think they can one-up God!

Let me back you up with a tad of history. The first cholesterol-lowering drug to hit the market was the statin called Mevocor® (generic lovastatin). Red yeast rice is a natural mixture of statins, the most prevalent one being lovastatin, the very statin that made the first leading prescription cholesterol-lowering drug, Mevacor. The difference is that **the natural statins of red yeast rice include 8-10 parts called monocolins in the pallet, just as they occur in real life, or nature. In contrast, the synthetic and very pricey statin Rx (prescription) medications contain only one monocolin.** Thus the prescription drug has all the side effects that you read about in the first chapter, in contrast to red yeast rice that has virtually no side effects.

Furthermore, red yeast rice treatment of cholesterol in general *costs about 1/5th of what the cholesterol-lowering statin drugs cost, but without the side effects.* In addition it has the benefit of being able to be titrated to lower doses for each individual (Perrreault). For studies show that the "one dose for all" mentality of the drug industry causes a greater avalanche of side effects and drug reactions (Cohen).

Another interesting fact is **the magnitude of cholesterol lowering by red yeast rice was greater in some studies than the synthetic pricey and side effect-laden prescription statins.** But that's not all. Additional benefits include the fact that red yeast rice is an antioxidant, which many natural products are, versus something made in the laboratory. As well, **red yeast rice lowers the CRP.** C-Reactive Protein, a blood test in your **Cardio/ION Panel** that we will discuss later is a potent indicator of dangerous inflammation raging in the body. **An elevated CRP is alarming, because it is more strongly predictive for an early heart attack than high cholesterol.**

In *The New England Journal of Medicine* "specialists" have recommended that doctors prescribe statins to lower CRP even if their patients do not have high cholesterol (Ridker)!   But this is ridiculous as you learned in the preceding chapter, because it is equivalent to killing the messenger and not correcting the underlying curable cause. You must find the cause of CRP, which can be anything from a silent tooth root infection that does not show on repeated x-rays, to an infected heart valve or hidden cancer. But more on this in subsequent chapters.

Besides containing lovastatin (the main ingredient in prescription Mevacor) red yeast rice contains eight other statin-type monocolins. This makes it much like a natural vitamin E that contains all eight components (4 tocopherols and 4 tocotrienols), versus the dangerous health-robbing synthetic "vitamin E". Many studies that bad-mouth vitamin E use only alpha-d,l-tocopherol (as found in cheap synthetic grocery store vitamins), containing only one of nature's 8 natural components, and in an unnatural and harmful synthetic form.

By the way, whenever you feel there's a big knowledge gap, terms you're not familiar with, or you feel overwhelmed, just keep plowing through. You will amaze yourself at how your knowledge and understanding start to build. Later on you may want to go to the other books and past years of **Total Wellness** *newsletter to fill in the blanks. I don't want to bore the faithful readers by repeating things that they have learned in the previous books and newsletters. Furthermore, because physicians read this as well, I often* *step out of my lay medicine mode to give them a little more in-depth information. So don't let it scare you off. Knowledge, like health or prowess in any sport, is built up over time and it would be extremely rare to get everything you need from just one book.*

Meanwhile, **Red yeast rice can raise HDLs (the good protective cholesterol) up to 16%.** This is important you now know, because many folks who never had high cholesterol got serious heart damage just because they had a low (or low normal, under 60mg/dl) HDL. And for those with high cholesterol, red yeast rice can drop cholesterol by 20%. Furthermore it has caused **regression or melting away of carotid artery** (the main artery from the heart to the brain) **plaque up to 40%** in experimental animals, even while they were fed a high cholesterol diet. There are no statin reports of melting away plaque by 40%.

Furthermore, red yeast rice **increased the number of LDL receptors** so the body could properly get rid of the "bad cholesterol". In addition, red yeast rice has **improved non-functioning calcium channels**. This is extremely important because calcium channel blockers are the number one prescribed category of drugs by cardiologists and they are usually prescribed for life, even though they are proven to shrink the brain and rot the intellect within five years use.

Since **red yeast rice is safer, cheaper, and more physiologic** (closer to the natural product than a synthetic drug), plus it **improves CRP, HDL, LDL receptors, calcium channels, and makes plaque melt away,** it's pretty clear that it would make another great starting point for cholesterol treatment. Or it may be all that you need. As opposed to drugs with lots of side effects including damaging liver function tests, red yeast rice has actually improved liver function tests, plus a dose of 50 times that which a human would use has been proven to be safe. And **it does not cause the potentially fatal rhabdomyolysis** (stealthily beginning with muscle weakness and pain) **that the statins do.**

From time to time you'll see it temporarily pulled off the market because pharmaceutical companies have successfully worked at eliminating their competition, but then it emerges once again, unscathed. And no wonder, when you recall **the magnitude of cholesterol lowering by red yeast rice was greater than the synthetic statins**. In addition, its benefits also include anti-oxidant effects, which are more likely with natural products than something made in the laboratory, plus it lowers the CRP and raises the HDL (Patrick)! But you know that just one brand of cholesterol-lowering drugs, like Lipitor, brings in over $10 billion a year. That's a lot of political clout.

Not All Red Yeast Rice Preparations
Are Safe or Even Effective

Unfortunately, an analysis of nine different red yeast rice over-the-counter products showed great variability. Some of them even **contained a toxic fermentation by-product called citrinin, which is a mycotoxin (mold toxin)** capable of causing kidney damage and genetic change leading to cancer, among other symptoms. You want a product free of citrinin. **Wakunaga's Kyolic Formula 107 Red Yeast Rice** is the only form I have found free of citron.

What's even better is that it is combined with Kyolic, which is a special proprietary form of aged garlic. I have written and referenced this extensively in *No More Heartburn*, *Detoxify or Die* and *The High Blood Pressure Hoax* because of its multiple benefits, all supported by over 300 research papers. As just a few examples, **Kyolic** itself can not only lower cholesterol, discourage plaque build-up as well as blood pressure elevation, but is an antioxidant, blood thinner, and kills some bacteria like H. pylori (that can cause coronary artery disease) and yeasts like Candida (which can mimic diseases like chronic fatigue, IBS, and fibromyalgia or trigger auto-immune thyroiditis that then raises cholesterol), and more. Odorless garlic protects cholesterol from becoming oxidized to the

form that causes deposits in arterial walls that then attract cholesterol patches (Munday). And garlic changes platelet function directly to decrease clot formation (Steiner).

Kyolic Formula 107 Red Yeast Rice contains 600 mg of Wakunaga's incomparable aged garlic extract, **Kyolic,** plus 600 mg of
red yeast rice, all rolled into one, and is on average nine times
cheaper than the prescription statin drugs. **Kyolic Formula 107
Red Yeast Rice** has no citrinins, but does have a healthful balance
of the rest of the monocolins. For now the most logical thing to
do is take two capsules of **Kyolic Formula 107 Red Yeast Rice**
twice a day with meals and check your cholesterol in a couple of
months (Wakunaga 1-800-421-2998). It can be combined with
Niacin-Time if you need.

The Sweet Solution

There is yet another easy, non-prescription solution for cholesterol.
Policosanol is a very unique natural product that is purified from
sugarcane wax and the wax of common honeybees (mainly a mixture of aliphatic alcohols, primarily octacosanol) or rice. It has
been studied extensively for over a decade, albeit mainly in Cuba
where the cane source is made. These researchers compared using
policosanol with many of the most popular prescription cholesterol-lowering drugs that cost infinitely more. Being synthesized
in a laboratory, unnatural and designed to poison enzymes in the
human chemistry, drugs are loaded with adverse side effects. On
the flip side, because policosanol is a product derived from natural
sources, it has no side effects and is cheaper. And get this. It's
doesn't do the same job as the prescription drugs, but **does a *better*
job than the prescription drugs in lowering cholesterol.**

Yes, you got that right. Policosanol at 20 mg, one twice a day (20-
40 mg per day total dose) has **outperformed the statin drugs**.
And it was compared with the three leading prescription drugs that
cost far more. Not only that, but it **lowered the LDL** or the bad

cholesterol significantly **more than the prescription drugs did**, and it **lowered the total cholesterol more than the prescription drugs did, sometimes twice as much**. And recall, **for every 1% reduction in total cholesterol there is a 2% reduction in the risk of fatal and nonfatal heart attack** (Pearson). So for example, when the UCLA study showed that policosanol dropped cholesterol levels 16%, that means they dropped the heart attack risk 32% (Heber).

More importantly, **policosanol elevated the HDL** or the good cholesterol, which a lot of prescription drugs doesn't touch. **For the HDL is one of the wheelbarrows that carry cholesterol away from the arterial wall and dumps it into the liver where it is made into detoxifying bile.** You also want a neutraceutical like policosanol that safely and naturally lowers cholesterol without forcing the body's cholesterol-controlling gene into submission, like statins do.

Because of policosanol's performance, safety, price, and rationale, to my way of thinking, it should be considered the unconscionable practice of medicine to put any patient on a prescription cholesterol-lowering drug before giving him a chance to evaluate **Policosanol, Kyolic Red Yeast Rice, Niacin-Time,** or any combination and the other natural cholesterol-lowering therapies that I'll show you here. Incidentally, some of the patients in the studies who were on the prescription cholesterol-lowering drugs actually had to drop out of the studies because they turned yellow (jaundiced) from dangerous damage to the liver from drugs. Nothing like that happens with policosanol.

You can get non-prescription, natural policosanol derived from either of two natural sources, your choice. The two sources of waxes include a 10 mg cane source of **Policosanol** (ProThera) and a rice source of **Policosanol** (Jarrow), although most of the research is on cane.

Who would ever think that compounds found in sugarcane could work in the exact same way as the statin drugs that turn off your liver's cholesterol production. Because **the liver makes 3 times as much cholesterol as you consume in your food, that's why diet is so unsuccessful for many people, since their liver is still cranking out cholesterol.** The interesting part is that in spite of a huge number of studies, rarely does the average doctor know anything about policosanol and its mechanism of action, or that it is cheaper and safer than the synthetic statin drugs. And it actually works better than the pricey prescriptions in many of the studies because **it lowered cholesterol, triglycerides and LDL cholesterol more than the Rx drugs, while increasing the good HDL cholesterol more than the drugs** (Castano 2001).

Let's take a peak at some of those studies. In one, when policosanol and pravastatin (Pravachol is the trade name of this statin Rx drug) were tested side-by-side, policosanol gave much better cholesterol lowering, plus it raised the good HDL cholesterol which the statin prescription drug did not do (Castano 1999).

In other studies comparing simvastatin (Zocor) or lovastatin (Mevacor) with policosanol, again the policosanol clearly outshined the statin drugs (Ortensi, Crespo). And policosanol does more than just lower cholesterol. It has improved the symptoms of severe leg pain cramps from arteriosclerosis when walking a short distance, called **intermittent claudication** (Castano). That implies it may have caused some of the plaque to recede from the arterial wall, perhaps via the **increased HDL wheelbarrow that carts cholesterol off the arterial wall,** but more on that later. Also it has **lowered the ability of platelets to clot**, another important mechanism to thwart heart attacks and strokes (Aarruzabala). This is important because the ability of statins to lower clotting has been used as another excuse to recommend it for millions of adults and children who don't even have high cholesterol.

But policosanol does it better, safer, and cheaper. As well, it improved the ability of patients with severe coronary artery disease to exercise (Stusser). Because it is natural, it avoids the arm's length list of side effects of the synthetic molecules that are in the *PDR (Physicians Desk Reference)*. The dose? Start with 10 mg **Policosanol** twice a day and move to two twice a day before adding anything else. Because policosanol and red yeast rice are also HMG CoA reductase inhibitors, I would recommend you add coenzyme Q10, at least until you check your CoQ10 status.

Always Look to Nature

I think it is rather ironic that most of the "invented" medicines have really been stolen from Mother Nature. But when real natural remedies become competitors, they are scoffed at and folks are ridiculed for using something so simple. Scientists have studied how God-given food components keep us in natural balance. When we stray from that natural balance by distorting the original molecules to create patentable drugs or processed foods and continually tank up on more environmental chemicals, we damage our chemistry. Fortunately Nature still has the answers for bringing us back to normal.

You now know more about natural treatments than probably 90% of physicians. If you don't believe me, just ask your doctor what he knows about Niacin-Time, Kyolic Red Yeast Rice or Policosanol. *You are already unbeatably terrific!*

Lycopene
What makes tomatoes red? A plant chemical or phytochemical called Lycopene. But God didn't just put it there so tomatoes could be red. It has a lot of other beneficial effects, one of which is to safely turn down (and not poison the gene that governs the enzyme like the statin drugs do) the enzyme that makes cholesterol, HMG CoA reductase. Lycopene is a carotenoid, a plant pigment, which *does not convert to vitamin A but does convert to beta-carotene.* It

is well known for its inhibition of prostate, breast and other cancers as well as improvement in diabetes (Monograph AMR). However it also can reduce lipids by inhibiting the enzyme in white blood cells HMG-CoA reductase (Fuhrman) and it also enhances the breakdown of the LDL bad cholesterol (Arab).

In one study, researchers looked at over a thousand individuals after they had had a heart attack. Only lycopene levels were found to be protective (Kohlmeier), while in other studies low lycopene levels were associated with early arteriosclerosis (Rissanen). In fact, among carotenoids, lycopene is the most efficient quencher of single oxygen, in other words **it is a very strong antioxidant, a major mechanism that can protect LDL cholesterol from doing its damage and gluing itself to your artery walls** (DiMascio). You see, cholesterol, no matter how high it is, is not damaging and does not normally adhere to arterial walls. It is only when the cholesterol has been oxidized by free radicals and the vessel wall has been damaged by acidity that the cholesterol bandage comes to the rescue. But more on this later.

Unfortunately the most popular source for lycopene is tomatoes, a nightshade category of vegetable. Nightshades are an unrecognized source of agony, for in 3 out of 4 folks who ache or hurt with any joint pain or tendonitis, nightshades are the hidden cause. But when folks don't know how to get rid of their arthritis or pain, they take NSAID drugs that damage the cartilage. This nearly guarantees they will eventually need a hip or knee replacement. For folks who want to get out of pain, read *Pain Free In Six Weeks* (prestigepublishing.com, Rogers). Fortunately, we have a tomato-free source of lycopene, but if you have arthritis, make sure none of your other nutrients contain a lycopene derived from nightshades.

For reducing LDL cholesterol, 60 mg of lycopene a day was the best dose (Fuhrman). Food sources include watermelon, pink grapefruit, papaya, red cabbage, beets, and other red foods, but you usually can't eat that much. Carlson 10 mg Lycopene is derived entirely from tomatoes while, for folks like myself who have nightshade-induced arthritis Carlson 15 mg **Lycopene** is tomato-free. Two Carlson **Lycopene 15 mg** twice a day could cut your cholesterol, LDL oxidation and development of arteriosclerosis.

Vitamin C

It sounds too simple doesn't it? After all, if ordinary vitamin C was good for high cholesterol that would be a lot cheaper and safer than the statin drugs. The truth is some of the research on vitamin C actually dates back more than 60 years. Does that give you further indication of the power of the drug industry? Let's look at some of the astounding facts.

For decades it has been known that **a vitamin C deficiency causes high cholesterol** (Ginter, Levy). Furthermore giving high doses of vitamin C (4 g daily in one study) has lowered high cholesterol. But there are numerous mechanisms by which ascorbic acid or vitamin C protects our arterial linings from hypercholesterolemia and arteriosclerotic plaque. Let's take a peek at just some of these:

(1) Vitamin C is necessary to finish **converting cholesterol into bile,** which then is stored in the gallbladder to be squirted out into the upper intestines to help us absorb our healthful fat-soluble nutrients like vitamins A, D, E, K, beta-carotene, CoQ10, lipoic acid, and the important fatty acids EPA and DHA, plus crucial phosphatidyl choline, all necessary in order to have a normal cholesterol level. But when folks are low in vitamin C, the pathway for normal cholesterol metabolism is blocked and it piles up inside the blood vessels, where it becomes a target for free radicals.

(2) On the flip side, with a vitamin C deficiency, the production of bile acids is markedly reduced. But bile acids include an enzyme needed to counter arterial plaque, **lipoprotein lipase**. Without enough, it is easier for cholesterol to get oxidized and glue itself onto arterial walls.

(3) **Vitamin C increases HDL levels,** which many statins do not (Salonen).

(4) Arteriosclerosis is an inflammatory disease. Cholesterol is only deposited on arterial walls that are damaged by infection or environmental toxins or lacking certain nutrients or when the cholesterol molecule itself is damaged by free radicals, creating oxidized LDL. Otherwise normal cholesterol will not attach itself to an undamaged vessel wall. That's another reason why vitamin C is so useful, because it is **anti-inflammatory and a detoxifier**: for inflammation is at the root of arteriosclerosis (Levy).

(5) **Cholesterol is also a Band-Aid**. It not only helps the body remove heavy metals and infectious organisms that eat holes in the blood vessel linings, but it patches these holes so that we don't bleed to death. Now you can begin to see the idiocy of killing the messenger, cholesterol. **When cholesterol is elevated, this means the body is vigorously attempting to put out the fires of inflammation or to detoxify itself or protect us from bleeding to death. Cholesterol is only the messenger, not the cause**. Because cholesterol is also a detoxifier, it screams that we had better find the underlying cause while we use large amounts of **vitamin C to quell the fires of inflammation and toxicity**. You'll learn more about the causes in subsequent chapters.

In essence, it has been known for decades that hidden unsuspected low levels of vitamin C cause high cholesterol and in humans you **can lower that cholesterol in many folks just by making their vitamin C levels normal** (Turely). Unfortunately like many nutrients, vitamin C is slowly going lower in the average American diet as people drink fruit juices that have been sterilized to kill vitamin C. Then a smattering of a synthetic ascorbate is added, so manufacturers can brag about the product being fortified with vitamin C on the label.

And vitamin C has a lot of other properties that the statin drugs do not and so when all of these are tied together, **vitamin C supercedes the statins in many parameters** (Kaul, Levy). You see the statins and vitamin C both can down regulate the peroxisomes (PPAR-alpha and -gamma, little organelles inside our cells) that are poisoned by phthalates or plasticizers from our diets. Therefore they both act like anti-oxidants in reducing LDL oxidation. But vitamin C also reduces lipid peroxidation (aging chemistry), platelet aggregation (abnormal clotting), and other cytokine factors that lead to arteriosclerosis as well as to cancers. Researchers show us that this makes vitamin C much more useful for prevention and treatment of coronary heart disease (Levine).

A major problem is that the levels of vitamin C to cause a deficiency are not so low that folks have the classic signs of scurvy that any doctor can diagnose. Instead most folks have what we call subclinical or marginal deficiencies. Their levels may even be "normal" on blood tests, but usually are on the low side of normal range. However, many folks need to be in the high normal range or even higher than normal in order to correct their hypercholesterolemia. But, frequently high oral doses are intolerable, first because they trigger diarrhea. One way around it is to cut the dose or try to fool the body by dividing it into two doses spaced several hours apart. And of course, there is a reliable blood test (part of the **Cardio/ION Panel**) to show your vitamin C adequacy. I prefer **Klaire Ultrafine Pure Ascorbic Acid**, but there are many other forms, like buffered ones, that some folks prefer.

Fire Your Cardiologist if He Doesn't Recommend Vitamin E

Studies from the most prestigious institutions, like Harvard have shown for over a decade that taking vitamin E and other antioxidants clearly lowers your chance of a heart attack, heart disease, stroke, dying of a heart attack and even keeps cholesterol from thickening the coronary artery wall (Rimm, Stampfer, Bonner,

Stephens, Kritchevsky). Yet where are the cardiologists who are recommending vitamin E as a first line of attack?

And you should scratch your cardiologist off your list if just tells you to "take some vitamin E". Preferably he would measure your vitamin E level (**Cardio/Ion Panel**) and then recommend a vitamin E that contains all 8 parts, 4 tocopherols and 4 tocotrienols. My favorite form is **E-Gems Elite** (Carlson), two a day. For if he tells you to take just any vitamin E, you'll probably pick the cheapest one which is synthetic d,l-tocopherol, proven to actually block and negate the good effect of natural d-alpha-tocopherol from foods and natural supplements. And only half of the synthetic form is absorbed as compared with natural vitamin E (Burton). Studies show that even **400 I. U. a day of vitamin E cuts the rate of nonfatal heart attack 77%** (Stephens), and multiple other studies support this (Swain), making it criminal to my way of thinking to neglect to recommend it.

E Stands for Essential

Before I tell you about the other parts of vitamin E, let's make sure you know what a miracle worker it is. In one study 900 I.U. of vitamin E nearly completely suppressed the uptake into the white blood cells of the bad cholesterol that normally deposits on the coronary lining. In fact, vitamin E has done such a great job in preventing the progression of plaque in coronary arteries that it has even done so in patients dumb enough to continue smoking!

In another study, 1200 units of vitamin E a day cut lipid peroxidation by 40%. Lipid peroxidation is one more important measure of deterioration and aging of the body, and is found in your **Cardio/ION Panel**. Alpha-tocopherol (also measured in there as vitamin E) is the principal and most potent fat-soluble antioxidant and is mainly located in cell membranes and in the LDL cholesterol molecule. White blood cells are the richest source of cytokines (infection and cancer killing substances that try to protect us, resulting in inflammation) like tumor necrosis factor and CRP. When the blood carries too much LDL cholesterol, it becomes attacked and oxidized by these cytokines that are really trying to protect us, hence an elevated CRP. And once the cholesterol is oxidized, it glues itself onto the blood vessel lining, resulting in arteriosclerotic plaque. Vitamin E protects against all of this. But **remember, the statin drugs lower your vitamin E.**

In addition, when animals were fed trans fatty acids to raise their cholesterol, researchers then compared the benefits of vitamin E with lovastatin versus lovastatin (Lipitor) alone. Needless to say, there was no money to support a study of vitamin E alone, which would have been the logical addition to this study. But suffice to say, the **coronary plaque size was much smaller in the vitamin E group** (Singh). But they got gutsy with another drug, Probucol, and compared it alone versus vitamin E alone in cholesterol-fed animals. The drug did not prevent arteriosclerosis but vitamin E did (Ozer)! And most importantly, in animals that already had arteriosclerosis, **8 months of vitamin E dropped the stenosis (plugging) from 33% to 8%** (Verlangieri). Do you need any more evidence on how misguided drug-driven medicine is?

The Eight Parts of Vitamin E to the Rescue

Lucky for us, the Master Biochemist has created **vitamin E for slowing down arteriosclerosis, calcifications, and unwanted clots**. If that were not spectacular enough, this vitamin **downregulates (decreases) the oxidation (or free radical change) of LDL cholesterol, so that it does not attach to blood vessel linings like Velcro** (Devaraj). Remember, it is the oxidation of LDL (by free radicals in our blood from fast foods and environmental chemicals) that makes cholesterol eager to grab onto our arterial blood vessel linings for dear life. This is the beginning of plaque that causes heart attacks. On the flip side, if we have enough antioxidants on board (from whole foods and nutrients that you are learning about), cholesterol remains harmless.

Alpha-tocopherol, one of the eight parts of vitamin E, not only lowers the bad LDL cholesterol, it turns down the damage from other inflammatory indicators, especially the tumor necrosis factor (TNF) and the CRP (Devaraj). But it only happens with vitamin E in the natural form of alpha-tocopherol, not the ineffective synthetic "vitamin E" (d,l-tocopheryl) in cheap grocery store nutrients (and the ones chosen for the negative outcome studies that make the press).

In one study a mere **800 IU of a-tocopherol reduced the heart attack and death rate by 33%** (Stephens). Wow! That means one in every three folks was spared from a heart attack just by taking one nutrient a day. There is no drug that has that type of power. And in spite of this being published in Britain's leading medical journal over six years ago, where are the cardiologists who should be recommending something so simple, safe, inexpensive, and lifesaving? Instead, most have fallen for the bad press that vitamin E is frequently subjected to as a result of flawed science.

This is unbelievably empowering information that all cardiologists should be telling their patients about. In another study **900 mg of vitamin E nearly completely suppressed the uptake of LDL onto the white blood cells so the white blood cells couldn't carry the bad cholesterol to glue it onto the coronary vessel lining**. Recall, that vitamin E has done such a great job at preventing the progression of plaque in the coronary arteries that it has even done so in patients who continued to smoke!

In another study, **1200 units of vitamin E a day cut lipid peroxidation by 40%.** Alpha-tocopherol is the principal and most potent fat-soluble antioxidant and is mainly located in cell membranes and **is also protective if enough of it is inside the LDL (bad) cholesterol molecule, as it was designed to be.** But the processing of whole grains into flour and the hydrogenation of vegetable oils into trans fatty acid vehicles has greatly reduced our food sources of natural vitamin E.

In fact, the hidden Vitamin E deficiency epidemic is scarier than I had imagined. In **one study of well-to-do kids ages 2-5, over 9 out of 10 or 91% of them were deficient in vitamin E!** (Drewel). And half of them didn't even have two-thirds of the RDA (recommended daily allowance). This is earth-shaking when you realize the RDA is a pathetic 11 international units or I.U., while the doses that cut many diseases including heart disease in half were 400-800 IU. I shudder for the future health of these kids.

White blood cells are the richest source of cytokines (infection- and cancer-killing substances) the body makes inside cells that protect us. When infection or some unwanted nasty chemical or heavy metal is in the body in amounts that stress the overworked detoxification system, this results in a warning, like elevated TNF (tumor necrosis factor designed by God to kill cancer cells), fibrinogen or hsCRP. When the blood carries too much of the bad cholesterol, LDL cholesterol becomes attacked and oxidized by these cytokines that are really trying to protect us, hence an elevated CRP. **Once the LDL cholesterol is oxidized, it easily glues itself onto the blood vessel lining, resulting in arteriosclerotic plaque**. **Natural vitamin E** with all of its original 8 parts, not some stripped down mimic or synthetic molecule made in a lab, **protects against this**. More on this to come.

For now, what form do I prefer? No contest. The only one I would give Luscious or use for myself, because it uniquely has all four tocopherols as well as all four tocotrienols, which I'll shortly tell you more about. Carlson's **E-Gems Elite** is the closest to God's design for vitamin E that we can get. Take 2 a day forever.

The Gamma Tocopherol Connection

So now you know, forevermore, that **vitamin E is 8 entities**, 4 tocopherols and 4 tocotrienols. Gamma tocopherol (one of the 4 tocopherols) is rarely talked about, but is very important (Himmelfarb, Jiang). What you shouldn't expect to see in a journal dedicated to drug-oriented medicine is that **alpha-tocopherol** (the most common form of vitamin E and the one you just learned about) **can lower CRP by not 21% (like a statin drug), but 52%. In essence, the primary form of vitamin E, alpha tocopherol, can more than double what a statin drug can do.** But remember, another part of vitamin E that conventional medicine totally ignores, **gamma tocopherol lowers CRP by 61%, almost triple the improvement and at 1/5 the cost of any statin drug and without the dangerous side effects.** But don't ever expect to read in the *New England Journal of Medicine* how **a nutrient like gamma tocopherol is three times better, safer and cheaper than a patented prescription drug.** Journals like that are half advertisements for pharmaceuticals by volume, and any time they report on a nutrient it is usually a negative study that has the (? intentional) faults I've told you about.

Toco --- What?

Some even more important components of vitamin E's 8 parts are the tocotrienols (pronounced toco tri' ee nol). The tocotrienols are particularly potent in regulating cholesterol and taming its potential damage to vessel walls. Remember, **statin medications work by damaging the gene** (turning off the RNA transcription of the gene) that controls the liver enzyme HMG-CoA. But **tocotrienols do not poison the gene that governs the liver's cholesterol synthesis like statins do** (Parker, Sun). They control the HMG CoA enzyme after it has been made, thereby **not poisoning its gene and synthesis** (Parker). Tocotrienols merely reduce the level of the HMG CoA enzyme, and this message can be over-ridden by interacting body chemistry as a safety valve measure. Not only do they effectively lower cholesterol in humans with elevated cholesterol, but are cheaper and safer than the drugs. No side effects were seen with up to 600 mg twice daily, but you only need 1-2 **Tocotrienols** (Carlson) 2-3 times a day.

And contrary to HMG-CoA inhibitor medications (Mevacor, Lipitor, etc.), **tocotrienols do not interfere with coenzyme Q10 production by the body.** Since dietary tocotrienols actually get incorporated into the human lipoproteins (proteins that carry fats to their workplace) in the blood, they are "Johnnie on the spot", ready to stop any free radicals from turning fats (lipids) into oxidized particles that then cling to and destroy blood vessel walls.

Tocotrienols actually get incorporated into the human lipoproteins in the blood so that they are ready to stop free radicals from turning lipids (like LDL) into oxidized particles, which then in Velcro-like fashion cling to and destroy blood vessel walls (Suarna). **Tocotrienols have not only reduced cholesterol, but they lower LDL, triglycerides and raise HDL** the good cholesterol that carries cholesterol piggyback out of the body (Ong, Qureshi). In some animal studies, tocotrienols reduced cholesterol by 30% and LDL by 67% (Iqbal). In another study of 90 humans, **100 mg a day of tocotrienols cut the cholesterol 20%, the LDL by 25%, the apo-B and triglycerides by 12%** (Qureshi).

Tocotrienols Lower Cholesterol

In rats fed a diet that creates rapid arteriosclerosis, when tocotrienols were added for 6 weeks, the diet was not as powerful in creating arteriosclerosis. Why? Because **tocotrienols are nature's HMG CoA reductase inhibitors**, **but without the side effects** of the HMG CoA reductase inhibitor drugs, like increased heart damage and cancer rates. **Tocotrienols turn out to be stronger antioxidants than the standard vitamin E form, a-tocopherol, and tocotrienols lower cholesterol better than the tocopherols ("regular" vitamin E)** (Pearce, Watkins). In addition, tocotrienols create more membrane fluidity (damaged by a lifetime of trans fatty acids in french fries and hydrogenated soybean oils), and they inhibit cancer cell growth (Nasaretnam, more in *TW*).

My favorite form is Carlson's **Tocotrienols** (from palm not rice source), 1-2 twice a day. Many tocotrienols are really made from rice, but the remarkable studies were done exclusively with Tocomin® (the form in Carlson's), coming from a palm source, which I feel is important to remember when you are trying to heal the impossible.

You can measure your cholesterol, but after it is normal, a much smarter assay is your lipid peroxides (also on your **Cardio/ION Panel**) because this will show if you are still drilling holes in vessel walls and cell membranes as well as aging prematurely, or whether you are on your way to creating a cancer. If lipid peroxides are elevated, you need more anti-oxidants to put out the fires of destruction. More on this to come.

Tocotrienols Make Coronary Artery Plaque Melt Away

This study was conducted at three research institutions, one of which was Elmhurst Medical Center in Queens NY, departments of neurology and radiology. They studied 50 patients with arteriosclerotic carotid artery plaque. For those on the tocotrienols, one-third of them (actually **32%**) **had regression or shrinking down of their arteriosclerotic plaque**, measured in the coronary arteries with ultrasonography. Those not on the tocotrienols had zero regression. On the flip side, **those not on the tocotrienols had a 44% progression or increase in arteriosclerotic plaque versus only 8% in the tocotrienol group progressed** (Kooyenga). Wow! Could there by any reason why all cardiologists are not prescribing this harmless non-prescription supplement?

In a study where animals were fed a very high cholesterol diet, those supplemented with palm tocotrienols had 98% fewer arteriosclerotic lesions. Palm **tocotrienols markedly prevented arteriosclerotic plaque or cholesterol deposits from forming** in the arteries. The mean lesion size was 3.7 times larger in the animals that just had vitamin E versus those with the palm tocotrienols (Black).

In addition, when folks are put on heart lung bypass machines to repair their clogged coronary arteries after a heart attack, sometimes the surgery is a success but the patient dies. As blood is pumped back through the heart after the heart lung machine is no longer needed, a condition called **ischemia/reperfusion injury** occurs. Translation? When the blood is rerouted through the machine, it runs out of antioxidants that are normally circulating through the living body. As this antioxidant-poor blood is sent back to the heart, because of its enormous anti-oxidant deficit, an injury sometimes leading to death or permanent heart failure or other problems occurs as the repaired heart is now flooded with blood loaded with free radicals that have accumulated while blood was restricted to the (dead) machine. Once this "spent" blood is released back into the heart at the end of the operation (reperfusion), the free radicals literally eat up heart muscle and membranes, their ion channels and receptors, a process we call lipid peroxidation. Reperfusion injury is often fatal. However, palm oil **vitamin E containing tocopherols and tocotrienols suppressed this reperfusion injury damage** (Serbinova). Yet this is not normally given for all bypass patients. Their free radicals are allowed to devour their heart tissues.

As well, in patients with arteriosclerosis of the major abdominal and leg arteries, called peripheral vascular disease or intermittent claudication, one of their main symptoms is severe pain in the gut or legs and shortness of breath with walking. Vitamin E with extra tocotrienols (as you would get with two **E-Gems Elite** once a day and 2 palm **Tocotrienols** twice a day) **doubled the patients' treadmill improvement within less than four months**, nothing that a medicine can do. Plus, it **decreased their lipid peroxidation (a measurement of accelerated rate of aging) 8.2 %** (Ong). And this improvement was double the improvement seen with aspirin, but aspirin is normally what cardiologists prescribe while tocotrienols are not. How can there be such a "disconnect" between medical science and clinical practice?

How can this be? I have no idea. But I do know that when you try to show many cardiologists this evidence they become adamantly defensive of their position, as though it's an insult that what they have been "taught" is wrong. What I don't understand is who is reading the medical journals? Can you imagine the frustration of the authors of all these wonderful studies? **Alpha tocotrienols possesses 40-60 times greater antioxidant activity than alpha-tocopherol and protect the major detoxification site, cytochromes P450, against oxidative damage 6.5 times better than alpha-tocopherol** does (Serbinova 1991). Now you understand one more reason why "scientists" chose to use just alpha-tocopherol as their solo form of vitamin E in studies to "prove" that vitamin E doesn't work. God designed vitamin E as an 8-component entity whose parts work in harmony. One part cannot be stripped from the rest and used as a solo act like a drug!

For resistant high cholesterol, I would suggest your daily vitamin E package consist of 1-2 E-**Gems Elite** and 1-2 **Gamma E-Gems** each daily, plus 1-2 **Tocotrienols** twice a day (all from Carlson). This formulation gives a great anti-oxidant, anti-aging, and anti-cancer boost, as well.

Fire Your Cardiologist if He Takes Aspirin

That's right. If your cardiologist takes aspirin to "thin the blood" and protect himself from a heart attack and recommends that you do the same, he is way out of the loop of information that is best for you. Two decades ago it was shown in the *Journal of the American Medical Association* that aspirin provides no benefit. In fact, since then over 8 other studies have shown **aspirin more than doubles your chance of having a stroke.**

Where did the error in thinking come from? Why do over 30% middle-aged white adults take aspirin in hopes of preventing a heart attack? A 1992 *Lancet* study funded by the Bayer Corporation (makers of Bufferin®) concluded that aspirin reduced the risk of heart attack. But why did this aspirin work when in all the other studies aspirin did not work? Bayer supplied them with Bufferin® which contains magnesium oxide. As you recall from *Depression Cured At Last!*, magnesium deficiency is extremely common since the American diet only gives you less than half the amount you need in a day. And magnesium deficiency leads very easily to sudden cardiac arrest. **So many study participants were getting enough magnesium in their Bufferin® to reduce the heart attack rate.**

That was not all. The researchers were trying to combine two studies in one, so **they also gave the subjects beta-carotene** to simultaneously study cancer prevention. But beta-carotene is a powerful antioxidant that lessens cholesterol deposition. In addition, they only took totally asymptomatic men with no previous illnesses for the study. Especially eliminated were any people with gut problems, because aspirin is known to cause leaky gut, ulcers, intestinal bleeding as well as kidney and liver problems. In fact even in this study, **aspirin users actually had double the normal number of strokes.** This should come as no surprise, since aspirin is an anti-inflammatory agent. But **the body uses inflammation as a defense to repair damaged vessels** so we don't bleed to death. If you turn off that protection, you are asking for acceleration of diseases due to damaged vessels. Hence, **a 200% increase in strokes in those on aspirin.** Many other errors were in this study and its data analysis.

And watch out for misrepresented studies. Many prestigious papers actually slant their abstract summaries away from the facts. I found this so hard to believe that I must quote for you directly from the paper lest you think I've made a mistake. As an example, I'll show you evidence from one study right out of the *Journal of the American Medical Association* in 2005.   I quote from the results in the summary: "No effect of aspirin was observed on total cancer".   However if you take the time to read this paper (whose authors included Harvard Medical School contributors) and look at the data clearly presented on page 51, it was clear that **for aspirin users there was a marked increase in cancers** of the pancreas, uterus, thyroid, lymphomas, leukemia, plus an increase in multiple myeloma in people who were taking 100 mg of aspirin daily (Cook).   But for a reporter or doc who just skims the abstract or summary, they will be left with the exact opposite conclusion.

Clearly**, aspirin is proven of no benefit, doubles your risk of stroke,** plus high cholesterol is not an aspirin deficiency.   Don't fall for such unfounded foolishness.   With this knowledge you have an easy and sure-fire test of your cardiologists' metal.   Just innocently ask if he recommends aspirin to prevent a heart attack. If he does, you know he is either grossly unknowledgeable about the very field he proclaims to be a specialist in, or that he knows the answer but does not think you are worth the few moments to explain it, or both.   In any case, you can do better.

When patients with leg pains from arteriosclerosis (claudication) were given **vitamin E, they doubled their treadmill improvement over what aspirin could do** in less than four months. This was done with a double-blind controlled study, randomized, considered among the most foolproof ways to prove medical facts. In fact, **100% of patients improved in the vitamin group versus only 40% improved who took aspirin.** For those on the vitamin E, 46% had "marked" improvement (defined as remarkably greater ability to walk without pain), versus only 21% for the aspirin group (Ong).   Which group would you rather be in?   And why didn't we hear of this great news on TV?   In spite of this study, cardiologists classically recommend aspirin but never tocopherols with tocotrienols as you are learning about. And remember this study was only for four months.   Can you imagine the improvement that occurs when nutrients are continued longer? Or when they are balanced with other nutrients, as you will learn to do?

One of the many mechanisms of how the complete form of vitamin E with tocopherol/tocotrienols and extra tocotrienols accomplishes clearing claudication is through **making platelets less sticky and less able to clot** (Colette, Salonen, Steiner). And even though much of this information has been known for over a quarter of a century, inferior aspirin synthesized from petroleum is more commonly recommended.

Nature to the Rescue

Besides vitamin E, what can you use in place of aspirin with all its side effects that would do a better job at keeping the blood from coagulating in arteries? Lots of things. Nature as usual has provided us with a host of possibilities. First, your old favorite, **Kyolic** aged garlic not only lowers blood pressure and cholesterol (two cardiovascular risk parameters), but also it makes blood less able to clot or agglutinate (less coagulable). So does quercitin, a bioflavonoid abundant in countless raw vegetables and fruits. That is why it is so healthful to begin meals with raw crudities or salads and snack on fruits between meals. The enzymes in raw foods also have anti-clotting action (Formic).

And remember the other half of E, **Tocotrienols**? They are powerful weapons against premature agglutination or clumping of red blood cells. CoQ10 (as in **Q-ODT**) is another nutrient that at 100 mg twice a day has caused a 20% decline in four factors involved in clotting of blood (fibronectin, thromboxane, prostacyclin and endotheilin-1). As well, having the correct ratio of fatty acids in the arterial cell wall membranes as well in the platelet cell walls (the cells responsible for clotting) decreased thrombosis or clotting (Andriamampandry). The oil change discussed in Chapter 4 fixes this. I think you get the picture and we haven't even scratched the surface. **Many natural products thwart hypercoagulability.**

We don't need to take an aspirin derived from a petrochemical, which doubles the risk of stroke and intestinal hemorrhage and encourages cancer.

Let's Get Rid of the Aspirin-Recommending Cardiologists

When a guy goes for physical and he is over 50, often the cardiologist recommends he take an aspirin a day to decrease his coagulability or clotting ability of the blood. Oftentimes the cardiologist himself is on aspirin and even more routinely recommends it for his high cholesterol patients. And once patients have had a heart attack, then they are admonished to take it forever.

I think you'll agree with me now that this is a hallmark of a horse and buggy level of knowledge. Researchers from Harvard, Tufts University and many other prestigious centers have shown clearly that **vitamin C and vitamin E retard the progression of arteriosclerosis**. They do so by a variety of mechanisms that I don't think you want to hear about (but which include increasing vasodilating nitric oxide synthesis and decreasing intercellular and vascular adhesion molecules…see, I couldn't control myself) that make cholesterol stick to vessel walls like Velcro. And the vitamins do a much better job than aspirin, the statin drugs, Plavix® and other commonly prescribed synthetic chemicals. The bottom line is that **with nutrients you get multiple good side effects.** You have already seen how vitamins C and E help cholesterol metabolism in many ways, and now you can add one more benefit. They are better than petroleum-derived aspirin.

For example, in one study of seriously ill folks who had had heart transplant surgery within the last two years, 400 units of vitamin E and 500 mg of vitamin C were taken twice daily (Fang). All patients had a standard treatment of statin drugs as well as three immune system suppressing drugs, corticosteroid and cyclosporine and azathioprine (the latter two are chemotherapy agents, capable of causing cancer). **Those who had just 2 vitamins had de-**

creased thickness of the artery studied and less plaque compared with those who just had standard medical treatment with no vitamins. And many other studies have shown that the two vitamins inhibit plaque growth. I showed you in April 2004 *TW* how just giving these two simple vitamins, C and E, made a difference of whether or not you died in ICU (intensive care unit of the hospital) after an accident. **Two inexpensive vitamins cut the chance of death in ICU by 57%.** What drug does that? I don't know of any.

Multiple studies in the most prestigious journals have shown that you can slow down the progress of arteriosclerosis, slow down clotting of vessels, in other words slow down aging and disease progression with mere vitamins C and E. The studies didn't even look at all the other crucial nutrients that work in harmony in the body. So to turn the poor patient loose by merely recommending he "Take some vitamin E", as many people have told me their cardiologists did is just as bad as not recommending it at all. For cheap grocery store supplements that list "vitamin E" in their ingredients mean that this is synthetic and actually works against any natural vitamin E you might get from your diet. In other words it becomes a negative.

My personal choice for Luscious is at least one **E-Gems Elite** (already part of the 3-part vitamin E program you learned about) and a quarter to half a teaspoon of **Pure Ascorbic Acid Powder,** each twice a day (that you already learned about). You can actually use the ascorbic acid (vitamin C) as part of your detox cocktail for one or both doses, to be described in Chapter 7. In fact glutathione, another component of your detox cocktail, is also proven to reverse the damage inside arteriosclerotic blood vessels. And as with the other nutrients, the reverse if true: **glutathione levels are lower in folks who have just had a heart attack.** Yet, it is my guess it will be another decade or two before this type of nutrient is recommended in medicine (more plus references in Chapters 5, 7).

And in case you forgot how to reply to the idiocy that vitamin E is proven not to help, remind the denigrators that Miller's study that vitamin E does not help reduce heart attacks is true, because he only used alpha-tocopherol. **That isolated part of vitamin E does not reduce platelet aggregation, but Gamma Tocopherol that you just learned about does inhibit platelet aggregation,** all while it also increases nitric oxide synthase and increases SOD in platelets. **It's the total of vitamin E with all 4 tocopherols and 4 tocotrienols that have anticoagulant effects better than aspirin,** Plavix, Coumadin and other pharmaceutical blood thinners. Another reason, therefore, for the rational of the inclusion of 2 **Tocotrienols** with a **Gamma E Gems** and 1-2 **E Gems Elite** in your program. Isn't it beautiful how it all compliments itself? Somebody up there knew we were going to be in deep biochemical trouble in this era, but cleverly designed our rescue.

Drug-oriented practitioners often limit their nutritional advice to solo, distorted nutrients, and without the benefit of measuring them in the patient. But there's no reason why you can't be ahead of the pack. There are many other nutrients you will learn about in the next chapters that also help stave off abnormal clotting, and together they are vastly more effective than aspirin, plus they have a multitude of other synergistic good effects.

Making the recommendation of a daily aspirin shows that these practitioners have failed to keep abreast of the molecular biochemistry literature, and instead rely on pharmaceutical company-directed practice guidelines. In addition, passing out a pill is far easier, quicker, and requires minimal thinking time. If you have a cardiologist whom you really like, get him out of the horse and buggy and on board the Starship Enterprise. He is so busy learning how to properly code for Medicare and insurance forms that there is little time to learn medicine anymore. Remind him: An inexpensive (a dollar a week) subscription to *Total Wellness* (prestigepublishing.com or 1-800-846-6687), written by a dedicated reference junky, will save him lots of time, keep him abreast of research he would never have the time to read and collate, and thus empower him to save many lives, the most important one being yours.

Don't Be Hoodwinked by RDAs

If you have chosen a multiple vitamin/mineral supplement as your only source of vitamin E, you are shortchanging yourself. The current RDA (recommended daily allowance) of vitamin E is 11-15 mg of alpha-tocopherol a day. This inferior standard shows clear lack of knowledge of the science of molecular biochemistry for the last two decades. *Never use the RDA as your guide.* First of all it totally ignores the fact that vitamin E has eight naturally occurring compounds, four tocopherols and four tocotrienols. Then it totally ignores the fact that processed foods, especially those with hydrogenated oils, have had the natural vitamin E stripped out or drastically reduced. Worse, "fat-free" foods containing olestra like Pringles and WOW potato chips actually inhibit the absorption of vitamin E (and other fat-soluble nutrients) from your foods.

Vitamin E clearly slows down the risk of developing vascular and heart disease, but the studies used 400-800 I.U. In many studies using *800 I.U. cut heart attacks by 30-50%.* In other studies using 400 I.U./day reduced the LDL (the bad cholesterol). In this era of unprecedented exposures to environmental chemicals and medications like **statin drugs that deplete vitamin E,** plus the fact that vitamin E is processed out of most foods, you can understand why **95% of children were deficient in vitamin E in that study of wealthy preschoolers**.

The Sytrinol Solution

Citrus fruits also have many God-given components that lower cholesterol like the tocotrienols you just learned about. Citrus fruits have a long history of reducing the incidence of cardiovascular disease by many mechanisms, which include (1) inhibiting oxidation of cholesterol, thereby discouraging its attachment to the vessel wall, (2) reducing inflammation of the vessel lining so that it doesn't eagerly grab onto cholesterol, and (3) reducing clotting ability (Maron, Monforte, Muramaki, Osiecki).   And citrus also contains other components called flavonoids (for physicians, these are primarily the polymethoxylated flavonoid tangeretin and the flavones hesperidin and naringin).

The dose of **Sytrinol** is one or two twice a day (Carlson).   Although it's not as powerful as some of the earlier alternatives you've learned about, it makes a great safe, non-toxic adjunct or addition to the others for a more potent package.

Pantethine

Pantethine is the biologically active form of vitamin B5 and it makes the substance called coenzyme A or CoA.   Many studies show that pantethine helps support healthy cholesterol metabolism by boosting many enzyme pathways needed for healthy cholesterol metabolism (Cighetti, McCarty, Donati, Arsenio).   I won't overload you with the chemistry.   Folks with high cholesterol would do well with a trial of **Pantethine 500 mg** once or twice a day (Carlson) added to their other choices.

Magnesium Acts Like a Statin

Last of all in this section of quick fixes, I must tell you about magnesium.   It's one of the most important minerals in the human body, since it **runs over 400 enzymes, including HMG Co A, the enzyme that governs cholesterol** metabolism.   As I have highly referenced in previous books and newsletters a multitude of facts about magnesium, I'll merely summarize some of the highlights here before I show you what a perfect example this one mineral is of how misguided medicine is in the 21st century.

Remember that most people are grossly deficient in magnesium because the **average American diet only provides 40%, less than**

half of the magnesium you need in a day. If that weren't enough, the June 13, 1990 *Journal of the American Medical Association* showed that in a study of over a thousand hospitalized patients in the medical Mecca of Boston, **95% of the doctors never even ordered a magnesium test.** When the researchers sneaked in and assayed the magnesium in these very sick hospitalized patients every time a doctor sent a blood specimen to the lab, the researchers chose to do the cheapest and least sensitive test, serum magnesium. Nevertheless, they found that **over 54% of the patients were grossly deficient in magnesium** and none of their treating doctors knew it. Unfortunately many of the patients in this study died from their undiagnosed magnesium deficiencies and no one ever recognized it.

Sadly the status of magnesium has yet to change in the medical world. If magnesium is measured, it's usually the serum value. But this is nearly worthless, because **less that 1% of the body's magnesium is in the serum,** yet this is the one that you see on your reports if it just says "magnesium". If your doctor is in the know, he will order the RBC (red blood cell or erythrocyte) magnesium. But I warn you; you had better look at the laboratory test yourself to be sure that he has ordered the correct one, because it's unusual that this is done.

So briefly, you get the picture that magnesium is (1) an extremely important mineral in the human body, (2) the diet never gives us enough, and (3) **doctors usually don't measure the proper form to determine if there's a deficiency**. Besides that, (4) stress, sweating (as in athletes and people doing detoxification saunas), high sugar and processed food diets and folks taking huge amounts of calcium are just some of the other ways that magnesium is driven even lower. When the body is missing magnesium, symptoms are anything from eye twitches, muscle cramps, muscle spasms, atrial fibrillation, back pain, migraines, headaches, cardiac arrhythmias, PVCs or the feeling that your heart has just skipped a beat, insomnia, irritability, rage, flying off the handle for no reason, spastic colon, or asthma, as just a sampling.

The sad part is that **magnesium is a major controller of the enzyme HMG CoA, the very enzyme that statin drugs poison.** In fact, **magnesium lowers the LDL-C 65%, better than any statin drug.** Also it **raises the enzyme lecithin acyl cholesterol transferase (LCAT) plus raises HDL,** the two most important items that carry cholesterol away from plaque (Rosanoff). They actually cause plaque to melt away, called **plaque regression.** Statins cannot do all this, plus statins lower your vitamin E, coenzyme Q10, selenium, and much more.

As well, **magnesium is nature's calcium channel blocker.** But calcium channel blockers (Norvasc, etc.), the most commonly prescribed classification of drugs by cardiologists, have been shown to actually shrink the brain and lower the intellect within five years (references in *Detoxify or Die*). Furthermore, magnesium is crucial in the **desaturase enzyme that makes possible the metabolism of omega-3 fatty acids that you will learn later also are critical in controlling coronary artery plaque and cholesterol** as well as triglycerides. So there you have it in a nutshell. **Magnesium deficiency is epidemic and it also can be one of the causes (and cures) of high cholesterol.**

Not only does magnesium lower cholesterol, but it corrects a lot of cardiac arrhythmias like atrial fibrillation, atrial flutter, superventricular tachycardia and it improves diabetes, Syndrome X, protects against unwanted blood clots, and much more. But in "modern" medicine we just throw drugs at these conditions. If that weren't bad enough, the official RDA is an inferior 280 mg, while the average American diet only provides 40% or less than half of that (Rosanoff, Nielsen). Clearly we will never run out of sick people.

Luckily you have lots of options with great magnesium products. The problem is most people need well over 600 mg a day, sometimes over 1000 mg, which is one more reason why it's great that we have so many options. The best form is a prescription form, **Magnesium Chloride Solution 200 mg/cc** (get a 12 oz. bottle and take ½ teaspoonful twice a day, available from the Windham Pharmacy, 518-734-3033). Alternative but less potent forms that do not require a prescription include **Magnesium Chloride Solution 85 mg/cc** (1 teaspoon twice a day), or **Natural Calm Powder 200 mg/teaspoon** (one tablespoon twice a day), or **Chelated Magnesium 200 mg** (2-3 tablets twice a day). You can use any form or combination of forms to give you around 800-1000 or more mg/day.

We're getting ahead of the story, but one amino acid in the body has multiple indispensable actions. It detoxifies our daily onslaught of chemicals that outgas from our homes, offices and traffic that trigger heart disease and cancer for starters. It also is a component of bile stored in the gall bladder, necessary for absorption of priceless heart disease-inhibiting vitamins A, D, E K, CoQ10, beta carotene, and phosphatidyl choline plus fatty acids like EPE and DHA. There are lots of other benefits of glycine that I've referenced in *TW*, some of which include being a calming or relaxing neurotransmitter in the brain, plus it has improved schizophrenia and calms the appetite. And it is a major component the body uses to make detoxifying glutathione that you'll learn more about. The good news is that Carlson **Chelated Magnesium** not only provides 200 mg of elemental magnesium, but 920 mg of glycine. This makes it do not double duty, but triple. You'll want to incorporate this form in with others. I'm a firm believer in several forms of magnesium, because it is so crucial and we are all so different in our assimilation. I only know this from measuring folks' magnesium levels over 3 decades on all sorts of magnesium preparations.

One caveat is that government supervision of medical laboratories has failed to appreciate the hidden epidemic of magnesium deficiency. So in re-establishing their norms, as with many nutrient values, they have allowed the cut-off of "normal" to slowly drop over the decades. For you see, to establish their "new up-to-date norms" they use one of two different types of populations. (1) People whose bloods have been sent to labs, which means they are usually sick and have some sort of disease or are on drugs (which is why they are having lab tests done in the first place), or (2) people who generally eat fast foods, take no nutrients, know nothing about nutrition, but do not yet have a disease label, so are considered "healthy". Even labs in the know are forced to use these government standards. As one pathetic example, **up until the end of 2006, the normal range for RBC magnesium was a 40-80 ppm packed cells. In 2007 it magically became 15-35.** That's a pretty enormous drop. So obviously when you see your result on a lab test, you want to be in the highest part of "normal", for mid-range "normal' is not sufficient.

Through the years we have been led to appreciate that **many people require far more than 1000 mg of magnesium a day** for a variety of reasons. Sometimes correcting persistently low magnesium is as simple as just correcting concomitantly low manganese. Adding **Chelated Manganese** one a day has improved the ability of their kidneys to save magnesium (not lose it through the urine). Another reason is that some people have a magnesium-losing nephropathy, in other words their kidneys leak magnesium. But once we chelate out the damaging heavy metals in the kidneys, the kidneys function more normally (directions for heavy metal chelation are in *The High Blood Pressure Hoax*).

Combination Fixes

As you can appreciate you have lots of options and in case you are not a purist and want to start with a shotgun approach with many of these nutrients and phytochemicals that have a history of lowering cholesterol, consider this. **CholestSure** (DaVinci) is an example of one product that contains small amounts of red yeast rice, policosanol, chromium, coenzyme Q10, and other additions like guggal lipids, artichoke leaf extract, EPA, and phytosterols, all known for their cholesterol-lowering properties. The dose would be 2-3, two to three times a day, depending on your cholesterol level. I hope you get the message that there are so many ways to more naturally and safely bring down your cholesterol and we have not even touched 1/10th of them. But as you'll find as you read further, the more you incorporate a more total and balanced program, the less of individual supplements you will need when they are allowed to harmonize with one another.

This is the Mere Tip of the Iceberg

There are lots of other ways to lower your cholesterol without drugs, and there will be many more new ones. I have in the past and will continue in the future to put them in the monthly subscription *Total Wellness* newsletter (1-800-846-6687 or prestigepublishing.com). It is my communication mode to keep you abreast of the latest things, especially subsequent to the latest books.

But you will need a multiple vitamin-mineral to balance your supplements as you learn about them. The sad news is there is no perfect one pill. It would be too large. So consider this. In one study in *Anticancer Research* (12: 599, 1992) they looked at folks with cancer of the lung. With everything medicine has to offer, 50% are dead in 6 months and 95% are dead in two years. But folks who used a multiple with a formula similar to Carlson's **Super 2 Daily** extended their six-month survival to 95% and two-year survival to 44%! **One multiple doubled lung cancer survival.** Of course, I have never met a lung cancer specialist who uses it. I like it for many other reasons: it contains EPA/DHA, it's made by a company I trust, has no iron (which is a free radical initiator in the heart), contains lutein that protects the eyes, and has no nightshades that trigger arthritis.

Not wanting you to have to rent a wheelbarrow to carry this book to the beach, let's stop here and correct some of the many myths about cholesterol that we physicians and I'm certain you also have been brainwashed with. After that, we will go into the many ways that you can actually get rid of your high cholesterol and not need to take anything. This is necessary because for many folks with high cholesterol nothing will work until they actually get to the root cause and correct it. As you can imagine, I have barely scratched the surface of natural ways to lower your cholesterol. But let's clear up some myths about cholesterol in the next chapter.

Busy Executive Summary

In the meantime, start with one or more of Niacin-Time, and/or Kyolic's Formula 107 Red Yeast Rice 600 mg, or Policosanol 10-20 mg or Sytrinol either once or twice a day. That may be all you'll ever need. Next repair your 8 parts of vitamin E with E Gems Elite, Gamma E Gems and Tocotrienols and be sure to repair your magnesium. Check your levels in a month and adjust doses. If need, use other adjuncts in this chapter like vitamin C. Meanwhile, there are so many other benefits from the Tocotrienols with Gamma Tocopherol and E-Gems Elite plus magnesium, that I would recommend using those forever, even without high cholesterol. I will in the subsequent chapters, show you how to find the actual cause and cure of your high cholesterol.

Sources for this Chapter's Recommendations

- Niacin-Time, carlsonlabs.com, 1-800-323-4141
- Kyolic Formula 107 Red Yeast Rice, wakunaga.com, 1-800-421-2998
- Policosanol, protherainc.com, 1-888-488-2488
- Policosanol, jarrow.com, 1-877-VIT-AMEN
- Lycopene, E-Gems Elite, Gamma E-Gems, Tocotrienols, Sytrinol, Pantethine, carlsonlabs.com, 1-800-323-4141
- Klaire Ultrafine Pure Ascorbic Acid, protherainc.com, 1-888-488-2488
- Magnesium Chloride Solution 200 mg/cc (prescription required), windhampharmacy.com, 1-518-734-3033

- Magnesium Chloride Solution 85 mg/cc (no prescription required), painstresscenter.com, 1-800-669-CALM
- Natural Calm 200 mg/tsp, supervites.net, 1-888-800-1180
- Chelated Manganese, Chelated Magnesium, Super 2 Daily, carlsonlabs.com, 1-800-323-4141
- CholestSure, DaVinci Labs, 1-800-325-1776
- Also 1-877-VIT-AMEN gives our readers a 25% discount on many products in this book, as does NEEDS, 1-800-634-1380, who carries nearly all products discussed here (needs.com). Check them out.

References

Niacin references:

Keenan JM, et al, Niacin revisited: a randomized, controlled trial of wax-matrix sustained-release niacin in hypercholesterolemia, *Arch Intern Med*, 151: 1424-32, 1991

Figge HL, et al, Comparison of excretion of nicotinuric acid after ingestion of two controlled release nicotinic acid preparations and man, *J Clin Pharmacol*, 28:1136-40, 1988

Carlson LA, et al, Pronounced lowering of the serum levels of lipoproteins Lp(a) in hyperlipidemic subjects treated with nicotinic acid, *J Intern Med*, 226:271-76, 1989

Gardner SF, et al, Combination therapy with low-dose lovastatin and niacin is as effective as higher-does lovastatin, *Pharmacother*, 16:419-23, 1996

Whelan AM, et al, The effect of aspirin on niacin-induced cutaneous reactions, *J Fam Pract*, 34; 2:165-68, 1992

Aronov DM, et al, Clinical trial of wax-matrix sustained-release niacin in a Russian population with hypercholesterolemia, *Arch Fam Med*, 5: 567-75, 1996

Altschul R, et al, Influence of nicotinic acid on serum cholesterol in man, *Arch Biochem Biophys*, 54:558-9, 1955

Jin FY, et al, Niacin decreases removal of high-density lipoproteins apolipoproteins A-1 but not cholesterol ester by Hep G2 cells: implications for reverse cholesterol transport, *Arterioscl Thromb Vasc Biol*, 17; 2020-28, 1997

Alderman JD, et al, Effect of a modified, well-tolerated niacin regimen on serum total cholesterol, high-density lipoprotein, cholesterol and the cholesterol to high-density lipoproteins ratio, *Am J Cardiol*, 64:725-29, 1989

Elam MB, Effect of niacin on lipid and lipoprotein levels and glycemic control in patients with diabetes and peripheral arterial disease, *J Am Med Assoc*, 248:1263-70, 2000

Shepherd J, et al, Effects of nicotinic acid therapy on plasma high-density lipoproteins subfraction distribution and composition and on apolipoprotein A metabolism, *J Clin Invest*, 63:858-67, 1979

Policosanol References:

Janikula M, Policosanol: a new treatment for cardiovascular disease, *Alt Med Rev*, 7; 3:203-17, 2002

Ortensi G, Gladstein J, Valli H, Tesone PA, A comparative study of policosanol versus simvastatin in elderly patients with hypercholesterolemia. *Curr Therap Res*, 58: 3941, 1997

Gouni-Bertold I, Bertold H, Policosanol: clinical pharmacology and therapeutic significance of a new lipid-lowering agent, *Am Heart J,* 143: 356-65, 2002

Castano G, Mas R, Menendez A, et al, Effects of policosanol and pravastatin on lipid profile, platelet aggregation and endothelemia in older hypercholesterolemic patients, *Int J Clin Pharm Res,* XIX (4): 105-116, 1999

Crespo N, Illnait J, Mas R, Fernandez L, Fernandez J, Castano G, Comparative study of the efficacy and tolerability of policosanol and lovastatin in patients with hypercholesterolemia and non-insulin-dependent diabetes mellitus, *Internat J Clin Pharma Res*, 19; 4:117-27, 1999

Rouse J, Policosanol: an exciting natural compound that lowers cholesterol and promotes cardiovascular health, *Appl Nutr Sci Rep*, pg 1-2, Dec 2001

Castano G, Mas R, Fernandex JC, Illnait J, Fernandez L, Alvarez E, Effects of policosanol in older patients with Type II hyperlipidemia and high coronary risk, *J Gerontol*, 56A: M186-92, 2001

Arruzazabala ML, Valdes S, Mas R, et al, Effect of policosanol successive dose increases on platelet aggregation in healthy volunteers, *Pharmacol Res,* 34: 181-5, 1996

Stusser R, Batista J, Padron R, Sosa F, Pereztol O, Long-term therapy with policosanol improves treadmill exercise-ECG testing performance of coronary heart disease patients, *Internat J Clin Pharmacol Ther*, 36: 469-73, 1998

Fernandezs JC, Mas R, Castano G, et al, Comparison of the efficacy, safety and tolerability of policosanol versus fluvastatin in elderly hypercholesterolemic women, *Clin Drug Invest*, 21: 103-13, 2001

Menendez R, Mas R, Amor AMA, et al, Effects of policosanol treatment on the susceptibility of low density lipoprotein (LDL) isolated from healthy volunteers to oxidative modification in vitro, *Brit J Clin Pharmacol*, 50: 255-62, 2000

Kyolic Formula 107 Red Yeast Rice References:

Heber D, et al, An analysis of nine proprietary Chinese red yeast rice dietary supplements: implications of variability in chemical profile and contents, *J Altern Complement Med*, 7; 2:133-39, 2001

Zhu BQ, Sievers RE, Parmley WW, et al, Effect of lovastatin on suppression and **regression** of atherosclerosis in lipid-fed rabbits, *J Cardiovascular Pharmacol*, 19:246-55, 1992

La Ville AE, Seddon AM, et al, Primary prevention of atherosclerosis by lovastatin in a genetically hyperlipidaemic rabbit strain, *Atherosclerosis*, 78:205-10, 1989

Wang J, Zongliang L, Chi J, et al, Multicenter clinical trial of the serum lipid-lowering effects of a *Monascus Purpureus* (red yeast) rice preparation from traditional Chinese medicine, *Curr Therap Res*, 58; 12:964-78, 1997

Heber D, Yip I, Ashley JM, Elashoff DA, Elashoff RM, Go VL, Cholesterol-lowering effects of a proprietary Chinese red-yeast-rice dietary supplement, *Am J Clin Nutr,* 69; 2231-36, Feb1999

Li C, Zhu Y, Wang Y, Zhu J-S, Chang J, Kritchevsky J, *Monascus purpureaus* fermented rice (red yeast rice): in natural food product that lowers blood cholesterol in animal models of hypercholesterolemia, *Nutr Res* 18:71-8, 1998

Patrick L, Uzick M, Cardiovascular disease: C-reactive protein and the inflammatory disease paradigm: HMG-CoA reductase inhibitors, alpha-tocopherol, red yeast rice, and olive oil polyphenols. A review of the literature, *Altern Med Rev,* 6; 3:248-71, 2001

Ma J, Li Y, Chang M, et al. Constituents of red yeast rice, a traditional Chinese food and medicine, *J Agricult Food Chem*, 48: 5220-25, 2000

Kyolic References:

Milner JA, Rivlin RS, Recent advances on the nutritional effects associated with the use of garlic as a supplement, *Journal of Nutrition*, 131; 35, Mar 2001, ISSN 0022-3166 (this whole issue was devoted to Kyolic and its molecular biochemistry with dozens of papers by outstanding scientists from medical schools throughout the United States and the world, detailing its cholesterol-lowering, antioxidant, detoxification boosting, cancer inhibiting, and many other properties:)

Budoff M, Aged garlic extract retards progression of coronary artery calcification, *J Nutr*, 136:741s-744s, 2006

Sivam GP, et al, Helicobacter pylori – in vitro susceptibility to garlic (Allium sativum) extract, *Nutr Cancer,* 27(2): 118-21, 1997

Davis W, *Track Your Plaque*, www.iuniverse.com, 2004, 414-456-1123

Budoff MJ, et al, Rates of progression of coronary calcifications by electron beam computed tomography, *Circul,* 98:1-656, 1998

Raggi P, et al, Progression of coronary calcium on serial electron beam tomographic scanning is greater in patients with future myocardial infarction, *Am J Cardiol*, 92:827-29, 2003

Raggi P, et al, Progression of coronary artery calcium and risk of first myocardial infarction in patients receiving cholesterol-lowering therapy, *Arterioscler Thromb Vasc Biol*, 24: 1272-77, 2004

Campbell JH, et al, Molecular basis by which garlic suppresses atherosclerosis, *J Nutr,* 131:1006s-9s, 2001

Steiner M, et al, Aged garlic extract, a modulator of cardiovascular risk factors: a dose-finding study on the effects of AGE on platelet functions, *J Nutr,* 131 (3s): 980s-4s, 2001

Lau BH, Suppression of LDL oxidation by garlic, *J Nutr*, 131:985s-8s, 2001

Budoff MJ, et al, Inhibiting progression of coronary calcification using aged garlic extract in patients receiving statin therapy: a preliminary study, *Prevent Med*, 39:985-91, 2004

Liu L, Yeh YY, Inhibition of cholesterol biosynthesis by organosulfur compounds derived from garlic, *Lipids,* 35:197-103, Feb 2000

Ide N, Lau HS, Aged garlic extract attenuates intracellular oxidative stress, *Phytomedicines*, 6; 2:125-31, 1999

Orekhov AN, Tertov VV, Pivovarova EM, et al, Direct anti-atherosclerosis-related effects of garlic, *Ann Med*, 27; 1:63-36, 1995

83

Steiner M, et al Changes in platelet function and susceptibility of lipoproteins to oxidation associated with administration of aged garlic extract, *J Cardiovasc Physiol*, 31:904-908, 1998

Steiner MA, Khan AH, Holbert D, I-San Lin R, A double-blind crossover study in moderately hypercholesterolemic men that compared the effect of age garlic extract and placebo administration on blood lipids, *Am J Clin Nutr*, 64: 8 66-70, 1996

Makheja AN, Vanderhoek JY, Bailey JM, Inhibition of platelet aggregation and thromboxane synthesis by onion and garlic, *Lancet*, 1979,1:781-2

Harenberg J, et al, Effect of dried garlic on blood coagulation, fibrinolysis, platelet aggregation and serum cholesterol levels in patients with hyperlipoproteinemia, *Atherosclerosis*, 1988; 74:247-9

Lau B, *Garlic And You: The Modern Medicine*, 1997, (over 100 references), Apple Publishing, 220 East 59th Ave, Vancouver BC, Can V5X 1X9

Pennsylvania State University and the National Cancer Institute, *Aged Garlic Extract, current Research Papers form Peer Reviewed Scientific Journals & Meetings*, 1998, Wakunaga, Mission Viejo CA, 800-421-2998

Neil HAW, Silagy C, Garlic: its cardioprotective properties, *Curr Opin Lipidol*, 1994; 5:6-10

McMahon FG, Vargas R, Can garlic lower blood pressure? A pilot study, *Pharmacotherapy*, 13:406-7, 1993

Santo OS, Grunwald J, Effect of garlic powder tablets on blood lipids and blood pressure. A six month placebo-controlled double-blind study, *Brit J Clin Res*, 4:37-44, 1993

Rietz B, Isensee H, Jacob R, et al, Cardioprotective actions of wild garlic (Allium ursinum) in ischemia and reperfusion, *Mol Cell Biochem*, 119:143-50, 1993

Orekhov AN, Pivovarova EM, Tertov VV, Garlic powder tablets reduce atherogenicity of low density lipoprotein. A placebo-controlled double-blind study, *Nutr Metab Cardiovasc Dis*, 1996, 6:21-31

Bordia T, Mohammed N, Thomson M, Ali M, An evaluation of garlic and onion as antithrombotic agents, *Prostaglandins, Leukotrienes and Essential Fatty Acids*, 1996, 54;3:183-6

Hamilton R, Fox A, *Discover The Power of Aged Garlic Extract*, 1999, Impakt Communications, Green Bay WI

Rahman K, Billinton D, Dietary supplementation with age garlic extract inhibits ADP-induced platelet aggregation in humans, *J Nutr*, 130: 2662-65, 2000

Munday JS, James KA, Thompson KG, et al, Daily supplementation with age garlic extract, but not raw garlic, protects low density lipoprotein against in vitro oxidation, *Atherosclerosis*, 143: 3 99-404, 1999

Yeh YY, Lin RIS, Evans, S, et al, Cholesterol lowering effects of age garlic extract supplementation on free-living hypercholesterolemic men consuming habitual diets, *J Am Coll Nutr*, 13: 545, 1995

Warshafsky S, et al, Effect of garlic on total serum cholesterol, *Ann Intern Med*, 199:599-605, 1993

Lycopene References:

Rogers SA, *Pain Free In 6 Weeks*, prestigepublishing.com, 1-800-846-6687

DiMascio P, Kaiser S, Sies H, Lycopene as the most efficient biological carotenoid single at oxygen quencher, *Arch Biochem Biophys*, 274:532-38, 1989

Arab L, Steck S, Lycopene and cardiovascular disease, *Am J Clin Nutr,* 71:1691S-1695S; discussion 1696S-1697S, 2000

Fuhrman B, Elis A, Aviram M, Hypocholesterolemic effect of lycopene and beta-carotene is related to suppression of cholesterol synthesis and augmentation of the LDL receptor activity in macro phages, *Biochem Biophys Res Commun,* 233: 658-62, 1997

Monograph AMR, Lycopene, *Altern Med Rev*, 8; 3:336-42, 2003

Kohlmeier L, Kark JD, Gómez-Gracia E, et al, Lycopene and myocardial infarction risk in the EURAMIC study, *Am J Epid*, 146:618-26, 1997

Rissanen T, Voutilainen, S, Nyyssonen K, et al, Low plasma lycopene concentration is associated with increased in some a-media thickness of the carotid artery wall, *Arterioscl Thromb Vasc Biol,* 20:2677-81, 2000

Ascorbate References:

Levine GN, et al, Ascorbic acid reverses endothelial vasomotor dysfunction in patients with coronary artery disease, *Circul*, 93:11 07-13, 1996

Salonen RM, et al, Six-year effect of combined vitamin C and E supplementation on atherosclerotic progression: the Antioxidant Supplementation in Atherosclerosis Prevention (ASAP) study, *Circul*, 107:947-53, 2003

Turely SD, et al, The role of ascorbic acid in the regulation of cholesterol metabolism and in the pathogenesis of atherosclerosis, *Atherosclerosis*, 24:1-18, 1976

Ginter E, Ascorbic acid in cholesterol and bile acid metabolism, *NY Acad Sc*i, 258:410-21, Sept 30, 1975

Ginter E, Marginal vitamin C deficiency, lipid metabolism and atherogenesis, *Adv Lipid Res,* 16:167-220, 1978

Levy TE, *Stop America's #1 Killer*, (overt 650 scientific references on vitamin C's role in preventing arteriosclerosis with or without hypercholesterolemia) 2006, LivOnBooks.com, 1-800-334-9294

Vitamin E References:

Parker RA, Pearce BC, Clark RW, Gordon DA, Wright JJ, Tocotrienols regulate cholesterol production in mammalian cells by post-transcriptional suppression of 3-hydroxy-3-methylglutaryl-coenzyme a reductase, *J Biol Chem*, 268(15) 11230-8, May 25, 1993

Swain RA, Kaplan-Machlis B. Therapeutic uses a vitamin E in prevention of atherosclerosis, *Altern Med Rev*, 4; 6: 414-423, 1999

Burton GW, Traber NG, Acuff RV, et al, Human plasma and tissue alpha-tocopherol concentrations in response to supplementation with deuterated natural and synthetic vitamin E, *Am J Clin Nutr*, 67: 669-684, 1998

Rimm EB, Stampfer MJ, Ascherio A, Giovanucci E, Colditz GA, Willett WC, Vitamin E consumption and the risk of coronary heart disease in men, *New Engl J Med,* 328: 14 50-56, 1993

Stampfer MJ, Hennekens CH, Manson JE, Colditz GA, Rosner B, Willett WC, Vitamin E and the risk of coronary disease in women, *New Engl J Med,* 328: 1444-49, 1993

Guy KF, Ten-year retrospective on the antioxidant hypothesis of arteriosclerosis, *J Nutr Biochem,* 6: 206-236, 1995

Bonner LL, Kanter DS, Manson JE, Primary prevention of stroke, *New Engl J Med,* 333:1392-1400, 1995

Stephens NG, Parsons A, Schofield PM, Kelly F, Cheeseman K, Mitchinson NJ, Brown MJ. Randomized controlled trial of vitamin E in patients with coronary disease: Cambridge Heart Antioxidant Study (CHAOS), *Lancet,* 347: 781-786, 1996

Kritchevsky SB, Shimikawa T, Dennis B, Eckfeldt J, Carpenter M, Heise G, Dietary antioxidants and carotid artery wall thickness: ATIC study, *Circulation,* 92: 2142-2150, 1995

Drewel BT, et al, Less than adequate vitamin E status observed in a group of preschool boys and girls living in the U.S., *J Nutr Biochem,* 17:132-8, 2006

Devaraj S, Jialal I, Alpha tocopherol supplementation decreases serum C-reactive protein and monocyte interleukin-6 levels in normal volunteers and type II diabetic patients, *Free Rad Biol Med,* 29:790-792, 2000

Devaraj S, Harris A, Jialal I, Modulation of monocyte-macrophage function with alpha-tocopherol: implications for atherosclerosis, *Nutr Rev,* 60; 1:8-14, Jan 2002

Thorand B, Lowel H, Koenig W, et al, C-reactive protein as a predictor for incitants of diabetes mellitus among middle-aged man, *Arch Inter Med,* 163: 93-99, 2003

Pirro M, Bergeron J, Lamarche B, et al, Age and duration of follow-up as modulators of the risk for ischemic heart disease associated with high plasma C-Reactive Protein levels in men, *Arch Intern Med,* 161: 2474-80, 2001

Kumpulainen JT, Salonen JT, et al, *Natural Antioxidants and Food Quality in Atherosclerosis and Cancer Prevention*, 1996, The Royal Society of Chemistry, Cambridge UK

Himmelfarb, et al, Alpha and Gamma tocopherol metabolism in healthy subjects and patients with end-stage renal disease, *Kidney Internat,* 2003 Sep, 64; 3:978-91

Jiang Q, Ames BN, Gamma tocopherol, but not alpha-tocopherol, decreases proinflammatory eicosanoids and inflammation damage in rats, *FASEB J,* 2003 May, 17; 8:816-22

Iqbal J, et al, Suppression of 7, 12-dimethyl benz(alpha)anthracene-induced carcinogenesis and hypercholesterolemia in rats by tocotrienol-rich fraction isolated from rice bran oil, *Europ J Cancer Preven,* 12; 6:447-53, Dec 2003

Qureshi AA, et al, Does-dependent suppression of the serum cholesterol by tocotrienols-rich fraction of rice bran in hypercholesterolemia, humans, *Atherosclerosis,* 161; 1:199-207, Mar 2002

Sun W, et al, Progress in tocotrienols, *Wei Sheng Jiu,* 33; 2:243-45, Mar 2004

Pearce BC, Parker RA, Deason ME, Qureshi AA, Wright JJK, Hypocholesterolemic activity of synthetic and natural tocotrienols, *J Med Chem,* 35; 3595, 1992

Watkins T, Lenz P, Gapor A, Struck M, Tomeo A, Bierenbaum M, g-tocotrienol as a hypocholesterolemic and antioxidant agent in rats fed atherogenic diets, *Lipids,* 28; 1113, 1993

Ong AS, et al, Palm oil: a healthful and cost-effective dietary component, *Food Nutr Bull,* 23; 1:11-22, Mar 2002

Suarna C, Hood RL, Dean RT, Stocker R, Comparative antioxidant activity of tocotrienols and other natural lipid-soluble antioxidants in a homogeneous system, and in rat and human lipoproteins, *Biochem Biophys Acta,* 1166(2-3)163-70, Feb 24, 1993

Kooyenga DK, Geller M, Watkins TRE, Gapor A, Diakoumakis E, Bierenbaum ML, Palm oil antioxidant effects in patients with hyperlipidaemia and carotid stenosis, 2-year experience, *Asia Pacific J Clin Nutr,* 61; 1: 72-75, 1997

Black TM, Wang P, Maeda N, Coleman RA, Palm tocotrienols protect ApoE +/- mice from diet-induced atheroma formation, *J Nutr,* 130: 2420-2426, 2000

Serbinova E, Khwaja S, Catudioc J, Ericson J, Torres Z, Gapor A, Kagan V, Packer L, *Nutr Res,* 12; supple 1: s203-s215, 1992

Ong ASH, Packer L (eds), *Lipid Soluble Antioxidants: Biochemistry and Clinical Applications,* Birkhauser Verlag, Basel Switzerland, pp. 606-621, 1991

Serbinova E, Kagan V, Han D, Packer L, Free radical recycling and intramembrane mobility in the antioxidant properties of alpha-tocopherol and alpha-tocotrienols, *Free Rad Biol Med,* 10: 2 63-2 75, 1991

Dutta A, Dutta SK, Vitamin E and its role in the prevention of atherosclerosis and carcinogenesis: a review, *J Am Coll Nutr,* 22; 4: 258-68, Aug. 2003

Wood LG, Fitzgerald DA, Garg ML, Hypothesis: Vitamin E complements polyunsaturated fatty acids in essential fatty acid deficiency in cystic fibrosis, *J Am Coll Nutr,* 22; 4: 253-57, Aug. 2003

Parker RA, Pearce BC, Clark RW, Gordon DA, Wright JJ, Tocotrienols regulate cholesterol production in mammalian cells by post-transcriptional suppression of 3-hydroxy-3-methylglutaryl coenzyme A reductase, *J Biol Chem,* 268:11230, 1993

Qureshi AA, Bradlow BA, Salser QZ, Brace LD, Novel tocotrienols of rice bran modulate cardiovascular disease risk parameters of hypercholesterolemic humans, *J Nutr Biochem,* 8:290, 1997

Qureshi AA, Bradlow BA, Brace L, Manganello J, Pererson DM, Pearce BC, Wright JJ, Gapor A, Elson C, Response of hypercholesterolemic subjects to administration of tocotrienols, *Lipids,* 30:1171, 1995

Nesaretnam K, Stephen R, Dils R, Darbre P, Tocotrienols inhibit the growth of human breast cancer cells irrespective of estrogen receptor status, *Lipids,* 33:461, 1998

Ozer NK, Sirikci O, Azzi A, et al, Effect of vitamin E and Probucol on dietary cholesterol-induced atherosclerosis in rabbits, *Free Rad Biol Med,* 24:226-33, 1998

Verlngieri AJ, Bush MJ, Effects of d-alphja tocopherol supplementation on experimentally induced primate atherosclerosis, *J Am Coll Nutr*, 11:130-07, 1992

Singh RB, Singh NK, Rastogi SS, Nangia S, et al, Antioxidant effects of lovastatin and vitamin E on experimental atherosclerosis in rabbits, *Cardiovasc Drugs Ther*, 11:575-80, 1997

Kumpulainen JT, Salonen JT, ed.s, *Natural Antioxidants and Food Quality in Atherosclerosis and Cancer Prevention*, 1996, The Royal Society of Chemistry, Cambridge UK

Sytrinol References:
Kurowska EM, et al, Hypolipidemic effects and absorption of citrus polymethoxtlated flavones in hamsters with diet-induced hypercholesterolemia, *J Agric Food Chem*, 52; 10:2870 9-86, May 19, 2004

Monforte MT, et al, Biological effects of hesperidin, a citrus flavonoid: hypolipidemic activity on experimental hypercholesterolemia in rats, *Farmaco*, 50; 9:595-59, Sept 1995

Maron DJ, Flavonoids for reduction of atherosclerotic risk, *Curr Atheroscler Rep*, 61; 1:73-8, Jan 2004

Murakami A, et al, Suppressive effects of citrus fruits on free radical generation and nobiletin, an anti-inflammatory polymethoxylated flavonoid, *Biofactors*, 12; 1-4: 187-92, 2000

Osiecki H, The role of chronic inflammation in cardiovascular disease and its regulation by nutrients, *Altern Med Rev*, 9; 1:32-53, Mar 2004

Pantethine References:
Cighetti G, et al, Pantethine inhibits cholesterol and fatty acid syntheses and stimulates carbon dioxide formation in isolated rat hepatocytes, *J Lipid Res*, 28; 2:152-61, Feb 1987

McCarty MF, Inhibition of acetyl-CoA carboxylase by cystamine may mediate the hypotriglyceridemic activity of pantethine, *Med Hypotheses*, 56; 3:314-17, Mar 2001

Donati C, et al, Pantethine improves the lipid abnormalities of chronic hemodialysis patients: results of a multicenter clinical trial, *Clin Nephrol*, 25; 2:70-4, Feb 1986

Arsenio L, et al, Effectiveness of long-term treatment with pantethine in patients with dyslipidemia, *Clin Ther*, 8; 5:537-45, 1986

Cighetti G, et al, Effects of pantethine on cholesterol synthesis from mevlonate in isolated rat hepatocytes, *Atherosclerosis*, 60; 1:67-77, Apr 1986

Magnesium References:
Rosonoff A, Seelig MS, Comparison of mechanism and functional effects of magnesium and statin pharmaceuticals, *J Am Coll Nutr*, 23; 5:501S-505S, 2004

Itoh K, et al, The effects of high oral magnesium supplementation on blood pressure, serum lipids and related variables in apparently healthy Japanese subjects, *Brit J Nutr*, 78:737-50, 1997

Rayssiguer Y, Role of magnesium and potassium in the pathogenesis of arteriosclerosis, *Magnesium*, 3: 226-38, 1984

Seelig MS, Rosanof A, *The Magnesium Factor*, New York: Avery, Penguin-Putnam, 2003

Rogers SA, *Detoxify or Die, Pain Free In 6 Weeks, Depression Cured At Last!, The High Blood Pressure Hoax, Total Wellness,* all from prestigepublishing.com or 1-800-846-6687

Aspirin Insanity References:

Andriamampandry MD, Leray C, Gachet C, Antithrombotic effects of (n-3) polyunsaturated fatty acids in rat models of arterial and venous thrombosis, *Thrombosis Research,* 93:9-16, 1999

Aspirin Myocardial Infarction Study Research Group, A randomized trial of aspirin in persons recovered from myocardial infarction, *J Amer Med Assoc*, 243:661-9, 1980
(Aspirin proven to be of no benefit)

Pierce JB, *Heart Healthy Magnesium*, Avery Publ, Garden City Park, NY, 1994

Juul-Moller, et al, Double-blind trial of aspirin on primary prevention of myocardial infarction in patients with stable angina pectoris, *Lancet,* 340:1421-5, 1992 (Rekindled notion of aspirin RX, but research was faulty).

He J, Whelton PK, Vu B, Klag MJ, Aspirin and risk of hemorrhagic stroke; A meta-analysis of randomized controlled trials, *J Amer Med Assoc,* 280; 22:1930-35, 1998

Ong ASH, Packer L (eds), *Lipid Soluble Antioxidants: Biochemistry and Clinical Applications*, Birkhauser Verlag, Basel Switzerland, pp. 606-621, 1991

Colette C, Pares-Herbute N, Monnier LH, Cartry E, Platelet function in Type I diabetes: Effects of supplementation with large doses of vitamin E, *Am J Clin Nutr,* 47: 2 56-61, 1988

Salonen JT, Antioxidant and platelets, *Ann Med*, 21: 59-62, 1989

Steiner M, Anastasia J, Vitamin E.: An inhibitor of the platelet release reaction, *J Clin Invest,* 57: 7 32-737, 1976

Esterbauer H, Dieber-Rothender M, Striegl G, et al, Role of vitamin E in preventing oxidation of low-density lipoprotein, *Am J Clin Nutr,* 1992:53:314s-21s

Steinberg K, Arthasarathy S, Witztum JL, et al, Beyond cholesterol: Modification of low-density lipoprotein that increase its atherogenicity, *N Eng. J Med,* 320:915-24, 1989

Cox DA, Cophen ML, Effects of oxidized low-density lipoprotein on vascular contraction and relaxation: Clinical and pharmacological implications in atherosclerosis, *Pharmacol Rev,* 48:3-19, 1996

Liu M, Wallmon A, Saldeen T, et al, Tocopherols inhibit platelet aggregation in humans: potential mechanisms, *Am J Clin Nutr,* 77:700-6, 2003

Ting HH, Timimi FK, Creager MA, et al, Vitamin C improves endothelium-dependent vasodilation in patients with non-insulin-dependent diabetes mellitus, *J Clin Invest,* 97:22-28, 1996

Gokce N, Keaney JF, Frei B, et al, Long-term ascorbic acid administration reverses endothelial vasomotor dysfunction in patients with coronary artery disease, *Circul,* 99:3234-40, 1999

Carr AC, Zhu BZ, Frei B, potential antiatherogenic mechanisms of ascorbate (vitamin C) and alpha–tocopherol (vitamin E), *Circ Res,* 87:349-354, 2000

Fang JC, Kinlay S, Beltrame J, et al, Effect of vitamins C and E on progression of translplant-associated arteriosclerosis: a randomised trial, *Lancet,* 359:1108-1113, 2002

Liu L, Meydani M, Mayer J, Combined and vitamin C and E supplementation retards early progression of arteriosclerosis in the heart transplant patients, *Nutr Rev,* 16; 12: 368-3 71, Nov. 2002

Salonen RM, Nyyssonen K, Poulsen HE, Six-year effect of combined vitamin C and E supplementation on arteriosclerotic progression: the Antioxidant Supplementation in Atherosclerosis Prevention (ASAP) Study, *Circulation,* 107:947-53, 2003

Hodis HM, et al, Serial coronary angiographic evidence that antioxidant vitamin intake reduces progression of coronary artery atherosclerosis, *Journal American Medical Association,* 273: 1849-54, 1995

Cook NR, et al, Low-dose aspirin in the primary prevention of cancer, *J Am Med Assoc*, 294; 1: 47-55, 2005

Chapter III

Fracturing the Myths About Cholesterol

I know how many of you readers battle with friends, trying to help them understand that they have control over their health. And I appreciate how frustrating it can be when you hear conflicting reports and then have the burden of deciding who is right. So I have created this chapter to arm you with the ammunition to take anywhere, to protect your credibility and good intentions, and to put these many cholesterol myths to bed, once and for all.

High Cholesterol Always has to be Treated

Wrong. There are families where the cholesterol is over 400 and folks have lived into their 90s with no medications and no medical problems. Plus research shows that **for folks over 70, those with a little higher cholesterol live longer than those with normal or low cholesterol.** And those **with higher cholesterol have less cancer and less suicide** than those with a normal level, 200 mg/dl or less. Furthermore, high profile articles in the *Journal of the American Medical Association,* for example, show that death rates actually go up, not down when efforts are made to lower cholesterol with drugs (Hulley 1992). Another study in the prestigious *Circulation* showed that **high cholesterol has no predictive value for who will have an early coronary death** (Hulley 1992). But I'll show you shortly some fantastic crystal ball tests that do predict, much better than cholesterol does, how soon you will have major trouble.

References:

Hulley S, et al, Childhood cholesterol screening: Contraindicated, *J Am Med Assoc,* 267:100-02, 1992

Hulley S, et al, Health policy on blood cholesterol, time to change directions, *Circul,* 86:1026-29, 1992

Schatzkin A, et al, Serum cholesterol and cancer in the NHANES I Epidemiologic Study. National Health and Nutrition Examination Study, *Lancet,* 2; 8554: 298-301, 1987

Kagen A, et al, Serum cholesterol and mortality in a Japanese-American population: The Honolulu Heart Program, *Am J Epidemiol*, 114; 1:11-20, 1981

Knekt P, et al, Serum cholesterol and risk of cancer in a cohort of 39,000 men and women, *J Clin Epidemiol*, 41:5 19-30, 1988

Kark JA, et al, The relationship of serum cholesterol to the incidence of cancer in Evans County Georgia, *J Chron Dis*, 33:311-32

Stemmerman G, et al, Serum cholesterol and colon cancer incidence in Hawaii and Japanese man, *J Natl Cancer Inst*, 67; 6:1179-82, 1981

Williams R, et al, Cancer incidence by levels of cholesterol, *J Am Med Assoc,* 245; 3:247-52, 1981

Behar S, et al, **Low total cholesterol is associated with high total mortality** in patients with coronary heart disease. The Bezafibrate Infarction Prevention (BIP) Study Group, *Heart J*, 1:52-9, Jan. 18, 1997

Cassidy AT, Carroll BJ, Hypocholesterolemia during mixed manic episodes, *Europ Arch Psych Clin Neurosci*, 252; 3:110-14, June 2002

Engleberg H, **Low serum cholesterol and suicide**, *Lancet*, 339; 8795:727-79, Mar 21, 1992

High Cholesterol is a Bad Guy
And a Major Cause of Heart Disease

Wrong. **High cholesterol is merely a messenger informing us that there is raging inflammation in the blood vessels.** That's all. Cholesterol is merely the patch for these damaged vessels. Cholesterol does double duty to protect us. It's (1) **like a fire hose putting out the flames of inflammation** as well as (2) **a patch for the holes that free radicals have burned into our arterial walls**. As you will learn, it can come from such triggers as hidden infection starting in the teeth, gut, vessels, or elsewhere and from undiagnosed nutrient deficiencies or accumulation of trans fats hidden in the diet. But the number one cause of inflammation in the arteries is our lifetime accumulation of chemicals, like pesticides, phthalates, Teflon, mercury and more. And how healthy your detoxification system is determines how fast you will tank up on damaging environmental chemicals.

For example, mice exposed to **pesticide poisoning** have more free radicals. Consequently, they also have **more plaque** in their arteries than exposed mice with healthier detoxification systems for the pesticide. Numerous studies and books show that there is an increase in heart attack risk as everyday pollutant levels go up. In fact **living in a polluted city gives you about the same 150% increased risk of death from heart attack or stroke as being an active smoker**. And over 30% of the US population lives in areas above the EPA's legal limit for pollution (which continually drops as they find that they have over-estimated the "safe" cut-offs, consequently an even greater percentage is at risk). Furthermore, for over 30 years it has been known that cholesterol levels are elevated by pesticides as well as by bacterial toxins.

The **LDL cholesterol plasters cholesterol onto the arterial wall, but only if the LDL cholesterol is oxidized.** LDL is only able to attach itself **when it has sustained too much free radical damage** from reactive oxygen species called free radicals (from infections, fast foods, and our daily accumulation of unwanted chemicals like pesticides, plasticizers, heavy metals, PCBs, flame retardants, and Teflon from our air, food and water, etc.). Once electrons have burned holes in the arterial wall and oxidized the LDL, it then glues itself as a patch so we don't bleed to death.

Fortunately, high levels of HDL and many nutrients that you will learn about here as well as detoxification protocols can act as the wheelbarrow to scrape cholesterol off from the arterial wall and dump it into the liver where it becomes protective and detoxifies bile (Moncada).

References:

Moncada S, et al, Symposium on regression of atherosclerosis, Review, *Europ J Clin Invest,* 23: 385-98, 1993

Watson K, et al, Functional role of cholesterol and infection and autoimmunity, *Lancet,* 1; 7902: 308-10, 1975

Bloomer A, et al, A study of pesticide residues in Michigan's general population, 1968-1970, *Pesticides Monitoring J,* 11; 3:111-15, 1977

Winstein KJ, Increased heart risk linked to air pollution, study of 58,600 older women finds a danger grows in cities with higher soot levels from autos and power plants, *Wall Street J,* D1, 4, Feb 1, 2007

Shih D, et al, Mice lacking serum paraoxonase are susceptible to organophosphate toxicity and atherosclerosis, *Nature,* 394; 6690: 284-87, 1998

Knowing My Cholesterol Level is the Most Important

Half the folks who die of a heart attack never had high cholesterol. Also studies prove that **having high cholesterol does not predict progression of arteriosclerosis**. In fact, **for many people high cholesterol is totally irrelevant to how much arteriosclerosis they have**. At least this is the result of a recent Johns Hopkins study published in *Atherosclerosis*. Patients who were already treated with cholesterol-lowering statins for their high cholesterol were then treated for their elevated homocysteine. As I showed in *The High Blood Pressure Hoax* it turns out that **having a high homocysteine is four times riskier for early death than having high cholesterol**. Yet to this day, when our readers ask their cardiologists to check their homocysteine levels, most are told they don't need to. This is the hallmark of a physician who is inferiorly equipped to correct biochemical abnormalities that are only correctable with nutrients.

Next researchers wanted to see what the progression of plaque accumulation in the arteries was really due to. The result? Way above whether or not the patients had high cholesterol was again, whether or not they had elevated homocysteine. But even though **elevated homocysteine has been known for decades to accelerate your risk of heart attack, stroke, macular degeneration, Alzheimer's,** and much more, many cardiologists to this day do not check it. Why? Because the treatment is vitamins and they don't deal with that type of chemistry; they like drugs. Even their practice guidelines, meetings and journals focus on drugs. **Since there is no drug for homocysteine, it has not become very popular even though it's four times riskier than having high cholesterol.** But because cholesterol drugs make so much money, you hear the puffed up dangers of high cholesterol, while even folks at cocktail parties brag about knowing their levels. Don't forget that **just one brand of the cholesterol-lowering drug,**

Lipitor, makes well over $10 billion (not a million, but billion) per year, which is over five times the annual budget of the FDA.

The **next most important indicator of yearly progression of coronary plaque was the hsCRP (high sensitivity C-reactive protein).** Both the hsCRP and homocysteine levels are in your **Cardio/ION Panel.** I'm utterly amazed at the number of people that I consult with who have been to top cardiologists for years, who have had coronary bypass surgery and the latest drugs, but have never had an hsCRP, fibrinogen or a homocysteine level checked, much less their vitamin, mineral and fatty acid levels. Without knowing this information from the Cardio/ION Panel, there is no hope of curing cardiology patients. The only recourse the physician has is to stifle symptoms with a drug that poisons one of God's molecular pathways. This is pretty scary.

The *American Journal of Cardiology* in 1995 strongly recommended that everyone, especially patients with high cholesterol, be measured for homocysteine. It's hard to believe that many physicians even read the leading medical journals in their fields when you examine the current status of dangerous medical practice. In 1991 it was clearly shown that having high homocysteine was an independent risk factor for early vascular disease, but that didn't make big news like some latest drug or the slamming of a vitamin (with shoddy science that I have shown you examples of) did (*TW* contains even more details and evidence).

Exciting news that never makes the press from other top line medical publications showed how the **vitamins used to treat homocysteine actually make coronary artery plaque regress or melt away.** Even for folks who were on the cholesterol-lowering drugs, **vitamins decreased the progression of plaque fivefold above and beyond what the drugs could do.** To quote from this scientific paper, "a major part of the regression was not due to lipid lowering therapy", since patients had been on the statins for "over two years before vitamin therapy". "The observations reported here support the causal hypothesis, in that **vitamin therapy was associated with the regression of carotid plaque.**" This, to my way of thinking, makes it malpractice for a cardiologist to ignore assessing and prescribing nutrients.

"It is of great interest that regression (melting away of arterial plaque) was observed even in patients with homocysteine levels below those conventionally thought to be high enough to warrant therapy." This latter statement is consistent with my suspicion that we've been **using the wrong cut-off** for years and that the true "norm" for homocysteine should be lower than 14. I firmly believe after looking at the data and patients' results for 38 years that the best levels should be less than 6-7, but given the history of medicine, it will be decades before the cut-off will be amended.

Homocysteine is a crystal ball test. The scary part is that when the **homocysteine level is above 12** μmol per liter, coronary plaque is proven by the electron beam tomography calcium score (Ultrafast Heart Scan) to increase by more than a third or 35% every year. That means **within three years you will have a grand slam heart attack.** And for a CRP level a little lower, over 8, coronary plaque progresses at a rate of 22% per year, giving you about five years before the big event. In the words of the Johns Hopkins investigators, "**Neither cholesterol** values, body mass index, gender, age nor presence of individual risk factors **predicted progression of coronary calcium.** Conclusion: presence of elevated **homocysteine (over 12 μmol per liter) strongly and independently predicts progression of coronary plaque burden". Translation: cholesterol is merely a bit player in the greater scheme of things.** Yet it is stressed and you're even asked to take cholesterol-lowering drugs when you don't have high cholesterol. And misleading, distorted studies and pharmaceutical PR (that you will learn about) leave your practitioner convinced he is right in prescribing statins for you.

You begin to lower homocysteine by checking and correcting vitamins B6, B12 and folic acid. When in doubt I would take 200 mg **Vitamin B6,** sublingual **B12 S-L** and one 5 mg sublingual **Folixor** daily. Many other nutrients like **DMG, Chelated Copper, Chelated Magnesium, NAC** and more also are involved if that doesn't do the trick (*TW 2006, TW 2007* and *The High Blood Pressure Hoax* have more details and evidence).

Meanwhile, **in my mind it's downright malpractice for anyone to fail to check homocysteine in everyone at least over 40 years of age**, since arteriosclerosis is the number one cause of death. At international medical seminars, although I've never yet met him, I've lectured on the same programs as Dr. Kilmer McCully. He is the brilliant Harvard researcher who brought homocysteine to the world's attention and wrote the landmark book, *The Heart Revolution: The Extraordinary Discovery that Finally Laid the Cholesterol Myth to Rest* (Perennial/Harper Collins, 2000). If that doesn't convince your doctor to order a homocysteine level and upstage the mundane and relatively useless cholesterol, it suggests it is time to move on to someone more open-minded, informed, eager to learn what is best for you, and knowledgeable.

References:

Raouli ML, Nasir K, Budoff MJ, et al, Plasma homocysteine predicts progression of atherosclerosis, *Atherosclerosis* 181: 159-165, 2005

Glueck CJ, Shaw P, Wang Y, et al, Evidence that homocysteine is an independent risk factor for atherosclerosis in hyperlipidemia patients, *Am J Cardiol* 75: 132-136, 1995

Hackam DG, Peterson JC, Spence JD, What level of plasma homocysteine should be treated?, *Am J Hypertension*, 13:10 5-110, 2000

Clarke R, et al, Hyper-homocystinemia: an independent risk factor for vascular disease, *New Engl J Med* 324:1140 9-1155, 1991

McCully K, *The Heart Revolution: The Extraordinary Discovery that Finally Laid the Cholesterol Myth to Rest*, Perennial/Harper Collins, 2000

Arteriosclerosis is a Problem of Old People

Autopsies of 18 year olds from auto accidents plus Korean and Vietnam wars have shown that arteriosclerosis begins in teen age. And why shouldn't it since they are weaned on trans fats, Teflon, fire retardants, plasticizers and other contributors to hypercholesterolemia as well as arteriosclerosis without high cholesterol. The umbilical cord blood of the average baby born in the US has measurable levels of all these chemicals and more. In fact an article in **The New England Journal of Medicine** showed kids born today are not expected to live as long as their parents. We are on the downhill side (references in *TW* 2006, 2007, *Detoxify or Die*). Consequently, we are now seeing diseases in younger ages that used to be reserved for old age, like hip replacements, cancer, and fatal heart attacks before age 40.

Reference:
Stary H, Evolution and progression of atherosclerotic lesions in coronary arteries of children and young adults, *Arteriosclerosis,* 9: 119-32, 1989

Statin Cholesterol-Lowering Drugs
Should be Used by Everyone to Reduce Heart Risk,
Even if They Don't Have High Cholesterol

In the American Heart Association's journal, *Circulation*, physicians were encouraged to aggressively prescribe statin drugs to lower cholesterol, even if their patients did not have high cholesterol. The premise was its anti-oxidant activity would reduce their cardiac risk (Grundy). Extending the use of statin drugs to folks who don't even have high cholesterol would dramatically increase (about triple) the number of patients in the United States on statin drugs to as many as 50 million (Herper).

What the journal conveniently forgot to mention, however, was that **six out of nine of the "expert" panelists making this decision received money from the pharmaceutical companies that make cholesterol-lowering drugs** (Ricks). So it shouldn't surprise you that an article in the prestigious *Lancet* detailed how one of the newest statin drugs, Crestor, was approved even when the FDA knew that it caused fatal rhabdomyolysis. And it did so more than any of the other forms on the market (except Baycol which was finally removed from the market after killing at least 31 people). Furthermore, Crestor caused kidney death in those it didn't kill (Wolfe). This deck appears to also be stacked with conflicts of interest.

Probably a good rule of thumb is that whenever you're advised to take any pharmaceutical for life, just ponder for a while whether you think that means your body has a deficiency of that chemical. After 38 years in medicine, I've never seen a deficiency of pharmaceuticals in the body, except for a few hormones like insulin and thyroid. And most of the time those glands stopped functioning merely because they were poisoned with environmental toxins and heavy metals that you'll learn about later. In fact, we have so polluted the world that the polar bears in the Arctic have osteoporosis and hypothyroidism from our chemicals! In other words, even peoples' glandular deficiencies could have been rescued if the underlying causes of glandular disease were looked for earlier. And many have successfully healed hypo-functioning glands using the detox and nutrient repairs that you are learning here.

References:

Wolfe SM, Dangers of rosuvastatin identified before and after FDA approval, *Lancet,* 363; 9427: 2189-90, June 26, 2004

Ricks D, Raven R, Panel's ties to drug makers not cited in new cholesterol guidelines, Newsday.com

Herper M, Cholesterol guidelines a gift for Merck, Pfizer, *Forbes Magazine,* July 12, 2004

Grundy SM, et al, The Coordinating Committee of the National Cholesterol Education Program. Implications of recent clinical trials for the National Cholesterol Education Program Adults Treatment Panel III Guidelines, *Circulation,* 110:227-239, 2004

Statin Drugs Lower Your Chance of Death

No. True, they do lower death from a heart attack. But what benefit you **gain is offset by dying at a higher rate from other things like suicidal depression**, accidents, aggression, violent crimes, and more. So **there is no overall gain in improved longevity**. It is just one of many ways you are deceived by not giving you the whole story. Yes, **statins lower the rate of heart attack, but at the expense of raising the death rate from other causes to offset this gain. Net gain is nothing.**

And you can understand why you increase your risk of dying of a multitude of seemingly unrelated diseases when you recall all the bad side effects of the statins that go essentially ignored by medicine (that you became an expert in via Chapter I). Clearly, statin drugs deprive the cell membranes of the cholesterol they need to function properly (Oliver, Hargreaves). Just look at how Vioxx more than quadrupled the heart attack rate. You can't take drugs that poison major pathways needed for health in the body and get away with it for too long. The bottom line is the gain from statin drugs is offset by increased deaths through other diseases, so there's no overall gain. But most of the unscrupulous studies look at only whether there is a decrease in heart deaths, and publish it that way. They discount other types of deaths so the drug treatment comes out looking far better than it really is.

For physicians: And if any doubt is left in any physician's mind about the devastating effects of statin drugs on the human biochemistry, their toxicity traces to statin-medicated inhibition of HMG CoA reductase activity that deprives cells of (1) essential components including cholesterol, crucial for all cell membrane functions; (2) ubiquinone, a component of the electron transport chain; (3) isopentenyl adenine, which is required for RNA function and (4) mevalonate-derived components, which are required for posttranslational processing like farnesylation, geranylgeranylation, dolichylation and (5) N-linked glycosylation (which trigger

Alzheimer's and more), and (6) for the membrane localization and (7) biologic functions of all cellular proteins (McAnally, references in Chapter III). Thus deranging of basic cellular communication, energy synthesis, genetic control, detoxification, protection against everything from cancer to Alzheimer's, plus induction of nutrient deficiencies occurs because of one prescribed poison. Is it worth it when there are superior alternatives?

References:

Golomb B, et al, Low cholesterol and violent crime, *J Psychiat Res,* 34; 4-5:301-9, 2000

Oliver MF, Is cholesterol reduction always safe? *Europ J Clin Invest,* 22: 441-2, 1992

Oliver MF, Serum cholesterol---the knave of hearts and the joker, *Lancet,* ii: 1090-5, 1981

Hargreaves AD, et al, Glucose tolerance, plasma insulin, HDL cholesterol and obesity: 12-year follow-up and development of coronary heart disease in Edinburgh men, *Atherosclerosis,* 94:61-69, 1992

Moncada S, et al, Symposium on regression of atherosclerosis, Review, *Europ J Clin Invest,* 23: 385-98, 1993

Also see references in section about having too low a cholesterol and cholesterol-lowering drugs raising cancer risk.

The Lower Your Cholesterol, the Better

Absolutely not. Too low of a cholesterol is just as dangerous as too high. Cholesterol is needed for all membrane structure and function, hormones, hormone receptors, and release of cytokines that fight off infection and cancers. And when the cell membrane is cholesterol-starved, it can malfunction and trigger autoimmune diseases, cancers, Alzheimer's and much more. In fact, folks with a **cholesterol under 160 mg/dL have double the risk of brain hemorrhage and increased risk of cancers of the liver, lung, pancreas, and leukemia, plus cirrhosis and suicide** (Behar). In another study, **low cholesterol folks had more than double the death rate** from non-cardiac conditions. **Besides doubling death, low cholesterol dramatically damages mental-health leading to depression, suicide, mania,** and more (Cassidy, Engleberg).

One of the fascinating things is that low **cholesterol has been well known to be associated with cancer** in scores of studies. Most of these studies were published well over 20 years ago, and in the most prestigious journals like *Lancet, Journal of the National Cancer Institute, Journal of the American Medical Association,* and much more. Oddly enough scientific data is conveniently ignored when it comes to prescription drugs.

References:

Schatzkin A, et al, Serum cholesterol and cancer in the NHANES I Epidemiologic Study. National Health and Nutrition Examination Study, *Lancet,* 2; 8554: 298-301, 1987

Kagen A, et al, Serum cholesterol and mortality in a Japanese-American population: The Honolulu Heart Program, *Am J Epidemiol,* 114; 1:11-20, 1981

Knekt P, et al, Serum cholesterol and risk of cancer in a cohort of 39,000 men and women, *J Clin Epidemiol,* 41:5 19-30, 1988

Kark JA, et al, The relationship of serum cholesterol to the incidence of cancer in Evans County Georgia, *J Chron Dis,* 33:311-32

Stemmerman G, et al, Serum cholesterol and colon cancer incidence in Hawaiian and Japanese men, *J Natl Cancer Inst,* 67; 6:1179-82, 1981

Williams R, et al, Cancer incidence by levels of cholesterol, *J Am Med Assoc,* 245; 3:247-52, 1981

Behar S, et al, Low total cholesterol is associated with high total mortality in patients with coronary heart disease. The Bezafobrate Infarction Prevention (BIP) Study Group, *Heart J,* 1:52-9, Jan. 18, 1997

Cassidy AT, Carroll BJ, Hypocholesterolemia during mixed manic episodes, *Europ Arch Psych Clin Neurosci,* 252; 3:110-14, June 2002

Engleberg H, Low serum cholesterol and suicide, *Lancet,* 339; 8795:727-79, Mar 21, 1992

My Doctor Wouldn't Prescribe Drugs That Would Worsen My Cholesterol

Beta blockers lower HDL. One of the most commonly prescribed categories of **medications for hypertension, arrhythmia, heart failure, and even for stage fright** lowers the good cholesterol, making you more vulnerable for a heart attack than you would be by having high cholesterol. And this was a study published in the *American Journal of Cardiology,* done on over 8,500 men throughout the United States who already had coronary artery disease. What they found was over half of them or 58% with coronary artery disease did not need statin drugs, because they did not have high cholesterol. But 41% did have a low HDL. They really needed nutrients to raise their HDL, the "good" cholesterol that actually carries cholesterol out of the bloodstream and into the liver to be dumped into the gut.

Remember, **having a low HDL is a better indicator of early coronary death than high cholesterol. Recall,** HDL is the wheelbarrow that carries cholesterol from the arterial wall and dumps it into the liver where it's made into healing and detoxifying bile. **HDL** is another crystal ball test that is an independent predictor of whether or not you can keep up with **cleaning plaque off your arteries** (Blankenhorn, Castelli).

And if the HDL is low and the triglycerides are high, this is an even better indicator of early coronary death than the standard cholesterol and LDL tests (Buring, Nikkila). But because there are drugs that make obscene profits (recall that single handed just one brand, like Lipitor brings in over $10 billion a year), you hear about reducing your cholesterol with drugs rather than emphasizing raising your HDL. There are however, drugs in the pipeline already to raise the HDL, but they still haven't figured out how to completely and safely one-up God's natural chemistry that does it better (as you learned in Chapter II).

If that were not scary enough, beta-blockers (basically most heart drugs whose names end in "–ol", like atenolol) are **known to increase triglycerides while they lower HDL cholesterol.** In other words, **one of the most popular classifications of heart drugs prescribed by all cardiologists, beta-blockers, actually makes sure you will die earlier of coronary artery disease** (Rubins, page 1199). If that were not enough damage, **beta-blockers also lower your thyroid that in turn raises your cholesterol!** Plus don't forget **beta-blockers also deplete nutrients like zinc** that are so crucial to tame inflammation and genetic damage in arteries that leads to arteriosclerosis.

So **this commonly prescribed category of cardiology drugs has four mechanisms, minimum, to make sure you will die sooner of a heart attack**. And there are many more. For example, they **lower coenzyme Q10.** And with a **low CoQ10 you then get an elevated Lp(a) which is another cardiovascular risk factor that is stronger than cholesterol** (Singh). There are many other drugs that accelerate aging and arteriosclerosis, as this is just one tiny example.

Let's look at another drug, the common **calcium channel blockers** (the brand names are in *Detoxify or Die)*. They **increase your chance of a heart attack and bring on a higher rate of heart attack than in folks not receiving them** (Waters). And why shouldn't they? Since they were prescribed to poison calcium channels versus repair them, as you will learn how here. And as I've shown in that book, MRI x-rays prove that within five years of using calcium channel blockers (which are usually prescribed for life), you **permanently shrink the brain and rot the intellect**. Such a deal! I could go on with every category of drug but that's not the focus of this book. I keep trying to show you how the medication merry-go-round is so self-perpetuating. Now you know why they give out so many samples.

Some of the common generic names for beta-blockers (with their brand names, usually much more expensive, in parenthesis) are below. Wow! Does that vegetable soup give you any idea that maybe no one wants you to really know what you are on, so you won't know the real side effects or what drugs actually do in your body to promote disease?

Beta-Blockers
Brand Names and Generic Names

Acebutolol (Sectral), Atenolol (Tenormin), Bentaxolol (Kerlone), Bisoprolol (Ziac), Carvedilol (Coreg), Labetalol (Normodyne or Trandate), Metaprolol (Lopressor or Toprol-XL), Nadolol (Corgard), Penandbutalol (Levatol), Pindolol (N/A), Propanolol (Inderal or InnoPran XL) and Timolol (Biocadren).

References:

Waters D, et al, A controlled clinical trial to assess the effect of a calcium channel blocker on the progression of coronary atherosclerosis, *Circul,* 82: 1940-53, 1990

Buring JE, et al, Decreased HDL 2 and HDL 3 cholesterol, apo A-I and apo A-II, and increased risk of myocardial infarction, *Circul,* 85:22-29, 1992

Nikkila M, et al, High-density lipoproteins cholesterol and triglycerides as markers of angiographically assessed coronary artery disease, *Brit Med J,* 63:78-81, 1990

Rubins HB, et al, Distribution of lipids and 8500 men with coronary artery disease, *Am J Cardiol,* 75:1196-1201, June 15, 1995

Kayser L, et al, The thyroid function and size in healthy men during three weeks treatment with beta-adrenoreceptor antagonist, *Horm Metab Res,* 23: 35-37, 1991

Blankenhorn DH, et al, Prediction of angiographic changes in native human coronary arteries and aortocoronary bypass grafts, lipid and neolipid factors, *Circul,* 81:470-76, 1990,

Castelli WP, et al, HDL cholesterol and other lipids in coronary heart disease, *Circul,* 55: 767-72, 1977

Singh RB, et al, Serum concentration of lipoproteins(a) decreases on treatment with hydro soluble coenzyme Q10 in patients with coronary artery disease: discovery of a new role, *International Journal Cardiology,* 68; 1:20 3-29, Jan. 1999

Nonprescription Drugs Can't Harm the Heart

There are no free rides on the drug trolley. Every drug not only uses up detox nutrients that could have been used to heal disease and keep you young, but by poisoning one of God's biochemical pathways in the body (that's how the vast majority work), **you eventually develop new symptoms and new diseases**. And these usually get treated with yet another drug. The average office visit of 7 minutes does not allow for any meaningful instruction. And that is why 50% of folks over 60 have 5 or more drugs, and it escalates each year thereafter.

The over-the-counter pain medicines called non-steroidal anti-inflammatory drugs (abbreviated NSAID) include common non-prescription medications like Motril, Ibuprofen, Aleve, Advil, while Celebrex, etc. require prescriptions. Needless to say showing you how to get rid of pain without using NSAIDs is beyond the scope of this book, but it is explained in *Pain Free In 6 Weeks* and important up-dates in *TW* 2006 and 2007 (prestigepublishing.com or 1-800-846-6687).

And do learn how to avoid all the **NSAID pain drugs**, for in addition to (1) **increasing the heart attack rate 36%,** (2) over 16,000 people die each year from them via intestinal hemorrhaging, and (3) they cause high blood pressure (see *The High Blood Pressure Hoax* on how to cure your pressure problems without drugs (prestigepublishing.com or 1-800-846-6687). And this is not all they do. (4) NSAIDs poison the chemistry of joint cartilage, guaranteeing that you'll need a hip or knee replacement in 10-20 years. Joint replacements used to be seen mainly in older folks. Nowadays, it is common in young folks in their 30s and 40s. Next, (5) **NSAIDs also damage the matrix chemistry**, which is the "stuff" between heart cells and arterial cells, **leaving you more vulnerable for coronary plaque** and a heart attack.

And in *Total Wellness 2006* I've shown you the dangers of the newer arthritis/colitis/psoriasis prescription drugs that you continually see hyped on TV advertisements (Remicade, Enbrel, Humira, and more), which are even scarier. (6) They actually kill your TNF, tumor necrosis factor; something the body makes to fight infection and cancer! No wonder there is increased incidence of fatal infections and cancer, like lymphomas, in those who take them. And last but not least, (7) NSAIDs cause congestive heart failure in over **100,000 people each year, which is more deadly than cancer**. Average survival from cancer (all types averaged together) is 6 years. For CHF, it's five years to death after diagnosis. Every drug has too high a price to be paid.

Reference:

Pain Free In 6 Weeks, Total Wellness 2006, *The High Blood Pressure Hoax* (prestigepublishing.com, 1-800-846-6687)

An Angiogram is the Best Way to See Coronary Calcifications

Wrong. "Many studies have shown that **coronary angiography frequently under-estimates the severity of coronary artery lesions and even misses significant narrowings**" (deFeyter). That is not good when you remember that you have to sign a release that says you know **you could die from the procedure**. As for an exercise or stress EKG, it can look totally normal, yet you can have a heart attack within the hour afterwards.

The cheapest, safest, and easiest way I have found for you is to get the Ultrafast Heart Scan (also referred to as EBCT or electron beam computerized tomography) complete with your **coronary calcification score**. In less than 10 minutes you can see the tiniest flecks of calcium in your coronary arteries. And it is done without even taking your clothes off, and of course, without injecting you with nasty radioactive materials that can actually kill you within seconds. Furthermore, an angiogram only looks at the calcifications in the coronary vessels, but if you add in a full body scan with your Ultrafast Heart Scan, you'll see calcifications in other important vessels as well throughout the body. After all, **calcification of vessels is a systemic problem, and not just limited to the major heart vessels.**

Just about everybody has some reason to go to Florida during the year whether it's a business meeting, visiting relatives, funerals, or taking the grandkids to Orlando's Disney World. And with the periodic off-season fare wars of the airlines, sometimes just flying down and back in a single day is a reality. You do not need a prescription, but merely call the 800 number and make your appointment. There is one facility in St. Petersburg, Florida that is less than an hour from Tampa or Sarasota and satellite facilities in the Orlando area. If you mention this book there is usually a discount as well. You'll receive a disk with the MRI pictures and a written report that you may share with your doctor, including your calcium score. Just call **D.O.C. (Diagnostic Outpatient Center)** 1-800-890-4452 or 1-727-896-0000 for probably the most important test you will ever schedule for yourself. Also check your local facilities (like New York Heart Center in Syracuse, NY).

Do you know your calcium score? It's ironic that people know the scores of famous teams and their favorite athletes, while they torture themselves with their own golf scores. They may know their cholesterol level and other conventional parameters of low significance, but they don't know **one of the most important scores to predict how long they will live, the coronary calcium score**. In a nutshell, if your score is 10 or under, you have less than 3% chance of a heart attack in the next year, but 30% over the next ten years (assuming the progression stays the same and does not accelerate).

If your calcium score is 101-400, your chance goes to 12% each year, or 120% in the next ten years. So in 5-10 years you will have a heart attack. **If your calcium score is over 400, you have a 50% chance of heart attack within the next year**, and you need to get very serious about your plans for reversing it, NOW (Davis). Although I have seen occasional folks who had no symptoms with a score over 1000 with 4 vessels badly calcified in many areas, they are a catastrophe waiting to happen. There are always exceptions, and this shows once more that nothing is the sole determining factor for having a heart attack. As **with every disease, there are multiple contributing factors.**

But just in case you are not entirely convinced of your need for an EBCT, consider these facts. In a large group of 274 patients with various cardiovascular risk factors **the annual rate of increase in**

the coronary calcifications score was a 39% per year if they were untreated (Budoff 1998). Progression of the calcium score more than 15% per year is associated with a 13-fold greater risk of having a heart attack each year Raggi 2003, Budoff 1998). An angiogram just shows your calcifications, you can die from it, you can get infection, the cannula could perforate the vessel causing you to bleed to death, you need anesthesia, it is very expensive, and you do not get your **crystal ball prognostic calcium score**. But the EBCT is safe and more diagnostic and prognostic (a better crystal ball test to reflect what your future holds in store.) The beauty is **you can change your odds** by doing many of the things you will learn here. We have followed folks for over a decade whose scores should have had them having bypass surgery or stents over 6 years ago, and they still have no symptoms and no medications.

Now when folks have coronary calcifications, most docs prescribe a statin cholesterol-lowering drug and a daily aspirin. Yet studies show that if you are on a statin drug plus an aspirin, your coronary score increases 22% (+/-18%) each year. BUT, taking **Kyolic** (a proprietary non-prescription aged garlic formula with over 300 research papers behind it) reduces progression to 7% (+/- 9%) per year, less than a third. **In essence, a huge swig of Kyolic Liquid twice a day is like a triple damper on the progression of your coronary artery disease**. How can you afford not to do it?

Likewise **if you are on a statin drug and an aspirin, your plaque volume increases 129% (+/- 102%) per year.** But if you add **Kyolic Liquid, it drops dramatically to a volume increase of 45% (+/- 57%) per year.** Remember that the large +/- variation is because there is a huge variability between individuals and the other contributory factors (diets, nutrients, toxins, knowledge, reading commitment and implementation, etc.).

So buck up. There is a non-prescription natural agent that can cut your chance of heart attack and death by more than half. In fact, this safe nutrient can cut your progression of coronary calcifications down to a third of the rate! A double blind study by a UCLA cardiologist showed that even if you are on a statin drug plus aspirin, **you could cut your chance of a heart attack down by two-thirds by adding Kyolic Liquid** (Budoff, 2006). How easy could that be? And you will learn of many more things you can do to axe your risk here, as well as to get you off drugs.

References:

deFeyter PJ, et al, Quantitative coronary angiography to measure progression and regression of coronary atherosclerosis. Value, limitations, and implications for clinical trials, *Circul,* 84: 412-23, 1991

Budoff MJ, et al, Inhibiting progression of coronary calcification using aged garlic extract in patients receiving statin therapy: a preliminary study, *Prevent Med*, 39:985-91, 2004

Budoff M, Aged garlic extract retards progression of coronary artery calcification, *J Nutr*, 136:741s-744s, 2006.

Budoff MJ, et al, Rates of progression of coronary calcifications by electron beam computed tomography, *Circul,* 98:1-656, 1998

Davis W, *Track Your Plaque*, iuniverse.com, 2004, 414-456-1123

Rumberger, et al, Electron beam CT coronary calcium score cutpoints and severity of associated angiography luminal stenosis, *J Am Coll Cardiol*, 29:1542-48, 1997

Greenland P, et al, Coronary artery calcium combined with Framingham score for risk prediction in asymptomatic individuals, *J Am Med Assoc,* 291:210-15, 2004

Shaw LJ, et al, Prognostic value of cardiac risk factors and coronary artery calcium screening for all-cause mortality, *Radiol*, 228: 826-33, 2003

Kondos GT, et al, Electron-beam tomography coronary artery calcium and cardiac events. At 37-month follow-up of 5,635 initially asymptomatic low-to intermediate-risk adults, *Circul,* 107:2571-76, 2003

Raggi P, et al, Progression of coronary calcium on serial electron beam tomographic scanning is greater in patients with future myocardial infarction, *Am J Cardiol*, 92:827-29, 2003

Raggi P, et al, Progression of coronary artery calcium and risk of first myocardial infarction in patients receiving cholesterol-lowering therapy, *Arterioscler Thromb Vasc Biol*, 24: 1272-77, 2004

Steiner M, et al, A double-blind crossover study in moderately hypercholesterolemia man that compared the effect of aged garlic extract and placebo administration on blood lipids, *Am J Clin Nutr*, 64: 866-70, 1996

Steiner M, et al, Aged garlic extract, a modulator of cardiovascular risk factors: a dose-finding study on the effects of AGE on platelet functions, *J Nutr,* 131 (3s): 980s-4s, 2001

Steiner M, et al, Changes in platelet function and susceptibility of lipoproteins to oxidation associated with administration of Aged Garlic Extract, *J Cardiovasc Pharmacol,* 31:904-8, 1998

Rahman K, et al, Dietary supplementation with aged garlic extract inhibits ADP-induced platelet aggregation in humans, *J Nutr,* 130:2662-65, 2000

Lau BH, Suppression of LDL oxidation by garlic, *J Nutr,* 131:985s-8s, 2001

Campbell JH, et al, Molecular basis by which garlic suppresses atherosclerosis, *J Nutr,* 131:1006s-9s, 2001

More Kyolic references in Chapter II

Statins are Safe for Breast Cancer Survivors

After having had surgery for breast cancer followed by implants, women are often found to have high cholesterol (from increased free radicals!) and are told they should go on a statin drug. This shows blatant ignorance of body and pharmacologic chemistry as well as the scientific literature. For they failed to get rid of the underlying causes that triggered the cancers in the first place (see *Detoxify or Die*, then *TW* 2007, 2006, 2005). Women blindly accept the false notion that cutting the cancer off and taking a few chemo and radiation treatments to poison the body will keep the cancer from surfacing again. This is dangerously naïve. They have done nothing to get rid of what caused the cancer in the first place. But it gets worse.

I quote for you from just one of several studies touting the benefits of statins to doctors. And by the way, this statistic was not mentioned in the abstract (summary) of the article, the only part of a scientific article that the majority of docs and reporters read. I quote from the *New England Journal of Medicine* (Sacks FM, et al, The effect of pravastatins on coronary events after myocardial infarction in patients with average cholesterol levels, vol. 335, pg 1001-9, 1996):

"Breast cancer occurred in <u>1</u> patient in the placebo group and <u>12</u> in the pravastatin group."

I personally would have strong reservations about recommending statins to a woman concerned about breast cancer. Statins appear to be fertilizer for breast cancer.

But there are far more dangerous recommendations being made. Because statins poison the ability of cells to make cholesterol, and cancer cells depend heavily on cholesterol for metastasizing (spreading through angiogenesis), the drug industry is capitalizing on this hypothesis as one more potential use for statins. But research shows that one of the isomers of vitamin E, delta tocotrienols, is much more potent and infinitely safer. It slows down angiogenesis (metastases or spread), makes cancer cells kill themselves (apoptosis), reduces protein kinase and improves the p53 cancer-fighting gene.

In animal studies of cancer, delta tocotrienols combined with a statin decreased the size of the tumors 50% and suppressed metastases 60%. But the levels of statin used were extremely toxic for humans since they are the ones that caused fatal rhabdomyolysis. It would be far smarter to combine **Kyolic Formula 107 Red Yeast Rice** (two twice a day) with 3 **Delta-Fraction Tocotrienols** three times a day. But this is out of the realm of this book, more on this in upcoming issues of *TW*. You will learn more about this fraction of vitamin E for your cholesterol levels and arterial health in Chapter VIII, because the **Delta-Fraction Tocotrienols** (Allergy Research Group) are also a safe HMG CoA reductase inhibitor.

References:
McAnally JA, et al, Tocotrienols potentiate lovastatin-mediated growth suppression in vitro and in vivo, *Exp Biol Med*, 232:523-31, 2007

Nakagawa K, et al, In vivo angiogenesis is suppressed by unsaturated vitamin E tocotrienols, *J Nutr*, 137: 1938-43, 2007

Cholesterol is the Best Blood Test
Indicator for Risk of Early Heart Attacks

Wrong. There are many tests that are much stronger indicators of early heart death. In fact, like every other disease, early heart attacks are a product of the total load to the body, and rarely if ever, due to just one thing. Even when you get the flu, it is not just the bug. It is the total body burden of your weakened and toxic immune system that determines whether you are one of its vulnerable victims, or whether you escape unscathed. You already learned about homocysteine, but there are others. (1) **The high sensitivity CRP (hsCRP) is a much better indicator than cholesterol of early heart death, and so is** (2) **an elevated fibrinogen.** In fact even if you don't have high cholesterol, an elevated CRP is an independent serious risk factor meaning you are slated for an early heart death (Ridker, Rutter). Clearly, as you'll learn here, **high cholesterol is one of the most meaningless indicators of early heart death**.

Likewise, (3) **a bad sign is a low level of the "good" cholesterol, HDL**. And as you'll learn here there are many other important indicators, and taken together, they create an awesome package that predicts whether folks will be plaque-free or dramatically slow down plaque progression, regardless of whether they have sky-high cholesterol or a normal one. Recall, the reason you have been focused on statin drugs is that just one brand alone, Lipitor brings in over $10 billion a year. Whereas indicators like homocysteine, fibrinogen, CRP, and even the HDL cholesterol are not all improved by statin drugs, but are improved and normalized by knowledge-based prescriptions of nutrients.

Luckily, as you learned in the last chapter, red yeast rice, niacin, policosanol, and vitamin C can raise HDL. Furthermore, you learned that **vitamin E could normalize the fibrinogen and CRP** (Devaraj), but remember that **statins lower vitamin E.** In one study, as little as 200 mg a day of **vitamin E has brought down** the CRP as much as 65% in some folks, and the fibrinogen was lowered by 24% (Leichtle). Likewise **when the bad LDL cholesterol is loaded with vitamin E, it is protected and cannot become oxidized. This means it can't grab onto the arterial cell wall to produce plaque,** no matter how high the cholesterol is. And needless to say vitamin E has been found to be infinitely safer than the statin drugs (Bendich).

And don't forget that **lipoproteins (cholesterol is one of them) are the main carriers of vitamin E.** So if you lower the cholesterol too much, as many are doing with the statin drugs, then you're also silently creating a vitamin E deficiency in yet another way by depriving it of its necessary carrier (Behrens). As another example, **knowing your levels of vitamins A, C, and E is strong enough to give 90% accuracy in forecasting your chances of an early death** (Gey, *The High Blood Pressure Hoax*). What a crystal ball! And don't let anyone forget, **statins lower your vitamin E** levels by themselves, so they contribute to earlier death by multiple mechanisms.

What is the best test that includes everything you need? The **Cardio/ION Panel,** for it contains all your cholesterol parameters including total, LDL, HDL, Lp(a), triglycerides, plus the dangerous indicators that cardiologists seem to ignore like homocysteine, fibrinogen, CRP, 8-OhdG, lipid peroxides, insulin, testosterone, as well as the indispensable RBC (red blood cell) minerals like magnesium, vitamins like E, fatty acids, heavy metals, amino acids, organic acids and more, that you'll learn about here.

How do you convince your doctor to order it? Call 1-800-221-4640 or go to metametrix.com to have information sent to your doctor, chiropractor, naturopath, or other health professional who can order this most important test for you. While you are at it, have MetaMetrix Lab also send your doctor the medical paper I published in 2006 showing why it really borders on malpractice to fail to at least look at a patient's organic acids, which are part of the **Cardio/ION Panel**. If you have no one to interpret it for you, I have scheduled non-patient phone consults. Here you and I can go over your 10+ page report of your molecular biology together and map out what nutrients would be indicated with which sources and doses, as well as which complementary nutrients need to be included that are not yet measured, dovetailing it all with your vast medical, surgical, dietary, dental, military, environmental and other histories that you can send.

References:

Ridker PM, et al, Established and emerging plasma biomarkers in the prediction of first atherothrombotic events, *Circulation,* 109; 4:6-19, 2004

Rutter MK, et al, The C-reactive protein, the metabolic syndrome, and prediction of cardiovascular events in the Framingham offspring study, *Circulation,* 110: 380-85, 2004

Cholesterol Treatment is Very Simple, I Just Need to Take a Drug to Lower It

Wrong. So what is the intelligent person's approach to high cholesterol? First realize that **cholesterol is a sign of overload, usually not of cholesterol, but of too many free radicals in the blood stream.** I'll tell you where they come from and how to get rid of them later. For now you merely need to firmly know that **Cholesterol is the body's smoke detector and band-aid**. It is the messenger screaming that much needs to be fixed. High cholesterol merely shows destructive free radicals (naked electrons) are eating holes in your blood vessel walls. Your body sends its protective Band-Aid to patch up the holes so you don't bleed to death. That Band-Aid is cholesterol. So killing cholesterol by turning off or actually poisoning the liver's ability to make it is just stupid. **For cholesterol serves multiple purposes, including being nature's antioxidant and patching up the leaks in damaged arterial walls**.

What fosters these wildly destructive free radicals or naked electrons? Predominately by three things (although there are more): (1) an environmental chemical overload (like the trans fatty acids and plasticizers in foods, heavy metals like mercury, cadmium, lead and arsenic that are unavoidably in our air, food, water and dental amalgams), pesticides, plasticizers that are in all of us, Teflon that even the newborn baby has, and more that you will learn about. (2) Bad bugs in the gut or teeth, and (3) undiagnosed nutritional deficiencies, like magnesium or vitamin E, are simple examples. The beauty of it all is that **it is correctable**, bringing most folks to levels of wellness they have never before experienced.

References:

Behrens WA, et al, Distribution of alpha-tocopherol in human plasma lipoproteins, *Am J Clin Nutr*, 35:691-96, 1982

Devaraj S, et al, Alpha-tocopherol supplementation decreases serum C-reactive protein and monocyte interleukin-6 levels in normal volunteers and type 2 diabetic patients, *Free Rad Biol Med*, 29:790-92, 2000

Bendich A, et al, Safety of oral intake of vitamin E, *Am J Clin Nutr*, 48:6 12-19, 1988

Leitchle A, et al, Alpha-tocopherol distribution in lipoproteins and anti-inflammatory effects differ between CHD-patients and healthy subjects, *J Am Coll Nutr*, 25; 5:420-28, 2006

My Doctor Says There is Nothing to Lower the CRP

CRP, is a blood test that measures the level of C-reactive protein, a marker of intense and dangerous inflammation raging somewhere in the body and that will eventually cause a serious problem, a heart attack being high on the list of possibilities. The high sensitivity CRP, hsCRP, is even a better test. Harvard researchers show that **a high hsCRP triples your risk of heart attack, even if you have normal LDL or bad cholesterol**, while if LDL is abnormal, your risk zooms up to 6-fold! (St. Pierre).

Many options are available for those who want to empower themselves. Whole foods diets like macrobiotics are extremely potent in not only knocking down CRP (inflammation), but also restoring the body's cancer-killing tumor necrosis factor (TNF) to normal. On the flip side, when potent drugs are used to cut inflammation (like Enbrel, Remicade, etc. as seen on TV ads for arthritis, psoriasis, and colitis) they also lower the TNF, thereby increasing your cancer risk; Remember TNF is a cytokine or protein that the body makes to fight off cancers as well as to control the inflammation that ushers in every disease. Killing your CRP with drugs also kills your cancer protection. Not a smart choice.

There's enormous evidence now to back up what we have seen for years: **diet has a huge bearing on health and in fact you can often reverse the most hopeless conditions with it.** See December 2006 *TW* for the case of a nurse bed-ridden, on oxygen, with wildly metastatic end-stage cancer with just days to live. She was completely cured with the macrobiotic diet, and is exceedingly healthy 12 years later (details in the next chapter). It is one of the best-documented cases the NIH has ever seen. If you're ever really stuck and cannot find the cause, a year or two of the macrobiotic diet could accomplish the same for you. Start with *You Are What You Ate* then proceed to *The Cure is in the Kitchen* followed by *Macro Mellow*. There are many reasons why this diet has enabled folks to heal the impossible regardless of what their medical label was (mechanisms described in *Tired Or Toxic?*).

So if you have elevated hsCRP (high sensitivity C-reactive protein), yes, it is a danger sign of early arteriosclerosis and many other degenerative problems. But the smartest thing is to find the source. Is it from infection in the blood vessels, as from H. pylori that has migrated from the gut, or a bad tooth that only occasionally nags you (details in Chapter V)? Is it from the inflammation pathways being turned on by your load of high fructose corn syrup hidden in everything from tonic water, sodas and fruit juices to all sorts of processed foods? Or is inflammation turned on by the plasticizers, pesticides, Teflon and fire retardants that permeate our foods (details in Chapters IV and VII)? In the meantime start 1-2 **Gamma E Gems** along with your 1-2 **E-Gems Elite** and two **Tocotrienols** twice a day that we talked about in Chapter II. This is a smart way to start to lower your CRP.

The bottom line is you are lucky you're so smart if you have a doc who found an elevated CRP. And you know that nutrient corrections can reverse it while you search for the cause. If all else fails, the macrobiotic diet gets rid of the trans fats, phthalates, Teflon, elevates the omega-3 oils, gets rid of the sugars and processed foods and corrects a whole lot of abnormal chemistry. In fact, it is so potent that **it has reversed not only coronary artery plaque, but also end-stage cancers.** What are you waiting for?

References:

St-Pierre AC, Bergeron J, Pirro M, et al, Effect of plasma C-reactive protein levels in modulating the risk of coronary heart disease associated with small, dense, low-density lipoproteins in men (The Québec Cardiovascular Study), *Am J Cardiol*, 91; 5:55 5-58, Mar 2003

Willett WC, et al, Intake of trans fatty acids and risk of coronary heart disease among women, *Lancet*, 341; 8845:581-85, 1993

Neustadt J, Western diet and inflammation, *Integrat Med*, 5; 4:14-18, Aug/Sept 2006.

Shulze MB, et al, Dietary pattern, inflammation and incidence of type 2 diabetes in women, *Am J Clin Nutr*, 82; 3:675-84, 2005

Gelman L, et al, An update on the mechanisms of action of the peroxisome proliferator-activated receptors (PPARs) and their roles in inflammation and cancer, *Cell Mol Life Sci*, 55: 932-43, 1999

Ridker PM, Cannon CP, Morrow D, et al, C-reactive protein levels and outcomes after statin therapy, *New Engl J Med*, 352; 1:20-28, Jan 6, 2005

Himmelfarb et al, Alpha and Gamma tocopherol metabolism in healthy subjects and patients with end-stage renal disease, *Kidney Internat*, 64; 3:978-91, Sep 2003

Jiang Q, Ames BN, Gamma tocopherol, but not alpha-tocopherol, decreases proinflammatory eicosanoids and inflammation damage in rats, *FASEB J*, 17; 8:816-22, May 2003

Devaraj S, Jialal I, Alpha-tocopherol supplementation decreases serum C-reactive protein and monocyte interleukin-6 levels in normal volunteers and type 2 diabetic patients, *Free Rad Biol Med*, 29; 8:790-92, Oct. 15, 2000

Rogers SA, *Total Wellness* 2006, *You Are What You Ate, The Cure is In the Kitchen, Macro Mellow, Tired Or Toxic,* (all from prestigepublishing.com or 1-800-846-6687)

Cholesterol-Lowering Drugs
Are Recommended for Elevated CRP

Yes, they are, but only by physicians who are not up on their molecular biochemistry of the bodies they were trained to treat.   If they rely chiefly on drug detail men and pharmaceutical-sponsored medical meetings and pharmaceutical-sponsored medical journals for their knowledge, then they will be drug-oriented and think they are correct to boot. Let's see why.

The *New England Journal of Medicine* published studies showing statin drugs cut the risk of heart attack by lowering CRP, the C-reactive protein. This at first glance would seem legitimate, because there was a 21% reduction in CRP (Nissen, Ridker 2005). And I was impressed that they used the CRP as a danger indicator. Because indeed, the **CRP is a greater risk factor for early death than having high cholesterol**, for it is stronger in predicting whether you will have an early heart attack or stroke (Ridker 2002, Krumholz, Rifai). However the researchers used very high doses of the statin cholesterol-lowering drug to accomplish this 21% reduction. The danger is that these high doses are more likely to also give a higher suppression of coenzyme Q10, resulting in more side effects like the fatal muscle disease, rhabdomyolysis.   And as usual, they totally dismissed looking at anything natural that could help you enormously better and infinitely cheaper.

What you shouldn't expect to see in a journal dedicated to drug-oriented medicine (they are easy to spot because you have to plow through the sea of pharmaceutical ads before you get to the actual articles that begin in the later half of the journal) is that **alpha-tocopherol (one of eight parts of natural vitamin E) can lower CRP by not 21% but 52%, or more than double what a statin drug can do, and without the lethal side effects** (now you understand why it had such bad press, based on defective science, a few years ago, since they wanted to wipe out any competition) (Devaraj). But hang onto your seats.   Another part of vitamin E that conventional medicine totally ignores, **gamma tocopherol lowers CRP by 61%, almost triple the improvement and at 1/5 the cost of any statin drug and without the dangerous side effects** (Himmelfarb, Jiang).

An additional nasty negative effect of this article was that information-challenged cardiologists thought it sounded so good that they even started pushing the statin drugs (and continue to this day) on innocent patients who did not even have high cholesterol, in the misguided attempt to stave off arteriosclerosis and coronary artery disease that the CRP is a warning of. But they overlooked the fact that **when you give cholesterol-lowering drugs to someone who does not have high cholesterol, you can get cholesterol that is too low.**

Too **low cholesterol is just as dangerous as too high**. Cholesterol is needed for all membrane structure and function, hormones, hormone receptors, release of cytokines that fight off infection and cancers. And when the membrane is cholesterol-starved, it can malfunction and trigger autoimmune diseases. In fact, folks with a **cholesterol under 160 mg/dL have double the risk of brain hemorrhage and increased risk of cancers of the liver, lung, pancreas, and leukemia, plus cirrhosis and suicide** (Neaton). In another study, low cholesterol folks had more than double the death rate from non-cardiac conditions (Behar). **Besides doubling the death rate, low cholesterol dramatically damages mental-health** leading to depression, suicide, mania, and more (Cassidy, Boston, Engleberg).

So if you have elevated hsCRP (high sensitivity C-reactive protein), yes, it is a danger sign of early arteriosclerosis and many other degenerative problems. I know I repeated this, but medicine is repeatedly brainwashing docs to Rx statins for CRP! The smartest thing is to find the source (this book will guide you and some will need to go further with *The High Blood Pressure Hoax*). Is it from infection in the blood vessels, as from H. pylori that has migrated from the gut, or a bad tooth that only occasionally nags you? In the meantime, start 1-2 **Gamma E Gems** along with your 1-2 **E-Gems Elite** and two **Tocotrienols** a day. This is the smart way to lower your hsCRP.

References:

Nissen SE, Tuzcu EM, Schoenhagen P, et al, Statin therapy, LDL cholesterol, C-reactive protein, and coronary artery disease, *New Engl J Med,* 2005 Jan 6; 351; 1:29-38

Ridker PM, Cannon CP, Morrow D, et al, C-reactive protein levels and outcomes after statin therapy, *New Engl J Med*, 2005 Jan 6; 352; 1:20-28

Ridker PM, Rifai N, Cook NR, et al, Comparison C-reactive protein and low-density lipoprotein cholesterol levels in the prediction of first cardiovascular events, *New Engl J Med*, 347; 20:1557-65, Nov 14, 2002

Krumholz HM, Seeman TE, Merrill SS, et al, **Lack of association between cholesterol and coronary heart disease mortality** and morbidity and all-cause mortality in persons older than 70 years, *J Am Med Assoc*, 272; 17:1335-40, Nov 2, 1994

Rifai N, Ridker PM, Proposed cardiovascular risk assessment algorithm using high sensitivity C-reactive protein and lipid screening, *Clin Chem*, 47; 1:28-30, Jan 2001

Wang XL, Rainwater DL, Mahaney MC, Stocker R, Cosupplementation with vitamin E and coenzyme Q10 reduces circulating markers of inflammation in baboons, *Am J Clin Nutr*, 80; 3:649-55, Sep 2004

Himmelfarb J, Kane J, McMonagle E, et al, Alpha and Gamma tocopherol metabolism in healthy subjects and patients with end-stage renal disease, *Kidney Internat*, 64; 3:978-91, Sep 2003

Jiang Q, Ames BN, Gamma tocopherol, but not alpha-tocopherol, decreases proinflammatory eicosanoids and inflammation damage in rats, *FASEB J,* 17; 8:816-22, May 2003

Devaraj S, Jialal I, Alpha-tocopherol supplementation decreases serum C-reactive protein and monocyte interleukin-6 levels in normal volunteers and type 2 diabetic patients, *Free Rad Biol Med*, 29; 8:790-92, Oct 15, 2000

Neaton JD, Blackburn H, Jacobs D, et al, Serum cholesterol level and mortality findings for men screened in the Multiple Risk Factor Intervention Trial. Multiple Risk Factor Intervention Trial Research Group, *Arch Intern Med,* 152; 7:1490-1500, July 1992

Behar S, Graff E, Reicher-Reiss H, et al, **Low total cholesterol is associated with high total mortality in patients with coronary heart disease.** The Bezafobrate Infarction Prevention (BIP) Study Group, *Heart J*, 1:52-9, Jan 18, 1997

Cassidy AT, Carroll BJ, Hypocholesterolemia during mixed manic episodes, *Europ Arch Psych Clin Neurosci*, 252; 3:110-14, Jun 2002

Boston PF, Dursun SM, Reveley MA, Cholesterol and mental disorder, *Brit J Psych,* 169; 6:682-9, Dec 1996

Engleberg H, Low serum cholesterol and suicide, *Lancet*, 339; 8795:727-79, Mar 21,1992

My Heart Specialist Will Order All the Tests I Need

Beware of the dangerous cardiologist, and there are a host of them out there, I can attest, for I am continually confronted with this scenario. After a heart attack, or unrelenting angina or shortness of breath, or recalcitrant arrhythmia, the victims usually have either bypass surgery or angioplasty or stent or repair of a cardiac valve, accompanied by a life sentence to a barrage of drugs. They are then turned loose to report back every 3 months. Some of them have been followed this way for over five years.

The horrifying part of the story is that when they finally convince someone (usually the local chiropractor) to order the **Cardio/ION Panel** for them, they were on death's doorstep with multiple dangerous high risk factors. The reason I am upset is because every one of these factors is 100% reversible. Yet these highly paid specialists never assayed the correct parameters. And this is in spite of the fact that the research behind all this has been in their own highly publicized journals. I'll bet the researchers and clinicians feel like tearing their hair out at being ignored and having millions of folks needlessly losing their lives. I know I stopped wasting my time publishing medical articles after about 20 of them. Instead, I devote my energies to focusing on super intelligent folks like you who want to take control of their health. Make sure you get a copy of all your lab work.

Some of the urgent tests that should be done include the hsCRP, homocysteine, lipid peroxides, fibrinogen, insulin, testosterone, fatty acids, RBC minerals, anti-oxidant vitamins, and much more. Some of these you've already learned about and others are coming.

My Doctor Wants Me to Take a New Drug to Raise My HDL

The HDL race is on. Not all cholesterol is bad. In fact, good cholesterol acts like a wheelbarrow and carts bad cholesterol right to the liver where it is dumped into bile and into our gut to be gotten rid of permanently. This HDL (high density lipoprotein) cholesterol has been known for decades, but like many things in medicine you didn't hear very much about it, merely because there wasn't a drug for it. But now that pharmaceutical companies finally have drugs to focus on it, expect to hear a lot more about the importance of raising your HDL. The first drug was rapidly removed from the market because of increased deaths, but others have followed.

HDL is much more important than how much of the bad cholesterol, LDL, you have. HDL is so important that many **people who have had serious cardiac valve replacement and heart attacks never had high cholesterol. They only had an HDL in the <u>normal range</u>, but less than 60** (Morgan). This also confirms that the current "normal" range for HDL is wrong and it should be well above 60.

Because HDL (high density lipoprotein) is the one form of cholesterol in the body that carries cholesterol away from the coronary arteries and dumps it into the bile, where we use it for detoxification of body chemicals, **HDL does double duty. It protects us against coronary artery plaque as well as helps us detoxify our daily onslaught of chemicals that trigger heart disease.** Of course, many natural nutrients and phytochemicals (parts of foods) help to raise HDL beautifully. In fact, the average person couldn't take all the natural things that raise HDL. For example, **vitamins C and B3 (Niacin-Time** that you learned about in Chapter II) **raise HDL** and minerals like **magnesium** do, as well as amino acids like **taurine** and **carnitine** (Hallfrisch, Handler, Mochizuk, Morgan, Rossi). The detoxifier and precursor to glutathione, N-acetyl cysteine or **NAC** also raises HDL, as do the **Tocotrienols**, part of vitamin E that you also learned about in Chapter II (Franceschini, Qureshi).

And this list of nutrients doesn't even begin to touch the surface. Wouldn't it be wonderful if someone put many of these nutrients into one product? Well they did. It's called **HDL Rx**. Take 1-2 twice a day (Integrative Therapeutics). You can start with two capsules three or four times a day and see if this is sufficient to raise your HDL. The constituents are much lower doses than those nutrients used in solo studies to raise HDL, but when you combine the symphony of nutrients you can usually get away with much lower doses of individual components. And if you need, you can certainly add your **Niacin-Time**, the 3 forms of vitamin E, and extra magnesium that you learned about in the preceding chapter that are so beneficial (Itoh). **Orchestrated natural solutions** certainly beat taking a prescription medication whose ingredients don't have all the other benefits that a proprietary blend of multiple nutrients like **HDL Rx** does.

References:

Morgan J, et al, High-density lipoproteins subfractions and risk of coronary artery disease, *Curr Atheroscler Rep*, 6; 5:359-65, Sept 2004

Hallfrisch J, et al, High plasma vitamin C associated with high plasma HDL-and HDL-2 cholesterol, *Am J Clin Nutr*, 60; 1:100-105, July 1994

Morgan JM, et al, The effects of niacin on lipoproteins subclass distribution, *Prev Cardiol*, 7; 4:182-7, Fall 2004

Itoh K, et al, The effects of high oral magnesium supplementation on blood pressure, serum lipids, and related variables in apparently healthy Japanese subjects, *Brit J Nutr*, 78:737-50, 1997

Rossi CS, et al, **Effect of carnitine on serum HDL-cholesterol**: report of two cases, *Johns Hopkins Med J*, 150; 2:51-4, Feb 1982

Mochizuki H, et al, Increasing effect of dietary taurine on the serum HDL-cholesterol concentration in rats, *Biosci Biotechnol Biochem*, 62; 3: 578-9, Mar 1998

Handler SS, Rorvik D, eds, Taurine In: *PDR® for Nutritional Supplements,* Montvale New Jersey, Medical Economics Co., 442-4, 2001

Franceschini G, et al, Dose-related increase of HDL-cholesterol levels after N-acetylcysteine in man, *Pharmacol Res*, 28; 3:213-18, Oct/Nov 1993

Qureshi AA, et al, Dose-dependent suppression of serum cholesterol by tocotrienols-rich fraction (TRF 25) of rice bran in hypercholesterolemia, humans, *Atheroscler*, 161; 1:199-207, Mar 2002

Cholesterol-Lowering Drugs
Only Work by Lowering Cholesterol

There are other "beneficial" effects of the statin drugs, for example, they increase nitric oxide inside arteries. But God designed a beautiful system where we make our own nitric oxide to dilate our arteries starting with the simple non-prescription amino acid **arginine** (all the protocols are explained in *The High Blood Pressure Hoax*). And if you're really into drugs, **nitroglycerin** is cheaper and does much the same thing. So why would you want to take a statin drug loaded with so many side effects when there are much more healthful options?

Sure, statin drugs also have anti-oxidant, plus anti-inflammatory activity, and they lower CRP (Karatzis, Morita, Zieden, Ridker). But that is still no reason to take them. You can normalize these elevated chemistries in far healthier ways and naturally, as you are learning.

References:

John S, et al, Increased bioavailability of nitric oxide after lipid-lowering therapy in hypercholesterolemia patients: a randomized, placebo-controlled, double-blind study, *Circulation,* 98; 3: 211-16, 1998

Karatzis E, et al, Rapid effect of pravastatin on endothelial function and lipid peroxidation in unstable angina, *Internat J Cardiol*, 101; 1:65-70, 2005

Morita H, et al, Fluvastatin ameliorates the hyperhomocysteinemia-induced endothelial dysfunction: the antioxidative properties of fluvastatin, *Circul J* (Jpn), 69; 4:475-80, 2005

Zieden B, et al, The role of statins in the prevention of ischemic stroke, *Curr Atherosclerosis Rep*, 7; 5:365-8, 2005

Ridker P, Rapid reduction in C-reactive protein with cerivastatin among 785 patients with primary hypercholesterolemia, *Circul*, 103; 9:1191-93, 2001

My Cardiologist is a Specialist and Highly Rated,
He Will Do All That I Need

Guard against the "clueless" cardiologist. The course of events in American medicine is really scaring me. I keep encountering folks who casually say they recently had a stent or two put in, as though they had merely gone in for a routine dental cleaning. The scariest part is now they are on multiple drugs, guaranteed to make them more ill. A common combination is a prescription is Zetia, Plavix, and Toprol-XL. We've talked about all of these separately in past *TW* issues (and you'll find the references for them within the last five years), but let's take a quick look at why these are so dangerous as a combination package.

Zetia is prescribed in attempt to lower their cholesterol even though most of them don't even have high cholesterol. As you recall, many people who have a heart attack never have had high cholesterol. But the studies clearly show that folks who have cholesterol less than 200 die sooner and have more medical problems. That is in part because they don't have enough cholesterol to repair cardiac cell membranes, nor to make their hormones, mitochondrial membranes (where heart energy is made), nor to make sufficient detoxifying bile, and much more.

And don't forget as I showed you in Chapter I, that most docs would cite the study that shows folks on cholesterol-lowering drugs dramatically cutting their heart attack rate. But the studies that looked at cholesterol-lowering drugs only looked at how many people on them died of a heart attack. They did not report the total death rate that includes how many people died from other things. Why? Because, as you recall, the **statistics clearly showed that the decrease in death from heart attack by statins was offset by increased deaths from other problems like suicidal depression, cancer** and more. These all stem from an actual uncorrected cholesterol deficiency produced by the drug. **There was no overall decrease in death rate with statin drugs.**

But that's not the worst problem. Zetia is not a statin, like Lipitor for example, but instead, as you learned in Chapter 1, works on a different mechanism. It actually inhibits your absorption of cholesterol from the gut. By interfering with absorption of fats, you also drastically cut your absorption of fat-soluble nutrients that you need for life, like vitamins A, D, E, K, CoQ10, beta-carotene, as well as the lipids and fatty acids like EPA, DHA, phosphatidylcholine and much more. **To stifle your absorption of these priceless fat-soluble nutrients is a slow death sentence.**

As far as the second commonly prescribed drug, Plavix, this dramatically confirms the unbelievable power of the drug industry in controlling the practice of medicine. As one example, a March 2006 *Wall Street Journal* article reported on a study presented at the annual scientific meeting of the American College of Cardiology in Atlanta, and I quote: "a large study found that **adding the blood thinner Plavix to aspirin wasn't significantly more effective than aspirin alone in preventing heart attacks, strokes or death** from cardiovascular disease in a broad group of high risk patients."

The article went on to explain that not only was this expensive $4 a capsule Plavix of little benefit, but that it was actually dangerous. "In addition, **for patients who have not had a heart attack or stroke, adding Plavix to aspirin was associated with a higher risk of death from cardiovascular causes than aspirin alone**." Even though this study was done on over 15,000 patients and published in a high profile journal plus the media, **Plavix continues to be the second-largest selling drug in the world after Lipitor.** In fact, most cardiologists continue to prescribe it and are totally unaware of the many alternatives that are not only safer, but also more effective and cheaper, as you will learn here. Don't ever underestimate the power of the largest for-profit industry in the world, the pharmaceutical.

If that were not enough reason to challenge his expertise before you let someone take control of the helm, **Lipitor blocks the anti-clotting activity of the blood thinner, Plavix** (Hensley). Did you get that? Most **cardiologists are prescribing an expensive combination of drugs where one negates or cancels out the other.**

And these are not cheap or without dangerous side effects. I'm warning you, you are about to know more chemistry about the body and prescription drugs than most cardiologists, so select carefully.

Our focus in medical school and most training thereafter for the rest of our careers is focused on drugs, not finding the causes and cures. And sadly most don't even know all the chemistry of the drugs they are licensed to prescribe. Most cardiologists, as an example, prescribe **Plavix and Lipitor together, yet one not only cancels the benefit of the other, but also perpetuates all the nutrient deficiencies that remain undiagnosed and uncorrected, guaranteeing an avalanche of new symptoms.** It is a scary world out there. So **since Lipitor blocks the blood thinning action of Plavix,** a guy who prescribes both is inadequately funded with knowledge to treat you.

Furthermore, I've shown you here and in *The High Blood Pressure Hoax* how vitamin E with all its eight parts is more effective than aspirin, while **aspirin doubles the rate of stroke!** In contrast, the membrane repair that you'll learn about in the next chapter decreases the ability of the body to make unwanted clots. Interestingly, for folks with high cholesterol and even many without it, the statin drugs are prescribed. But remember, the **statin drugs for lowering cholesterol actually increase platelet aggregation and increase fibrinogen.** In other words they actually make sure you will have an earlier heart attack or clotting of your new stents or vessels.

And as far as the addition of **beta-blockers** goes, I showed you many of their nasty effects and how they accelerate death. **(1) They poison your body's ability to make thyroid, which of course, raises your cholesterol which then encourages depression, constipation, exhaustion, weight gain that won't budge. Meanwhile, (2) they also increase your triglycerides, and (3) lower the good cholesterol, HDL that carries the bad choles-**

terol away from the arterial wall. **(4) Beta-blocker drugs also lower zinc (which fuels inflammation and increases your cancer risk for starters), (5) raise triglycerides that promote arteriosclerosis, and they (6) bring on diabetes.** They do more, as you learned, but I think you get the picture.

For the average person who has not been a steady reader of the books and *TW* newsletters, they don't have the back-up evidence to show their cardiologist. Instead he remains adamantly dedicated to his drug program. He surprisingly remains totally clueless regarding how he might even begin to determine the underlying causes and cures for your coronary artery disease. So he likewise **remains clueless that he is actually accelerating death and that the medical literature even supports and proves it.** Because if he goes by what he learns at his meetings, which are sponsored by pharmaceutical companies, he feels comfortable and committed to prescribing what he thinks is the best for you.

You think your cardiologist is worth salvaging? Then go for it. There is such a huge knowledge gap that the best place for him to start would probably be *The High Blood Pressure Hoax*, since it's highly referenced and shows him how to improve the health of blood vessels. Then he needs to catch up on at least the last half-dozen years of the referenced *TW* newsletter, to learn the dangers of the elevated fibrinogen, CRP, homocysteine, and insulin, low testosterone, and many other indicators of early heart attacks that are all beautifully assayed in the **Cardio/ION Panel**. You may well save his life in the process of trying to save yours.

I'm really very concerned, because millions of people are needlessly subjected to accelerated decline and earlier death, as well as the exorbitant expense of these medications. The ball is definitely in your court, because nobody else will pick it up for a long time. One of the first things you can do to start to heal your coronary vessels is to repair the cell membrane of your coronary artery cells, as described in the next chapter (and in more detail in *The High Blood Pressure Hoax*).

One of the most crucial nutrients that you should begin taking, but does not yet have an assay, is phosphatidylcholine. In one study of 30 patients for four months, adding three capsules twice a day of **PhosChol** (or 2 tbs/day) was far **more effective than being on the cholesterol lowering statin** alone. As well, it allowed folks to cut their dose of statins in half, thus markedly reducing the side effects of the drug. The addition of **PhosChol** also corrected the abnormal liver enzyme elevations that came about as another side effect of the statins. But that is not all, as **PhosChol decreased the hyper-coagulability or the platelet aggregation that was induced by the statins**. Of course these folks who did the study had no idea of the things you have learned about, like **Niacin-Time** twice a day can be even more effective than a statin drug. Combined (as God has magically designed us in the first place), the healing power of nutrients is awesome.

Now you begin to understand why I'm so concerned, because their **knowledge gaps are so egocentrically dismissed.** Most have no idea of the importance of the fatty acids except to recommended people eat fish, and then in the next breath to tell them to cut down on fish because of possible mercury toxicity. They have no clue about measuring the actual EPA, DHA, DGLA, trans and other fatty acids, or properly adjusting and balancing the doses. They've no clue about getting the heavy metals out of the coronary arteries, or such rudimentary things as the proper RBC assay for magnesium. Remember the *Journal of the American Medical Association* article that showed 90% of physicians admitting over 1000 patients to a Boston hospital never even checked magnesium levels in their patients, and many of them died from magnesium deficiency causing cardiac arrhythmias or sudden cardiac arrest.

If you have a cardiologist whom you feel is really interested in your longevity, then try to get him/her on board starting with this book, or *Detoxify or Die* and then *The High Blood Pressure Hoax* and at least the *Total Wellness* newsletters from 1999 to present (they have actually been in existence for over 18 years). If he's interested in your longevity, he will read these and prescribe the **Cardio/ION Panel** for you. If you need help with interpretation, you can schedule a non-patient phone consult with myself and you can have your doctor on the line as well, as you prefer. My gosh! He should at least be concerned about his own cardiac health! We're talking super serious stuff here, because if you can't find a cardiologist who's interested in your longevity, you'll have to take the bull by the horns all by yourself. When will the time come when folks will hold physicians accountable for their lack of knowledge?

References:

Winslow R, Loftus P, Plavix plus aspirin shows few benefits. Study of blood thinner in heart patients marks a setback for Bristol-Myers, Sanofi-Aventis, *Wall Street J*, B3, March 13, 2006

Gurevich V, et al, Polyunsaturated phospholipids increase the hypolipidemic effect of lovastatin, *Europ J Intern Med*, 8: 13-18, 1997

Illingworth DR, et al, Long-term experience with HMG-CoA reductase inhibitors in the therapy of hypercholesterolemia, *Atherosclerosis Rev*, 18:161-67, 1988

Hensley S, Drug problem: When one pill cancels another, *Wall St J*, D1, April 23, 2003

Since I Don't Have Symptoms or Diabetes, High Insulin is Not a Concern

High insulin is a dangerous promoter of early arteriosclerosis. When you need energy, a sugar molecule comes knocking at the door of the cell. Insulin is the key that opens the door to let the sugar in. When it doesn't work, the body says, "What are you, deaf?" and sends even more insulin. The reason insulin doesn't work is the insulin receptors in the cell membrane have been damaged. It can be from trans fatty acids from french fries, commercial breads and salad dressings, pretzels and chips, pizza and other processed foods, plasticizers that leach from food containers and packaging, fatty acid deficiencies, and lots more.

High insulin can also trigger the body to make high cholesterol and/or high triglycerides, which further promote arteriosclerosis. And high insulin can trigger chronic fatigue, depression, mood swings, alcohol dependence, and **weight gain that just will not budge**. The next chapter will guide you.

There is much more I could tell you about high insulin, also called **insulin resistance or metabolic syndrome or Syndrome X.** The information could fill many books, so let me just remind you to always keep in mind your total load or the total package that you bring to the table. The more "good stuff" you are doing for your-self, the greater your chances of healing. As a simple example, exercise and the lipoic acid that's in your detox cocktail are impor-tant in improving insulin resistance and keeping you from further deterioration. Make sure you at least get minimum 300 mg of **R-Lipoic Acid** twice a day (more to come on this in Chapter VII). The plastics that are the highest pollutant in the human body now also trigger insulin resistance. Chapter VII shows you how to get them out (and *Detoxify or Die* has even more detail).

References:

Klein-Platat, et al, Plasma fatty acid composition is associated with metabolic syndrome and low-grade inflammation in overweight adolescents, *Am J Clin Nutr*, 82:1178-84, 2005

Torres N, Torre-Villalvazo I, Tovar AR, Regulation of lipid metabolism by soy protein and its im-plication in diseases mediated by lipid disorders, *J Nutr Biochem* 17:365-73, 2006

Henriksen EJ, Exercise training and the antioxidant alpha-lipoic acid in the treatment of insulin resistance and type 2 diabetes, *Free Rad Biol Med,* 440: 3-12, 2006

There is Nothing to Reduce an Elevated Fibrinogen

Elevated fibrinogen is very dangerous. It means your blood is in a hypercoagulable state. Translation: **it's ready to throw clots at any moment.** There are wonderful enzymes that I've written about and referenced in past *TW*s that can lower the fibrinogen, like **Wobenzyme, Lumbrokinase** and **Nattokinase**. Then there is a sublingual form, **Ananese**, absorbed under the tongue. Use the directions in *Wellness Against All Odds* or 2006 *TW*. No one has compared all four side by side to determine which is superior. More on these in subsequent chapters. Meanwhile, it goes without saying that you want to find the underlying cause of elevated fibrinogen so that you don't need a lifetime of enzymes. The first place I would look is with (1) an Ultrafast Heart Scan for asymptomatic coronary artery disease, then (2) look for a hidden cancer, then (3) look for low grade infection as in a tooth or sinus that only occasionally bothers you yet nothing is found on x-ray.

Worst if all, it often means that plaque in arteries is what we call "vulnerable" and ready to rupture, producing a heart attack. Having a clean Ultrafast Heart Scan is no guarantee you don't have plaque, for it can migrate deep into the vessel wall and be uncalcified, rather than sticking out into the vessel opening and be calcified. **It is imperative to heal endothelial dysfunction to normalize the fibrinogen.** Vitamin C and many other nutrients you will learn about here can do it. It can sometimes be as simple as half a teaspoon of **Arginine Powder** twice a day. But it deserves the most careful follow-up until it has been normal at least a year, and then I would check it annually, since it has become one of your weak areas (much more is even described in *The High Blood Pressure Hoax*). Elevated fibrinogen is very serious (more on this later).

References:
Sumi H, Hameda H, Hiritani H, et al, Enhancement of the fibrinolytic activity in plasma by oral administration of Nattokinase: Natto VR 501, *Acta Hematologica*, 84:139, 1994

The FDA Will Protect Me from Dangerous Drugs

As I showed in multiple examples in *TW*, the FDA is grossly under funded. Their annual budget is less than 1/5th of what one brand of cholesterol-lowering drug makes in a year. There are scores of books cited in *The High Cholesterol Hoax* detailing the FDA's problems. And there are countless examples that did not come to light until millions of people were forced to take drugs for decades.

Just recall how women's hormones turned out to actually potentiate cancers, blood clots and heart disease by more than 25%.

As one of multiple examples, Dr. S. Nissen of the Cleveland Clinic published an analysis of a diabetes drug in the *New England Journal of Medicine,* 2007, using all the data the FDA had available to it from 42 clinical trials. It turns out Avandia increased the rate of heart attack a walloping 43%, and of course is still on the market (Frieden). Diabetics often cannot be improved until the vascular chemistry is repaired, and the deficiencies that promoted it (more described in *The High Blood Pressure Hoax)*. Or look at how medications to turn off stomach acid, like Prilosec, can increase the rate of stomach cancer death not 8-times normal, as it has risen for the general populace over the last couple of decades, but 43-fold. And why shouldn't it when they never looked for the underlying causes (described in *No More Heartburn*)?

Or look at the over 1600 folks who die in the hospital each year just from intestinal hemorrhage from pain drugs. Or look how long it took to remove Vioxx from the market when it more than quadrupled the rate of heart attack (Topal, Fitzgerald, Whelan, Rogers). Or look *at The New England Journal of Medicine* study that showed that folks who had a sham knee arthroscopy fared just a well as folks who had the real surgery (Lieber). And why shouldn't they since surgery is not necessarily the total answer for chronic pain (folks have to find the underlying causes, as described in *Pain Free in 6 Weeks)*. As multiple examples confirm, there is no money in folks finding the curable causes of their problems so that they are no longer dependent on drugs.

References:

Frieden J, FDA gets brunt of criticism at house Avandia hearing, *Skin & Allergy News*, 54, July 2007

Harris G, As a patent expires, drug firm lined up pricey alternative, *Wall St J,* A-1, June 6, 2002

Naik G, Carroll J, Glaxo medicine for bowel illness is allowed to return to market, *Wall St J*, B3, June 10, 2002

Kolata G, Petersen M, Hormone replacement study a shock to the medical system, *The New York Times*, A1, A16, July 10, 2002

Gorman C, Park A, The truth about hormones, *Time*, 32-36, July 22, 2002

Begley S, Are tainted vaccines given to baby boomers now causing cancer?, *Wall St J*, B1, July 19, 2002

Lieber R, The $5000 surgery your knees don't need; rethinking "scoping", D1, D3, *Wall St J*, July 11, 2002

Cohen JS, *Overdose.The case against the drug companies: prescription drugs, side effects, and your health*, Tarcher/Putnam/Penguin Books, New York, 2001, available from 1-800-669-CALM.

Cauchon D, **FDA advisers tied to industry**: Approval process riddled with conflicts of interest, *U.S.A. Today*, Sept. 25, 2000

George CF, Adverse drug reactions and secrecy, *Brit Med J*, 304; 23: 1328, 1992

Angell M, **Is academic medicine for sale?**, *New Engl J Med*, 342: 1516-18, May 18, 2000

Angell M, *The Truth About the Drug Companies*, Random House, 2004 (Written by former editor of *The New England Journal of Medicine*)

Lazarou J, Pomeranz BH, Corey PN, Incidence of adverse drug reactions in hospitalized patients: a meta-analysis of perspective studies, *J Am Med Assoc,* 279; 15: 1200-1205, April 15, 1998

Stelfox HT, Chua G, Detsky AS, **Conflict of interest** in the debate over calcium-channel and agonists, *New Engl J Med,* 338; 2:101-6, Jan. 8, 1998

Haley D, *Politics of Healing*, Potomac Valley Press, Wash DC, 2000

Fitzgerald GA, Coxibs and cardiovascular disease, *New Engl J Med,* 351: 1709-11, Oct. 21, 2004

Topal EJ, Failing the public health – Rofecoxib, Merck, and the FDA, *New Engl J Med*, 351: 1707-9, Oct. 21, 2004

Whalen J, Study by Vioxx critic links drug to extra coronary cases, *Wall St. J*, D3, Jan 25, 2005

Killing Cholesterol Saves Lives

Several serious medical studies and entire referenced books show that lowering cholesterol with medications did not reduce the number of deaths by stroke nor the amount of sickness, including heart attacks and (Atkins, Herbert, *TW*, Suurbula, Ravnskov, Smith).   In addition, some commonly prescribed cholesterol-lowering drugs actually lowered the good HDL cholesterol as well (Johansson), putting you at higher risk of an early heart attack.

In Rubins' study of **over 8500 U.S. patients with documented coronary artery disease, only 42% of them had high cholesterol.** But 41% had low HDL, 33% had a high triglycerides, while **87% had an elevated LDL** or the bad cholesterol. But recall that **LDL is not dangerous until it is oxidized.** Sufficient antioxidants keep LDL harmless. More on that as we roll along. As you are learning there are much safer, cheaper and healthier ways to improve these parameters than with statin drugs. The bottom line was however that **58% of these men with coronary artery disease did not need statin drugs,** although current recommendations are extended to people who do not even have high cholesterol and perhaps have only an elevated CRP. And now statins are recommended prophylactically for preventing colon cancer! (See *TW* for rebuttal and evidence beyond the scope of this tome).

Furthermore many studies show that when folks do lower their cholesterol with medications, they have just as many deaths. Unknowledgeable or unscrupulous (I have no idea which they were) researchers only counted the cardiac deaths. But recall that non-cardiac deaths from suicide and accidents offset the decrease in heart related deaths from cholesterol lowering drugs (Golomb). Could it be they were so ignorant of these side effects of the drug?

As reported in the *Journal of the American Medical Association* in 1998, **drug reactions in the hospital are the sixth leading cause of death.** But this study only looked at (1) people in the hospital who (2) had recognized drug reactions, and (3) whose deaths were admitted to be due to the drug. It did not include the over 2 million people who are seriously injured by a prescription drugs each year, making **drugs, the number one cause of medical problems** (Lazarou).

Once you have developed high cholesterol, it means you have suddenly stopped metabolizing cholesterol the way your body used to. If your cholesterol is not high from eating an enormous amount in the diet (and remember the liver makes 80% of your cholesterol irrespective of your diet), there must be a nutrient deficiency in your enzymes that process cholesterol. And minerals, vitamins, amino acids, and fatty acids are the main nutrients that control or drive this chemistry. Our nutrient levels get lower as we age for many reasons. For one, processed foods (the ones with a list of chemical names) in the grocery store are notoriously low in trace minerals needed for proper cholesterol metabolism.

Therefore, **it's unconscionable to treat high cholesterol with a drug without at least bare minimum checking for these missing minerals** that drive normal cholesterol metabolism, as included in your **Cardio/ION Panel.** Because once your nutrient levels are low enough to cause high cholesterol, this also makes you more vulnerable for the nasty and sometimes deadly side effects of the drugs that you just learned about in Chapter 1. In addition, as you will learn, **stockpiling of environmental chemicals also is a reversible cause of high cholesterol.** Once again, if this is ignored and covered up by just prescribing a drug, it leads to numerous side effects and ushers in a lifetime of seemingly unrelated diseases.

As you are learning, **cholesterol is much more of a good guy than a bad guy.** It protects the body from infections and toxins. **Cholesterol is a messenger giving you a last ditch warning. You should not poison him because he brought you the message that you are in trouble.** For that trouble is totally correctable. He is a hero, not to be crucified with a statin.

Remember, **50% of the people who have a heart attack don't make it to the emergency room**. They are dead and had no warning. If you think you're off the hook because you don't have high cholesterol, **half the people who have a heart attack never had high cholesterol.** And having an angioplasty (putting in new blood vessels after a heart attack) or even just an angiogram (injecting dye to see if any of the vessels are in danger) are great free radical initiators and require hefty doses of antioxidants before and after either of those procedures (more on how to protect yourself in Chapter VIII). Furthermore **within six months of having angioplasty, 50% of the people are already re-plugging their "new" arteries. Our medical system is geared to drive you toward drugs, keeping the pharmaceutical industry the number one for profit industry in the U.S.**

References:

Lazareau JB, et al, Incidence of adverse drug reactions in hospitalized patients: A meta-analysis of prospective studies, *J Am Med Assoc*, 279; 15:1200-05, 1998

Golomb B, Cholesterol and violence: Is there a connection?, *Ann Intern Med*, 128; 6:478-87, 1998

Rubins HB, et al, Distribution of lipids in 8500 men with coronary artery disease, *Am J Cardiol*, 75:1196-1201, June 15, 1995

A Mere Vitamin Deficiency Cannot Cause High Cholesterol

Many nutrient deficiencies can cause high cholesterol. As one brief example, a vitamin C deficiency can cause high cholesterol, and vice versa, high cholesterol can lower vitamin C, thus perpetuating and exacerbating your problem. Even more importantly, **a deficiency of vitamin C can cause coronary artery disease without even having high cholesterol**. The good news is that in some folks, as little as **300 mg a day of vitamin C can lower cholesterol 34%.**

References:

Ginter E, Ascorbic acid in cholesterol and bile acid metabolism, *Ann NY Acad Sci*, 258:410-21, 1975

Ginter E, Marginal vitamin C deficiency, lipid metabolism, and atherogenesis, *Adv Lipid Res*, 16:167-220, 1978

Ginter E, et al, Hypocholesterolemic effect of ascorbic acid in maturity–onset diabetes mellitus, *Internat J Vit Nutr Res*, 48; 4:368-73, 1978

The Signs of a Heart Attack Are Easy to Recognize

Wrong. I know two surgeons who treated themselves for "heartburn" for a month, and a chiropractor that treated his "chest muscle strain" before getting bypass surgery. Then there are the folks who have a silent infarct and never know they even had a heart attack, or it was misdiagnosed as reflux from a hiatus hernia, indigestion, heat stroke, left shoulder bursitis, bad tooth, or hypochondriasis. When I was a full-time emergency room physician, I recall a young man in his early forties presenting to the admitting desk in a sweat, holding his left shoulder and complaining of bursitis. I had the nurses whisk him into a bed. An immediate EKG confirmed my suspicion that he was in the throws of an acute heart attack. But you should nonetheless memorize the common classic signs of a heart attack: unusual chest tightness, chest heaviness, chest pain, radiation into the left arm, left jaw, left shoulder, unusual sweating, faintness, sudden arrhythmia, or loss of consciousness.

Another interesting fact is that when you question men who have been the lucky 50% who survive their first heart attack, they didn't quite feel right the week before. In fact, I would be particularly protective of yourself after any illness. Why? Because the mere fact that you got *anything* shows your immune system reserves are down and vulnerable. Second, even just having **a common cold triples your risk of a heart attack within the next 10 days** (Meier). So boost the nutrients that you learn about here for your safety net during that period.

Reference:
Meier C, et al, Acute respiratory-tract infections and risk of first-time acute myocardial infarction, *Lancet,* 351; 9114:1467-71, 1998

Impotence or Erectile Dysfunction
Has No Bearing on a Heart Attack

Erectile dysfunction can save your life. It's no secret that there's an epidemic of erectile dysfunction and of course, it is being clobbered with the latest drugs that include Viagra, Cialis, or Levitra. Unfortunately, these have caused heart attacks. And we know why. Even medicine is finally starting to realize that erectile dysfunction is an early warning sign of serious heart disease that is going to raise its ugly head within the next 3-13 years, as an article in the *American Journal of Medicine* pointed out this year. For the vessels that govern the blood flow to the penis merely reflect disease that's going on throughout the body, including the coronary and brain vessels.

Lots of things contribute to erectile dysfunction, like the trans fatty acids, plasticizers, heavy metal toxicity and nutrient deficiencies. Of course, as a side effect any of these can and do cause high cholesterol, which is then clobbered with another drug loaded with an arm's length of side effects, some of which have included death.

Meanwhile, the most important thing you can do is make sure your erectile dysfunction is treated just as though it were angina or high blood pressure. For **erectile dysfunction is a disease of damaged blood vessels** (and the nerves and other tissues supplied by these blood vessels are merely secondarily impaired). As the director of male sexual health at New York University School of Medicine has said, "**The penis is a barometer of the health of the vascular system**". Start with the magnesium and arginine protocols, since they are extremely easy and may be all you have to do. (If you need to go even further, use the protocols in *The High Blood Pressure Hoax* to heal the arteries wherever they are.) Whatever you do, do not ignore this gift. It is a warning of far more serious trouble down the road that is completely reversible now.

Reference:
Parker-Pope T, A surprising risk factor for heart disease in men, *Wall St J,* D1 Feb 20, 2007

After Bypass Surgery, I'll Be as Good as New

Not only do the new vessels start collecting "cholesterol" plaque, but you have to remember that you only had two or three vessels dealt with. Do you really think those are the only vessels among the miles of blood vessels in your body affected by the generalized process of arteriosclerosis? That's one reason why you want to go back to *The High Blood Pressure Hoax*, even though you don't have high blood pressure, so that you can make your vessels as healthy as possible. Furthermore, **75% of the people who have bypass surgery lose brain function.**

Reference:

Newman MF, Longitudinal assessment of neurocognitive function after coronary-artery bypass surgery, *New Engl J Med*, 344; 6: 395-402, Feb 8, 2001

Medications to Lower Triglycerides Will Improve My Health

Omacor is often prescribed for high triglycerides. As you will learn in the next chapter, the proof is overwhelming that an oil change for many folks is the only thing needed to bring down elevated cholesterol or triglycerides, both of which can lead to earlier vascular disease and heart attacks.

Elevated triglycerides can come from numerous causes as from (1) a low thyroid (the plasticizers stuck in our bodies or beta blockers prescribed by your cardiologist can cause hypothyroidism, and without damaging thyroid tests, see *Detoxify or Die*), (2) diabetes (they also cause this, as does the epidemic of undiagnosed vitamin D deficiency, trans fats, arsenic toxicity (from eating chicken, etc. and more), (3) liver damage by alcohol, (4) lack of phosphatidyl-choline, (5) eating trans fats, as just a few examples. **The trans fatty acids and the plasticizers in the diet are the major culprits for damaging lipid metabolism and raising cholesterol and triglycerides**.

Luckily, **cod liver oil can bring down the triglycerides by as much as 30%, more than most medications**. But the last thing you want in your body is synthetic oil, especially when you can have the finest quality natural cod liver oil available. Contrast Carlson's natural **Cod Liver Oil** with the prescription Omacor that is 1gm of synthetic cod liver oil (880 mg EPA/DHA as omega-3-acid ethyl esters) with a miniscule 4 mg of synthetic vitamin E as a preservative. Nobody in their right mind would prescribe a synthetic one when we already know there's enormous data showing that every time we use a synthetic nutrient versus something natural, we get undesirable side effects that the natural agents do not possess. Even when Omacor was combined with a dangerous statin, it did not touch LDL or HDL. But you do get improvement in those parameters with real **Cod Liver Oil** and **Niacin-Time**, like lowering LDL 21% and raising HDL 29%. There is no comparison. And if your chemistry dictates, you may add **Kyolic Formula 107 Red Yeast Rice** (that does not contain dangerous toxic monocolins), then other nutrients if needed. These have superlative benefits over a synthetic laboratory mock-up of God's provisions.

References:

Durrington PN, et al, An omega-3 polyunsaturated fatty acid concentrate administered for one year decreased triglycerides in simvastatin treated patients with coronary heart disease and persisting hypertiglyceridemia, *Heart,* 85:544-48, 2001

Harris WS, n-3 Fatty acids and serum lipoproteins: Human studies, *Am J Clin Nutr,* 65(5suppl); 1645-54s, 1997

Wahrburg U, What are the health effects of fat?, *Europ J Nutr*, 43(suppl 1) 1:6-11, 2004

Keiffer D, Omega-3 fatty acids and hyperlipidemia, *Alt Med Alert*, AHC Media, Atlanta, July 2005

If There is Something Important That
I Should Know About Cholesterol, It Will Be On TV

There is a huge amount of news that never makes TV or other media, but could have an enormous impact on the health of the nation. There is voluminous data showing that folks with high levels of EPA/DHA have significantly reduced coronary disease and in fact many other diseases, even Alzheimer's. Fish certainly contains these, but **Cod Liver Oil** is much more concentrated and therefore corrects life-threatening deficiencies faster.

Fish oil levels are so important in preventing heart attack that researchers and other experts now suggest in *The New England Journal of Medicine* that **low levels of omega-3 fatty acids in the body should be considered a new risk factor for sudden car-**

diac death (Von Schaky). But where are the cardiologists, internists and family docs who should be measuring the levels, just as they measure cholesterol? And why didn't this make the evening news like other *NEJM* articles slamming vitamins did?

Likewise, **in the *Journal of the American Medical Association* they show the C-reactive protein should really be checked in everyone,** including women, as it is a major risk factor for early heart disease if a level is over 310 mg/l. Again, why is it not standard and done routinely as the major medical journals instruct? It is not stressed because it entails (1) finding the cause, then treating it with the nutrients you are learning about here. (2) Could it also be because physicians would have to learn God's magnificently orchestrated molecular biochemistry of the body in order to fix it? (3) Drugs are so much quicker and easier. They help you maintain that average office visit time of 7 minutes and you don't bog down your day with copious instructions and questions about how to heal. Plus (4) medicine's focus on drugs makes the pharmaceutical industry happier and more powerful, which in turn provides more perks and funding for physicians, medical schools, drug research, and medical journals. It's a marriage made in hell.

References:

Harris WS, et al, Blood Omega-3 and trans fatty acids in middle-aged acute coronary syndrome patients, *Am J Cardiol*, 99; 2: 154-8, Jan 15, 2007

Ridge PM, et al, Development and validation of improved algorithms for the assessment of global cardio-vascular risk in women: the Reynolds Risk Score, *J Am Med Assoc*, 297; 6:611-9, Feb 14, 2007

Blumenthal RS, et al, Further improvements in CHD risk prediction for women, *Am Med Assoc,* 297; 6:641-3, Feb 14, 2007

Von Schaky C, et al, Fish consumption and the 30-year risk of fatal myocardial infarction, *New Engl J Med*, 336; 15:1046-53, Apr 10, 1997

Lim GP, et al, A diet enriched with the Omega-3 fatty acid docosahexaenoic acid reduces amyloid burden in an aged Alzheimer mouse model, *J Neurosci*, 25; 12:3032-40, Mar 23, 2005

My Doctor Said a Medical Study Proved
Correcting Homocysteine is Not Important

Remember, homocysteine, even though it is a proven risk factor for early diseases like arteriosclerosis, is treated with nutrients, not drugs. That is one major score against it. So in order to thwart the efforts of the few physicians who do read and understand the medical journals and then implement the findings in their practices to actually cure folks, pharmaceutically driven medicine goes one step further with **intentionally sloppy "science"**. Here is an example of just one study published in the high profile *New England Journal of Medicine* (354:1578-88, 2006 and 354:1567-77, 2006) to illustrate how **drug-sponsored medical journals manipulate the media to denigrate nutrients so you and your doctor will think vitamins are worthless.** This study focused on folks who were seriously ill for a long time and also had elevated homocysteine. Researchers merely gave the patients B12 and folic acid to try to lower their homocysteine levels and then reported that giving these two nutrients in trying to correct homocysteine did not improve the medical status of folks who were desperately ill.

You don't have to go to medical school to know that by the time somebody gets sick enough to have had a heart attack, diabetes or documented heart disease, they are not going to be turned around with only two vitamins. But apparently these researchers were not so logical or knowledgeable about the workings of the human body. But they were experts in manipulating the media, since it was plastered all over the TV and newspapers that giving (only 2) vitamins in attempt to correct homocysteine provided no health benefit. The patients didn't magically get better. The conclusion was correcting homocysteine (which they failed to do) and giving vitamins (only two) did not help these folks who very seriously and chronically ill. Do you find that as astounding as I do?

In fact, their study beautifully illustrates how ridiculous the medical model is. For these scary researchers never mentioned how the multiple drugs that these very ill people were on also (1) further seriously depleted their nutrient levels, plus (2) interfered with their nutrient absorptions, and especially (3) limited the absorption of the very 2 nutrients that were being given. For starters, they didn't even take them off drugs like diuretics that are notorious for raising homocysteine levels or off acid inhibitors that are notorious for creating B12 deficiencies, or off beta-blockers that create zinc deficiency that then impairs B6 conversion, necessary to lower homocysteine.

Furthermore, since the clinicians did not bother to assay or correct the underlying defects that gave these poor patients their serious diseases to begin with, of course, they got worse and snowballed faster. Furthermore, if the patients had elevated methylmalonic acid (which is in any lab, but also on the **Cardio/ION's Organic Acids**), this would suggest they had high probability for inability to even orally absorb B12. So even if B12 deficiency was the cause of their elevated homocysteine, it would not be corrected with oral B12. They needed to bypass the stomach and use a form absorbed under the tongue that goes directly into the bloodstream, just like nitroglycerin. Either **Methylcobalamin 5 mg** or **B12 SL** or **Betalin 12** would have been preferred. For sublinguals bypass the stomach, important because Candida, H. pylori, and other bugs that are common in the stomach can destroy the intrinsic factor in the stomach lining. A damaged stomach lining can make it impossible to absorb B12 by mouth until the condition has been cured (see *No More Heartburn* for the diagnoses and treatments). Consequently the person needs either the sublingual form or injections to get the B12 into the bloodstream. But these "researchers" did not look at this very fundamental chemistry. I would have been very ashamed to have had anything to do with this study, for it screams biochemical ignorance.

Nor did they measure the formiminoglutamate to see if the very ill patients needed sublingual folic acid. For if the formiminoglutamine is high (also on the **Cardio/ION**), there is a block in the chemistry, producing a folic acid deficiency. The best substitute is **Folixor** 1 or 5 mg sublingual, one dissolved under the tongue daily. If the normal intestinal bugs that are needed to transform folic acid into the form that is useable by the body for preventing heart disease and cancers, as one example, are over-run by undesirable bad bugs, conversion is axed. Once again you can bypass the damaged gut through the sublingual route.

Both B12 and folic acid are crucial in homocysteine metabolism. Now you can appreciate one more reason why heart disease and strokes constitute the number one cause of death. Eating out a lot, eating processed foods, having undetected nutrient deficiencies, undiagnosed heavy metal toxicity, taking prescription drugs, needing frequent antibiotics all contribute to damaged guts. This in turn impairs B12 and folate conversions that in turn can lead to elevated homocysteine, which triggers early vascular disease in the form of heart attack, arrhythmias, heart failure, claudication, strokes, Alzheimer's and more.

Meanwhile, **to expect two vitamins to turn around a lifetime of damage in very sick and heavily medicated patients is extremely naïve and shows dangerously deficient rudimentary biochemical knowledge of the human body. Then to not even measure to see if the form you gave was sufficient, is unspeakable.**

As another example of how irresponsible this study was, they never mentioned checking the levels of vitamin B2 in these articles, yet that also can correct homocysteine. **They acted as though homocysteine is strictly a deficiency of only B12 and folic acid.** To think that these two vitamins alone are responsible for heart attacks and strokes doesn't even compute. The researchers demonstrated they must be extremely deficient in knowledge of the chemistry of the body by trying to use merely two simple nutrients either alone or together like a drug. Surely they cannot be that ignorant of God's beautifully orchestrated molecular biochemistry.

It would be interesting to check what their pharmaceutical connections were.

When the two nutrients failed to correct their homocysteine, and failed to turn around these patients' lifetime of heart diseases, the erroneous conclusion blurted through the media was that homocysteine is not that important! But as I evidenced in *The High Blood Pressure Hoax*, it is more important an indicator of accelerated disease on the fast track than having a high cholesterol. Furthermore, they appeared totally ignorant of the many other nutrients that are often needed to correct a high homocysteine, like **Chelated Copper, DMG, NAC, Vitamin B2, Zinc,** and more.

Let's look at some of the other important cures for an elevated homocysteine that have been proven besides the two B vitamins used in this paper. One nutrient that is rarely thought of to correct high homocysteine, even among nutritionally trained physicians, is **copper.** (For physicians: copper is important for the enzyme **methionine synthase**, the enzyme needed to pull methyl groups off folic acid precursors and put them on homocysteine to generate methionine.) The safest way to correct that is with **Chelated Copper**. Balancing copper with **Chelated Zinc** is crucial for it avoids creating a copper-induced zinc deficiency later on.

And if you run into a nutritionally naïve physician who can't understand why you might be copper deficient in the first place, remind him that lead toxicity is ubiquitously unavoidable, plus the cut-off for "safe" levels (as we have fully documented in previous issues and books) is alarmingly high. Furthermore, a little known fact about **lead is that it creates a silent copper deficiency. This leads to not only elevated homocysteine, but high cholesterol, impaired ability to detoxify (via low SOD), increased risk for diabetes, heart disease, metabolic syndrome X ("insulin resistance") with inability to lose weight,** and much more.

The bottom line is the physician who is unaware of his patient's copper status (and other associated minerals, vitamins, fatty acids, etc.) is powerless to find the correctable cause and cure of disease. His only resort is to mask symptoms with drugs that merely poison a pathway in the body chemistry. This invariably leads to further dysfunction and drugs. The patient ends up on the drug--new symptom--new drug--new symptom--new drug merry-go-round and can never get off the **medication merry-go-round** until he falls into the hands of a physician who will look at the chemistry of the body to determine what needs fixing.

Also refer back to 2007 *TW* on how **NAC** also lowers homocysteine while it also reversed Alzheimer's in folks in their 80s so well that some got their driver's licenses back and were able to live independently again! Now that is worthy of the media! (Does it surprise you hat it never got media mention?)

From now on, you are now too smart to be fooled. **When you're stuck, there is always a biochemical explanation.** That's the beauty of your **Cardio/ION Panel**. It takes a lot of the guesswork out of diagnostic problems and focuses you on the road to recovery, but more on that as we move along.

References:

McNulty H, Dowey LRC, Strain JJ, et al, Riboflavin lowers homocysteine in individuals homozygous for the MTHFR 677CT polymorphism, *Circulation*, 113:74-80, 2006

Tamura T, Turnland JR, Effect of long-term, high-copper intakes on the concentrations of plasma homocysteine and B vitamins in young men, *Nutr,* 20: 757-59, 2004

Kwok T, Cheng G, Pang CP, et al, Use of fasting urinary methylmalonic acid to screen for metabolic vitamin B12 deficiency in older persons, *Nutr,* 20: 764-68, 2004

Klevay LM, Copper deficiency, lead, and paroxonase, *Environ Health Persp,* 115; 7:A341-2, 2007

Tamura T, Turnland JR, Effect of long-term, high-copper intakes on the concentrations of plasma homocysteine and B vitamins in young men, *Nutr,* 20: 757-59, 2004

Kendall RV, *Building Wellness With DMG,* 1-800-959-9797, 2003

Lipoprotein(a) is Not An Important Risk Factor

Elevated lipoprotein(a) or Lp(a) is a special protein (also found on your **Cardio/ION Panel**, that acts a lot like the CRP, since it is strongly correlated with early coronary artery disease. But we have to remember that these were also designed by our Maker to be protective. Just as an elevated cholesterol is protective in that it patches up holes drilled in our arteries (from free radicals, *H. pylori*, etc.), these indicators of early coronary problems merely designate that nature's protection is at work overtime and we had better find out why.

Lp(a) is a lot more dangerous if you are under 60, because then it is a much a stronger predictor of early coronary artery disease. On the flipside, there are people over a hundred years old with elevations for which it obviously is not a risk factor. It makes platelets more eager to clump and hooks onto the bad cholesterol LDL, but it appears to be focused on housekeeping or cleanup of oxidized LDL. The best start is **Niacin-Time**, the slow released form of niacin or vitamin B3 for reducing it (see Feb. 2007 *TW* for references). Take one twice a day and recheck the level. Also **CoQ10 lowers lipoprotein(a)**. Use 2-3 **Q-ODT** under the tongue daily (references above in another myth).

The American Heart Association Tells Us to Eat More Fish

What a disconnect there is. The American Heart Association and the Mayo Clinic tell folks to eat fish twice a week. On the flip side, as though they don't know of cach other, the government's EPA warns about mercury. In fact, studies confirm **the mercury exposure cancels the benefits from a fish diet**. The optimal solution is to (1) know your actual levels of the most important fatty acids in the brain and heart, EPA and DHA, (2) correct them, then maintain healthful levels with the lowest mercury level and highest-quality that I know of, **Carlson's Cod Liver Oil**, a tablespoon three times a week. Meanwhile, (3) enjoy non-farm raised, wild salmon once or twice a week for dinner, or sardines on whole grain organic toast for lunches, or smoked salmon for breakfast.

References:
Guallar E, et al, Mercury, fish oils, and the risk of myocardial infarction, *New Engl J Med*, 347:17 47-54, 2002

Budtz-Jorgensen, et al, Separation of risks and benefits of seafood intake, *Environ Health Perspect*, 115; 3: 323-27, 2007

A Low Fat Diet is the Best Diet for High Cholesterol

Wrong. Research shows that a Mediterranean-style diet with olive oil and nuts has more benefit compared with the torture of a low-fat diet that is generally recommended by hospital dietitians (Estruch). In fact, the low-fat diet is intolerable for many people and does not raise the good HDL cholesterol. Instead, the low-fat diet lowers the HDL. On the flip side, the Mediterranean-style diet tastes good and does not lower the good HDL. Unfiltered virgin olive oil, **macadamia nut oil** and walnuts are beneficial for not only cholesterol levels but improving blood pressure, insulin resistance, and inflammatory molecules that all lead to earlier heart disease. There are so many myths that I could make a whole book out of them, but let's get on to food. There is much on the fun fat foods you can eat in the next chapter. So let's go!

Reference:
Estruch R, et al, Effects of a Mediterranean-style diet on cardiovascular risk factors, a randomized trial, *Ann Intern Med*, 145: 1-11, 2006

Executive Summary

There are so many more myths that I could fill two books with them. You now understand that there is a wealth of data to prove you are being misled in a multitude of ways, which insidiously destroy your health while they fuel the coffers of the medical/pharmaceutical industry. So let's get on with teaching you more. I want to empower you with so many proven options that you can't fail in finding one or more to bring you to better health.

Sources for this Chapter's Recommendations

- Coronary calcium score, Diagnostic Outpatient Center, 1-800-890-4452
- Gamma E Gems, E-Gems Elite, Niacin-Time, Tocotrienols, Cod Liver Oil, Chelated Copper, Chelated Zinc, Chelated Magnesium, B6, Vitamin B2, B12 SL, Arginine Powder, carlsonlabs.com, 1-800-323-4141
- NAC, Methylcobalamin, jarrow.com, also 1-877-VIT-AMEN
- HDL Rx, integrativeinc.com, 1-800-917-3690
- Cardio/ION Panel, metametrix.com, 1-800-221-4640
- Kyolic Formula 107 Red Yeast Rice, Kyolic Liquid, wakunaga.com, 1-800-421-2998
- DMG, NAC, davincilabs.com, 1-800-325-1776
- PhosChol, nutrasal.com, 1-800-777-1886
- Folixor, Betalin 12, R-Lipoic Acid, intensivenutrition.com, 1-800-333-7414
- Wobenzyme, 1-877-VIT-AMEN, or needs.com, 1-800-634-1380
- Lumbrokinase, allergyresearchgroup.com, 1-800-545-9960
- Nattokinase, allergyresearchgroup.com, 1-800-545-9960
- Macadamia Nut Oil, realfoodgrocery.com, 1-877-673-2536
- Delta-Fraction Tocotrienols, allergyresearchgroup.com, 1-800-545-9960
- Q-ODT, Ananase, intensivenutrition.com, 1-800-333-7414
- New York Heart Center, 1000 E. Genesee St., Syracuse, NY 13210, 315-471-1044
- Anasese, intensivenutrition.com, 1-800-333-7414

Chapter IV

The Diet Connection –The Good, Bad, and the Ugly

The Cause of High Cholesterol Has Been Known for Decades

You have done a great job so far. In the first chapter you learned about the dangerous side effects from killing cholesterol that happens to be a main building block for the entire body's chemistry. In the second chapter you learned about a number of safer, better and even cheaper substitutes. And in the third chapter you busted a lot of the myths about cholesterol treatment and the field of medicine as well. So from here on to the end of the book we are now going to look at what actually causes high cholesterol and arteriosclerotic plaque, and how you can cure your high cholesterol and even reverse its damage. Gone are the days when high cholesterol is a deficiency of statin drugs.

Would you believe for starters that one of the main causes of high cholesterol was intentionally created by the food industry, okayed by the FDA, and it has been known for decades? And even though Harvard physicians and other respected public health advocates and scientists have warned about this for decades, the medical/pharmaceutical communities have consistently and successfully turned a deaf ear. **A major cause of high cholesterol is the trans fats that permeate the American diet. This is in spite of the fact that Harvard researchers have warned for decades that trans fats are a major cause of high cholesterol** (Mensick, Enig, Koletzko).

Over 60 years ago food chemists learned that if you expose cooking oils to extremely high temperatures over 400°F and add hydrogen, oils will not go rancid and will last much longer, even without refrigeration. The process is called **hydrogenation**. With the high temperature of hydrogenation, this chemical processing of oils **twists the oil molecule and actually changes it into a shape that**

damages the human body chemistry. One of the things that it does is damage the ability of the body to properly metabolize cholesterol and therefore **trans fats create high cholesterol.** I still find it difficult to even conceive that Harvard researchers and others could warn about this for over half a century, yet they have continually been ignored.

The abnormal change in the molecule makes it so that no self-respecting bug would be caught dead eating the stuff. That's why that bottle of vegetable oil in your pantry lasts longer. Remember in the good old days, when oils went rancid after a few weeks? But we don't have to worry about that happening any more because of hydrogenation, which in turn creates trans fatty acid chemistry. In fact eating trans fats is more dangerous than saturated animal fats that have received so much adverse publicity (see *Detoxify or Die* and *The High Blood Pressure Hoax* for an enormous amount of references). In other words, **a fat juicy steak is less damaging by far than the french fries or grocery store salad dressing**.

The wording you want to avoid like the plague on every food label is anything that contains **hydrogenated or partially hydrogenated oils, just plain unidentified "oil", soy oil, soybean oil, vegetable oil, shortening, margarine, or oils that do not specify** they are expeller-pressed or cold-pressed (organic unfiltered extra virgin olive oil is an exception and is great, and never hydrogenated). Sadly, some of the worst foods in terms of trans fats have no labels, namely the standard French fries and salad dressings at restaurants. Other common sources are margarines, breads and most baked goods, fake coffee creamers, pizza, but much more. You really have to become a dedicated label ingredients reader to protect yourself and your family. Why? Because...

The Bar Has Been Raised

It is not bad enough that you have been duped for decades, but now it has been made legal. Harvard scientists have published for decades the proof that the major cause of high cholesterol is the trans fatty acids that permeate the food industry. Finally, folks are getting a little savvier, and consumer groups have demanded getting rid of trans fats. Consequently, the FDA has legalized raising the cut-off for "safe". In spite of **Harvard's research showing there is no safe level**, the FDA has decided they know how much of each type of food each one of us will eat and how much trans fats our systems can handle. Why do I say this? **If a food contains an enormous 500 mg of trans fats in a puny one half-cup serving, the manufacturer may plaster in huge letters over the front of the food that it contains "No Trans Fats" (Federal Register, 2006).**

This ruling was made and published in the Federal Register after food manufacturers lobbied the FDA in 2005, crying that there was no way they could get rid of the trans fats all together in foods, and that if they had to put how much was on the label it would discourage people from buying their products. So the solution was to make a "serving" unrealistically small and put a cap on any mention in an arbitrarily and capriciously conceived amount. The result was that if there was less than 500mg in a tiny ½ cup serving they could claim "No trans fats". A legal lie?

Subsequently, in 2007 many of the fast food establishments made a big deal about publicly saying they were getting rid of trans fats. Some were even substituting oils, but the facts about the proposed substitutes are nebulous as oftentimes canola oil, which is genetically modified, was mentioned. Has the FDA legalized lying to you? Meanwhile, I guess they have also become clairvoyant, because this ruling implies they know that you and I will wisely restrict ourselves to a tiny ½ cup serving, plus they know just which foods we will eat that have 500 mg of trans fats legally disguised as "no trans fats". For if you think about it, this is the only way they could now protect us from innocently consuming too many damaging trans fats. The control has been removed from the unknowledgeable consumer.

The Poisoning of America's Kids

For the average parents who do not know what a trans fatty acid is, they are slowly being paid back for this lazy "leave it to the doctor" attitude. I'm often frustrated at seeing grocery shopping carts loaded with trans fatty acids, pushed by mothers who look 10 years older than their ages and are trying to control obviously hyperactive kids. As well, I'm baffled when I see children of parents of obvious means expensively dressed, sitting in a high tech stroller that costs hundreds of dollars eating from a 25 cent fast food box of animal crackers or some other trans fat vehicle.

But then I have only to reflect how physicians who are key in the Harvard School of Public Health must feel, having tried to get the message across for decades. They know it's not easy to fight the financially powerful lobbying of not only the huge food manufacturing industry, but drug-dominated medicine as well. But let's face it. **If parents gave up one hour of television 1-2 nights for just one week and read about trans fatty acids, they could become a master of how to get them out of the diet and out of their children's bodies.** They could learn how to do a proper oil change which requires no prescription, yet can dramatically change the health and future of the entire family. Is it not worth it? For trans fats do far more than cause high cholesterol. They **trigger allergies, cancer** and just about every **degenerative disease** you can name, for they damage the fundamental chemistry of the human body where cholesterol is such a crucial part, the cell membrane. Remember, there is no safe level of trans fats.

As an example of how far this insanity goes, the *Wall Street Journal* had a section cover article showing how **upper middle class parents fed their kids chicken nuggets 3-5 times a week.** The parents had some inkling that there might be something unhealthful about them, but they were eager to be duped by the hope that they contained high-quality protein in the form of chicken. And unfortunately there will not be huge changes after this *WSJ* article,

155

since it did not show people (as *Detoxify or Die* does) that **trans fatty acids are able to trigger all disease** and how to bring about a permanent oil change for the entire family.

The good part of the article was they did indeed show how things like chicken nuggets are made. They start with chickens that are fed a nearly continual diet of antibiotics throughout their pesticide-exposed lifetimes and are notoriously ridden with many bacteria and cancer viruses. The meat is finely ground while including as much skin as possible. Now recall that skin holds much more pesticides, antibiotic residues, heavy metals like arsenic from the pesticides and other environmental chemicals than does the meat. For **chickens** are grown in such close quarters that their feathers drop off and they get lice easily. Hence, **arsenic-containing pesticide powders are sprayed directly on their bodies** to kill the bugs. This is **absorbed through their skin and into their meat.**

Meanwhile back to the recipe for chicken nuggets, they add spices like MSG (that fosters food addiction and cravings); add breading and the batter, more chemicals, and their favorite, *partially hydrogenated soybean oil*. This is where the *trans fatty acids* come from. And as if they do not have enough trans fatty acids already, they then fry this batter/paste in more hydrogenated soybean oil or vegetable oil to make an even higher level of the health-damaging and cancer-causing trans fatty acids. Of course it's usually served with even more trans fatty acids disguised as french fries.

The protein content of this is alarmingly low, while the fat content is unhealthfully high. What was the *WSJ* solution or take-home message for yuppie parents? Mind you, grinding up all of the skin, adding addictive spices like MSG, and then twice adding hydrogenated soy or vegetable oils leads to a fast food that promotes disease. And furthermore, stealth trans fatty acids in the diet make a beeline to the cell membranes, contributing heavily to metabolic syndrome, also called Syndrome X, with heightened sugar cravings, marked obesity, arteriosclerosis, diabetes, and inability to lose weight, all of which are epidemic (Enig 2000, 1993, Koletzko, Mensinck). Still the solution was not to tell folks how to do the oil change that is needed. Instead they gave a little recipe for mothers to make their own chicken nuggets at home, using genetically modified canola oil (which turns into trans fatty acids when it is used for frying) and bread crumbs (which usually also contain hydrogenated oils with trans fatty acids).

American Heart Association is a Day Late and a Pound Short

Harvard Medical School professors have warned of the dangers of trans fatty acids for over 2 decades. Regardless, after reviewing over 90 medical studies, the American Heart Association has actually set a limit of trans fats to less than 1% of the diet (Assoc. Press, *WSJ*, 6/20/06). Well what layperson knows how to calculate that? Why couldn't they just come out and say what has been proven, that **there is no safe level of trans fats?** Furthermore, why are they not advocating that doctors measure the levels of trans fats in their patients (so easy in the Cardio/ION) so they can counsel them in how to get rid of them? That may come in another couple of decades if we are lucky.

The average American is loaded with damaging trans fats that can trigger most chronic maladies of the human body, from high cholesterol to heart disease, cancer, arthritis, colitis, brain rot, and more. Folks get trans fatty acids from french fries, salad dressings, mayonnaise, cookies, chips, and most all processed foods. **Anything that says hydrogenated oil, soy oil, soybean oil, vegetable oil, partially hydrogenated oil of any type, or cottonseed oil is a tip-off.** And a big sign splashed across a label that says "No trans fats" will never hoodwink you again, now that you know the FDA lets food manufacturers lie to you (sorry to repeat this for those with great memories, but too many folks' healing will be stalled indefinitely until they indelibly learn this). Each miniscule ½ cup (2 oz.) serving in the container can contain 500 mg of trans fats! Why isn't the AHA telling you that?

The research keeps pouring in, but continues to be ignored. In the prestigious cardiology journal, *Circulation* (Sun Q, 115:1858-65, 2007), **folks with the highest trans fats consumption** from fried foods, baked goods, salad dressings, mayo and margarine **were more than three times more likely to develop heart disease.** But when was the last time your cardiologist measured the level or counseled you about a trans-free diet?

Trans fats are part of the "cholesterol" plaque (Waddingon, Kuhn). Don't be fooled by saying, there is so little in the amount that it will not make a difference. Just **one tablespoon of oil** (that hydrogenated type of polyunsaturated oil you get in the grocery store with trans fats) **delivers over 100,000 trans fatty acid oil molecules to <u>every</u> cell in your body**. That's right! **Every one of your 100 trillion body cells gets a dose of 100,000 dead, toxic molecules** that put a monkey wrench in normal cholesterol metabolism (Peskin, www.BanTransFats.com).

Give Yourself and Family an Oil Change

Deficiencies of essential fatty acids have been known as a cause of arteriosclerosis since even prior to 1956 in the prestigious *Lancet* (Sinclair). But until a drug is invented, such as the latest one that is actually a processed form of cod liver oil (Omacor) that you learned about in the preceding chapter, healing oils remain a secret.

So one of the first things you can do is give yourself an oil change. It takes 3-6 months to get the trans fats out of your cell membranes and replaced by good wholesome organic fats. You can measure your trans fats levels easily because they are part of the indispensable **Cardio/ION Panel** that you have already learned about. **For some folks, just getting the trans fats (that act like a broken monkey wrench in the cellular chemistry) out of the body, is enough to permanently correct their hypercholesterolemia.**

How do you do an oil change? Never again eat a trans fatty acid. This includes those low animal-fat foods so often recommended like **margarine, shortening, polyunsaturated or unspecified source vegetable oils, soy oil and soybean oils.** In fact, they all contribute to high cholesterol as well as to other degenerative diseases of "old age". And so do those foods that contain them like most **TV dinners and boxed breakfast cereals, many commercial breads, muffins, cookies, crackers, chips, dips, pretzels, many restaurant desserts, french fries, fried foods, and salad dressings, mayonnaise, margarine, prepared foods, fast foods, pizza (they skip olive oil for cheap vegetable oil) synthetic coffee creamers, roasted nuts, "healthful" granolas**, candies, and more. Start to read labels of everything before you buy and **never again buy anything with partially hydrogenated oil, soy oil, soybean oil, unspecified oil, vegetable oil, or hydrogenated oil** of any sort. Choose to stop being part of the trans travesty.

But the oil change involves two parts: (1) getting the trans fats out, and (2) replacing them with good healthful fats and phosphatidyl choline. So next, you need to restore the health of your cell membranes.

Oil Those Arteries so Plaque Slips Off

So what do we replace the trans fats with? We know from hundreds of blood analyses via the **Cardio/ION** that the most commonly low fatty acids are in the omega-3 category, especially EPA (eicosapentaenoic acid) and DHA (docosapentaenoic acid). Now free radical damage to arterial walls is really a lot like rust, since they are both oxidative radical problems. How do you keep your iron skillet or wok from rusting? You oil them. Well, you need to do the same with your arteries to keep them young, supple, and free from rust (oxidation).

The cheapest and best way to restore this is with a teaspoonful of cod liver oil a day. But not any old oil will do, since rancid oils can be hidden in capsules, plus some cheaper sources can be heavy with mercury and other contaminants. My research has led me to Carlson's **Cod Liver Oil**. If you are afraid of the taste because of past experiences (you are in for a surprise because fresh uncontaminated oil is really quite pleasant), it comes lemon-flavored. Also an alternative dose is to take a tablespoon every 3 days or twice a week instead of a daily teaspoonful, since the body stores fats. It does come in capsules (and I have seen the independent laboratory analysis showing no detectable heavy metals). As a last resort they also make remarkably tasteless **Fish Oil** (we've even used it on popcorn at meetings to prove its lack of taste), but it does not have the vitamins A and D. That's why I prefer the whole product, closest to what God created, **Cod Liver Oil,** which contains also vitamins A and D. Cook with extra virgin unfiltered olive oil or better yet, macadamia nut oil, **MacNut Oil**, because of a better fatty acid ratio and higher smoke point than olive oil, and use butter whenever you want.

In one study, just a daily teaspoon of cod liver oil plus a borage oil capsule altered the blood lipids enough to project a 43% reduction in heart attack rate over the next ten years. What a monstrous savings in lives and money. Furthermore another study by doctors at Harvard showed a daily intake of **cod liver oil was associated with a 24% decrease in the risk of metastatic cancer** in men with prostate cancer. And we know we shouldn't be recommending more fish (unless you know your source), because of frequent warnings about the high mercury content, not to mention PCBs, cadmium and more.

Even the Mayo Clinic found that men could significantly drop their risk of heart attack by using cod liver oil. The problem is nobody out there is recommending that fatty acid levels be measured to determine who needs it, how much, for how long, and whether it needs balancing with the other fatty acids. **Health is a balancing act**, not a mere dumping of nutrients into the body.

But hang on. The fish oil solution does more than restore the membrane structure. **Fish oil controls the gene for HMG CoA reductase, the very gene that controls the enzyme statins are designed to poison.** And cod liver oil also **controls the genes for the LDL receptor,** the place where the bad cholesterol does its damage to the cell wall. **It also down-regulates LDL particle size** (making it less likely to produce arterial plaque and damage). Whereas fructose, the corn sugar sweetener in most processed foods and sodas, plus omega-6 oils (grocery store oils) worsen the above.

For physicians: EPA, omega-3 fatty acid, also controls insulin signaling (that also controls cholesterol), protects from insulin resistance by serving as a PPAR ligand and induces peroxisomes (increases hepatic peroxisomal content two-fold), doubles lipoprotein lipase 2.2-fold (an enzyme needed to control cholesterol), improves diabetes, boosts detoxification (via **induction of cytochrome P450 (CYP4A2),** in addition to EPA down-regulating HMG CoA reductase and increasing LDL particle size (Lombardo). In essence **cod liver oil** not only lowers cholesterol, but **counters a lot of the bad chemistry of plasticizers and other environmental toxins** common in the body.

Clearly it would be beneficial to eat more fish, starting for example, with salmon in the morning on whole-grain toast with sliced onion. But make sure you read the package carefully. You want wild salmon, not farmed salmon. For studies clearly show that in addition to the known higher levels of mercury, farmed fish have significantly higher levels of dioxins, chlorinated pesticides, and PCBs compared with their free-swimming relatives (Easton, Iacobs, *TW*). These all can trigger high cholesterol, or create cardiovascular damage without raising cholesterol, as well as promote cancers. Furthermore, farmed fish don't have as high health-restoring omega-3 levels since their commercial feed is often predominately omega-6. The farmers actually change the chemistry of the fish by feeding them what they wouldn't get in nature.

Meanwhile, if your cardiologist doesn't measure your fatty acids or at least prescribe **Cod Liver Oil**, you should fire him. The evidence is overwhelming that the right **fatty acids do a better job in lowering the cholesterol, make arterial plaque less able to form, make plaque stable so that it doesn't rupture, decrease arrhythmias, increase the good HDL cholesterol, act as nature's calcium channel blocker (along with magnesium), repair sodium channels, and decrease sudden death from heart attack by more than 50%** (Jacobson, Reiffel).

Carnitine Moves the Fats to the Right Place

The **normal heart gets 70% of its fuel from fat** (Sinatra). So we also have to be concerned with how that fat gets moved into heart cells and further into the little mitochondria inside the cells. For this organelle inside our cells is where God's miracle actually changes the fat we eat into energy that runs the cell. **Carnitine is the nutrient we make that moves these fatty acids into the mitochondria to be turned into energy.** But its production is poisoned by plasticizes that are unavoidably in our foods (Chapter VII). Therefore you will want to add the best form on which the most convincing research has been done, **GPLC** (glycerinated propionated l-carnitine) (Gomez-Amores). Another good form is ALCA.

And there are other benefits, because **carnitine also lowers the dangerous Lp (a), triglyceride levels, and cholesterol levels, while slowing down arteriosclerosis** (Dayanandan, Sayed-Ahmed, Arockia). It has decreased the death rates by as much as tenfold. There is much more that it does, like **decrease the size of an infarct** (damage from a heart attack), decrease angina, but more will be on this in Chapter VIII (DeFelice, Jacoba). Use one twice a day. Then check so you can know if your dose is enough (the organic acids on your **Cardio/ION** adipate, suberate, ethylmalonate will tell you). But there is more to your membrane repair than just cod liver oil and carnitine.

PC, the Forgotten Nutrient

As we age, the red blood cell lining or membrane becomes stiff and is no longer flexible enough to bend itself into a shape that fits inside the smaller blood vessels called capillaries. Once the cell membranes become too old and stiff to squeeze into pretzel-form so they can fit inside tiny capillaries, you deprive the cells on the other end of oxygen and nutrients plus detox clean up. That is the beginning of all disease and seriously accelerated aging.

What is the limiting factor that allows for RBC pliability or flexibility? The old "meat" of the membrane sandwich is the stuff in between the "bread" (which is cod liver oil). For you can think of all cell membranes as being like a double-layered sandwich. You can think of the bread as being cod liver oil and the meat of the sandwich as phosphatidylcholine. **PhosChol** is the most potent form I have yet to find after 38 years. That's why it's so crucial for folks who have not only high cholesterol, but any heart disease, vessel disease, organ disease, "poor circulation," poor memory, or deterioration of any sort, or any "incurable" symptoms at all. With any disease, be sure to do this membrane repair.

And you remember from *Depression Cured At Last,* when the body runs out of phosphatidylcholine (PC), it steals it from other areas, robbing Peter to pay Paul. If it steals from the brain you get Alzheimer's type symptoms beginning with memory loss, or if it steals from the heart you can have coronary artery disease, congestive heart failure, cardiomyopathy, arrhythmias, high blood pressure, and much more. That's why PC is so crucial in repairing any diseases. Folks with alcoholic cirrhosis or liver damage from drug addiction or colitis take a particularly long time to correct this nutrient deficiency, but it dramatically repairs liver and colon as well as heart, and cell membranes in general throughout the body.

If that weren't enough, phosphatidylcholine has another super important role to play in the body. As you now know, cholesterol is not the bad guy but is merely a Band-Aid to patch up free radical damage inside of our blood vessels. So that we don't completely plug off all of our arteries and end up dead from a stroke or heart attack, the body continually carries this cholesterol off the arterial wall. The body uses HDL and various nutrients, like PC, to dump cholesterol into the liver where it can be made into hormones or into bile, which is then used to detoxify the body's chemicals. **PC is another wheelbarrow**.

And phosphatidyl choline does even more. It **lowers cholesterol, primarily the "bad" LDL cholesterol, while it raises the good or HDL** cholesterol (which we also use to wheelbarrow the cholesterol off the wall to then dump it into the liver). **PhosChol** lowers triglycerides and raises fat dissolving enzymes like lipase and it **makes the blood less eager to form unwanted clots**. It also fosters the production of anti-inflammatory compounds. If that were not enough, clinical studies show that giving **PhosChol** has improved EKGs, decreased angina and the amount of medications needed as well as the frequency and severity of attacks, **has improved exercise tolerance, running times and strength in athletes,** as well as vitality and even increases the glutathione in the vascular wall.

Because it lowers the viscosity or stickiness of platelets, it **decreases platelet aggregation (ability to clot) and makes the red blood cell more fluid**, more like a rubber pretzel, than an old plastic pretzel. In short, **PC improves circulation**. Also as a crucial part of the cell membranes, **PC heals damaged calcium channels and hormone receptors** that didn't work in the past. It's also often the forgotten nutrient when folks are repairing the kidney bean system of membranes inside of cells where energy is created, the **mitochondria**. In fact I'm dumbfounded when I see that many "specialists" in mitochondrial diseases totally forget to prescribe phosphatidylcholine, as though they are ignorant of the chemistry they are dealing with. Supplementing **PhosChol** literally rejuvenates and regenerates body tissues by restoring membrane function.

Because no commercial lab has yet to make a test of PC available, we have to infer its need. But it's pretty simple when you see, for example, someone has "starving" cell membranes on the **Cardio/ION** with serious deficiencies of the fatty acids EPA, DHA, or DGLA. **If the bread" of the membrane sandwich is missing, it is a sure sign that the "meat" of the sandwich is missing too,** since there is not sufficient bread to hold it. So for starters, **whenever you have to correct fatty acid deficiencies, you know most likely you had better correct the PC deficiencies as well.** Start with a tablespoon daily for a month or two and then reduce it to a teaspoonful of **PhosChol** indefinitely. If you're looking for one of the rarely appreciated secrets of anti-aging as well as reversing disease, this is it.

Stuck? Think PC

Are you stuck with resistant cholesterol? **PhosChol** is a nutrient that you must always think of because we constantly use it up and insufficiently replace it. If that were not enough, recall there's no readily available laboratory test to detect its deficiency. And we have changed the diet so that we eat progressively less of it.

Regardless of what you are trying to heal, addressing the health of the cell membrane is vital. **If you have poor circulation**, it's probably because your red blood cell membranes are too stiff to squeeze themselves into the tiny little capillaries of the fingers, toes, heart, and brain to supply oxygen and nutrients to the tissues. If you cannot correct an **angina or arrhythmia** it may be that the cardiac cell membranes are too stiff to release the mediators that allow the healing flow of magnesium into the cell and to pump out the calcium. If you have **resistant hypertension** it may because you have not restored the PC that enables the arterial wall to relax. And if you continue to dump cholesterol into the arterial wall you probably don't have sufficient PC in the walls to carry it off (Foster).

If you **don't metabolize fats properly**, it may be because you don't have enough of this nutrient in the bile to help you assimilate and metabolize the fats. The big problem is that **we lose lots of this underappreciated nutrient every day just in the amount we throw away in the gallbladder's bile.** We also lose a significant amount every moment we detoxify a chemical, which is perpetual. Chronic colitis or bronchitis or allergies especially use it up with wasting of mucus, which is high in PC.

Why are we low in **phosphatidylcholine,** the predominant phospholipids in all cell membranes? Decades ago people grew, dried and ate beans. Now they are considered peasant food, or are inconvenient because you have to soak them and actually cook them. Liver and eggs are also top sources, but the **cholesterol conundrum** has damaged their reputations. In fact daily beans in the **macrobiotic diet** is one of the scores of reasons why it has been able to more than **triple survival in cancer patients** (see *You Are What You Ate, The Cure is in the Kitchen, and Tired or Toxic?*).

Phosphatidylcholine however is more important than just for crucial lifesaving membrane repair. It also **dissolves cholesterol off the blood vessel wall and attaches it to the good HDL cholesterol to drag it out into the bile** (Bielicki). This process is called **reverse cholesterol transport.** We are in our infancy in understanding how to best use this to reverse coronary calcifications without surgery. I will leave this subject here, but please join us as a subscriber to the *Total Wellness* monthly eight-page referenced newsletter because we have more in store for you on this. It's our only way of communicating with folks to keep them up-to-date with newer findings since the publication of the over dozen books.

But you need to know that an enzyme abbreviated **LCAT** (lecithin-cholesterol-acyl-transferase) is what actually moves the phosphatidylcholine to the cholesterol. It's important to have high levels of this enzyme for another reason, since folks who have survived heart attacks have higher levels of LCAT. This enzyme increases the levels of HDL as it catches the cholesterol for removal from the vessel wall. From there PC carries cholesterol to the liver where it becomes part of detox bile. Folks who have survived their heart attacks have higher levels of this enzyme than those not surviving (Dobiasova). **A most important nutrient for protecting the LCAT enzyme from oxidation is vitamin C** (Chen).

Unsaturated lecithin was twice as effective at increasing the rate of absorption of cholesterol out of implants as well as protecting the aortas of cholesterol-fed animals from developing arteriosclerosis (Adams). So it shouldn't be surprising that lecithin from beans lowers cholesterol while it also stimulates the liver's uptake of HDL cholesterol (Mastellone, Polichetti). **PhosChol**, containing 3000 mg (3 g) of phosphatidylcholine per teaspoon is a much more potent form of phosphatidylcholine than beans or lecithin. I would strongly urge you to take a teaspoon the rest of your life or 1-3 capsules a day if you don't like the licorice flavored liquid. For my way of thinking, however, anytime you can relieve your body of the work of detoxifying another capsule you might as well do it, so liquids are great. For faster healing, many start out with a table-spoon a day for a month or two before reducing it to a teaspoon.

PC the Cholesterol-Dissolver

Meanwhile animals fed a high cholesterol diet normally develop atheromatous plaques (cholesterol collections) in their arteries. But when you feed them **phosphatidylcholine and vitamin C** not only do they not develop them but there's **regression or melting away** of some lesions (Altman).

Whole books are devoted to the effects of PC (Gundermann, Archakov, Peeters, Schlettler). For starters, it makes the cell envelope or membrane strong and function its best, making it not only resistant to ROS (reactive oxygen species or free radicals, the biochemical cause of disease), but infection by making strong the area of the cell that engulfs or swallows bugs in the blood stream. PC is also important in other membranes where detoxification of ROS occurs, and increases the action of cholesterol-metabolizing enzymes like **cholesterol esterase**. Active in making it much harder for cholesterol to attach to arterial walls, **PC makes cholesterol patches melt away** (Wojcicki). In fact in one study, **giving PC reduced cholesterol plugs that occluded arteries from 37% to 4% in less than 4 months.** And many others have duplicated this.

In addition to **causing plaque to dissolve away, PC reduces the ability of blood to clot** (reduces platelet aggregability), facilitates cholesterol metabolism in a variety of areas, **decreases the LDL or bad cholesterol,** and improves blood flow, even that of the microcirculation. Furthermore, **PC reduces the damage done by LDL, or the "bad " cholesterol** (Avogaro). **Phosphatidylcholine also lowers homocysteine 18%** (Olthof). And **PC reduces cholesterol** (Vroulis). How can you go wrong? In fact how can we survive without it?

Why are we low in PC? You guessed it. The processed fast foods diet is the culprit. Foods like eggs, liver, and beans, all great sources of PC, are pretty much ignored these days. The safest and best source is a steady diet of "G, G, & B" (grains, greens and beans), for there are multiple other factors in such a whole foods diet or macrobiotic diet that make heart or vessel disease obsolete.

The 4 big things that make cell walls plastic instead of pliable or flexible as they were designed to be are (1) trans fatty acids, (2) lack of oils (omega-3 oils like EPA and DHA and omega-6 oils like DGLA), (3) lack of PC, plus (4) toxins (Chapter VII). Memory and mood improve with restoration of PC plus the dissolving away of a myriad of symptoms, including high cholesterol. **PhosChol** is a major underappreciated nutrient that **protects and rejuvenates hearts and arteries**.

So I've told you about the membrane sandwich. Do you know what the "salt and pepper of the sandwich is? Vitamins and minerals strategically located on the membrane to trap free radicals and make the membrane conduct the electricity of life better. Start with the vitamin E and magnesium you learned about in Chapter II.

Epidemic of Women Killing Their Husbands

I'm always heart broken to hear of a young woman whose husband has died of a heart attack. But then the tide shifts when I ask, "Was it challenging to get him off his trans fatty acids?" and she gives me a blank look revealing she hasn't the faintest clue of what trans fats are! Call me old-fashioned, but I believe if the husband is out making a living, it is the woman's responsibility to nurture the family to the best of her abilities. However, since both partners work in many marriages, a decision has to be made as to who will be responsible for the health knowledge and its implementation. To choose to be ignorant about the care and feeding of your family is to beg for premature disease and death.

If she has been feeding him crackers, pretzels, potato chips, commercial salad dressings and breads, french fries, margarines, mayonnaise, boxed breakfast cereals, and other processed foods that clearly say they contain hydrogenated and partially hydrogenated products (or unspecified oils that are not cold-pressed) in their ingredients, then she has failed in her major duty as the caretaker of the family's health. I firmly believe it is the cook who should become knowledgeable about the selection, purchasing and preparation of healthful foods, as well as reading and convincing her husband about crystal ball items such as the incomparable **Cardio/ION Panel** and the **DOC Ultrafast Heart Scan** with coronary calcium score, that you learned, about. And, of course, the healthiest families will be sure that everyone shares the knowledge, not just one person. Then no one has to be viewed as a "nag" either. Everyone should know the score and help.

Furthermore, teen sodas and fries super-charge the fat formula for obesity, the diabetes epidemic in kids, as well as contribute to the

169

brain drain of our youth. Parents who think they're smart for giving kids high fructose corn syrup fruit juices and trans fatty acid salad dressings are grossly undereducated and clueless.

Stop Torturous Low Cholesterol Diets

As soon as high cholesterol is diagnosed, it seems that someone wants to take away your favorite foods and torture you with tasteless tidbits. I guess it makes you more eager to resort to a drug. They've done it for decades with low salt diets for folks with hypertension. The key is once you correct the damaged sodium channels, there's no longer any problem with the way the body handles salt. Then you can have as much salt as you want (directions in *The High Blood Pressure Hoax*). The same scenario goes for low-fat diets that are recommended for folks with high cholesterol. Only the situation is doubly dangerous, for without sufficient cholesterol we cannot make our hormones or the membranes that are crucial for the functioning of every cell in the brain, heart, and even the mitochondria (little factories inside of every cell where energy is made). In essence, **on a low cholesterol diet, you accelerate aging while you torture the person with a tasteless low fat diet.** We need fat and we need a variety of fats because that's the way the body is designed. Don't worry. A diet of torture is not necessary or even helpful.

First of all, studies show that diet alone is rarely successful in lowering cholesterol, because **the liver can make three times as much cholesterol in a day as you could eat**. The liver makes 80% of our cholesterol regardless of our diet. Furthermore, you need not give up delicious eggs, for example, for they provide cholesterol that you need for your brain and all cell membranes, as well as for making your sex and adrenal stress hormones and for preventing Alzheimer's, cancer and heart disease. More importantly, eggs are a great source of phosphatidylcholine that the body cannot live without. In fact, as you have learned, sometimes replenishing phosphatidylcholine is all it takes to correct high cholesterol! It is not only the "meat" of the cell membrane "sandwich", but a component of the HDL wheelbarrow and the bile for getting rid of excess cholesterol.

The Whole Foods Fix

The good news is you can eat all the whole foods you want: grains like brown rice, millet, quinoa, kasha, corn; beans like split peas, lentils, great northern, lima, adzuki; any nuts and seeds (raw better than roasted), anything green, any vegetable (above ground or below ground root veggie) or fruit. In fact, if you already have calcifications of your coronary arteries, **the grains, greens and beans, seeds and weeds, roots and fruits** of the macrobiotic diet have melted coronary calcifications and stopped angina, even when all that medicine has to offer has failed. And it has even gotten folks off heart and cholesterol medications (Ornish 1998, Rogers). The macrobiotic diet is so healing that folks have completely cured end-stage metastatic cancers when they were given only a few days to live and had failed everything medicine had to offer (see *Total Wellness* December 2006). Granted a macrobiotic diet is not easy for some, so luckily there are alternatives. However, keep in mind if you are ever really in big trouble, it has been the ultimate rescue for many, and beyond their wildest dreams!

Mediterranean Madness

Instead of a tasteless low cholesterol diet, research shows that the best (and easiest) diet for most people is what's referred to as the **Mediterranean diet** (LaPointe). Basically you have a lot of fresh vegetables, herbs, fruits as well as good-quality extra-virgin unfiltered olive and nut oils, plus clean seafood and rare meats. Peasant foods like beans and whole grains will be never neglected, nor is good old-fashioned cooking where you use the entire part of the animal and not just muscle meat. And yes, this diet includes polyphenol-rich red wines and plentiful raw salads, fresh herbs in cooking and crudities (raw vegetables).

So for a quick start, switch to a whole foods diet which is satisfyingly delicious, because it allows meats and wine, beans, whole grain breads, nuts, seeds and lots of vegetables, fruits, and **especially fresh herbs**. Research clearly shows that it's **diets high in antioxidants and polyphenol bioflavonoids that keep cholesterol (no matter how high it is) from becoming the bad type that glues itself onto arterial walls**. That's why **oxidized LDL (becomes bad cholesterol after being exposed to free radicals) is a more sensitive marker of heart disease risk than total cholesterol** (Toshima).

Or if you prefer, frequent fresh juices (not packaged or bottled) like carrot juicing plus raw foods diet with only about 20% of foods cooked is a preferred option for others. This includes the highly nutritious "birdseed cereal" breakfast and crudities with bean dips for lunch (spelled out in even more detail in *The High Blood Pressure Hoax* and *Macro Mellow).*

The truth is there are lots of highly nutritious and delicious diet types to choose from, and you can mix and match. Clearly, *the closer you eat to nature, the more healing power you have.* The **Price-Pottenger Nutrition Foundation** (P.O. Box 2614, La Mesa, CA 91943-2614, ppnf.org or 1-800-366-3748) is a great place to start learning more about how to properly prepare foods, especially high fat meats, which can be an important part of your diet. For example, Sally Faloon and Dr. Mary Enig's *Nourishing Traditions* fills this bill. And where you live is never an excuse for a poor diet. For a quick start, get the **Natural Lifestyle** catalogue (natural-lifestyle.com) for organic, non-GMO whole grains, beans, condiments, nuts and seeds, and other whole foods cooking essentials that create the backbone of any type of healing eating.

Follow the Fiber Trail to Lower Cholesterol

The closer you eat foods to nature, especially fresh raw salads, crudities, whole grains and raw fruits, the more fiber you get. **The**

more fiber, the more you lower your risk of heart disease and all disease (Pereira). So make it easy on yourself. Start off the morning with the birdseed cereal (overnight soak buckwheat groats, sunflower seeds, and almonds) with your choice of fruits, yogurt, etc. added in the morning (*The High Blood Pressure Hoax*). Carry hummus and vegetables for lunch, adding a hunk of cheese, hard boiled eggs, nuts or fruits if desired, and have a big salad at dinner plus some whole grains with fruit for snacks or dessert. Make a **powerhouse antioxidant salad dressing** in a blender. A large handful of fresh herbs is essential, with the high quality oils we discussed, plus fresh garlic, fresh lemon, grated ginger, and or maple syrup are easy starts. And you can add your favorite rare meats with a glass of wine.

Don't forget when your nutrient levels are corrected and your body is detoxified (see Chapter VII), you can pretty much eat what you want. It's only when we are nutrient-deficient and pollutant toxic that we don't properly metabolize. Undoubtedly you've read popular books about adjusting your pH. Well, eating like this automatically alkalinizes you without all the hassle (for folks who are struggling to become alkaline, bear in mind that taking any medications, alcohol, and sodas, coffee, and sometimes even nutrients will make it impossible for you to get alkaline).

The Fiber Fallacy

Many studies reaffirm that folks who eat whole foods have lower cholesterol levels. Researchers used to think that the fiber just made food truck through the intestine faster, so the cholesterol didn't have time to get absorbed. Because of this erroneous hypothesis, they thought that any old fiber would do. This is not true. Then how does real fiber lower cholesterol? It is actually first fermented by bacteria in the colon to short chain fatty acids. These intestinal short chain fatty acids then turn down the action of the enzyme HMG COA reductase, thereby suppressing cholesterol synthesis in the body (Anderson). Thus having **abundant natural fiber turns off the cholesterol enzyme naturally and safely**.

Fiber does a lot of other good things like **increasing insulin sensitivity and supplying IP6, which tames cancer cells** (*TW*). But fake fiber, as found in processed foods and prescription or over-the-counter medications, does not have this benefit. For example, methyl-cellulose is often an ingredient to stop foods like grated cheeses from sticking together. But this is sawdust or wood fiber. Our stomachs are not geared to break this down. In fact neither are any of the four stomachs of a grass-fed cow able to ferment this to boost gut health.

The bottom line is there is no substitute for fiber from real foods like whole grains, greens and beans, seeds and weeds, roots and fruits (which are also the foods of the macrobiotic diet, which you would benefit greatly from learning about even if you never need to go on it). I doubt whether any self-respecting intestinal bacteria would want to ferment Metamucil® when he can have a real food. Also it points up another important fact, that if you don't have the right probiotics or "good bugs" in the gut for this fermentation, then your food fiber may be wasted. More can be found on this in Chapter V.

Fight Disease With Food Power

Since **high cholesterol is a sign of overload, usually not of cholesterol, but of too many free radicals** in the blood stream, it's important to eat a diet high in free radical fighters. Remember, **cholesterol is merely the body's smoke detector and band-aid**. It is the messenger screaming that free radicals (naked electrons) are eating holes in your blood vessel walls. Your body makes a protective Band-Aid to patch up the holes so you don't bleed to death. That Band-Aid is cholesterol. So killing cholesterol by turning off or poisoning the liver's ability to make it is just counter-productive. Never forget cholesterol serves multiple other purposes, above and beyond being nature's antioxidant, like making our detoxifying and fat absorbing bile, and patching up the leaks in damaged arterial walls.

To prove how powerful a whole foods diet is in sopping up free radicals that trigger the body's cholesterol to rise, in one study they just had folks eat good wholesome foods and eliminate the junk. Their daily diet contained 2 tbs. of sesame butter, 2 slices whole wheat toast, raisins (3 small boxes) and 2 tbs. almonds or pecans for snacks, ginger tea and (2 cups) green tea, 1 tbs. wheat germ oil, 6 servings of fruits and vegetables (1/2 cup each), beans, whole grains and an optional 3 oz. meat, fish or poultry, eggs and nonfat dairy. Disallowed were white flour, processed foods, sugars, hydrogenated oils (trans fats), and whole milk products.

The results? Dietary fiber, vitamin E, vitamin C, and carotene levels in the blood increased 160, 145, 160, 500%, respectively. **Cholesterol dropped 13% on a whole foods diet,** and the bad cholesterol, **LDL dropped by 16%.** As well, the crystal ball laboratory tests that are indicators of free radical damage in the body improved dramatically. (For you physicians, the erythrocyte superoxide dismutase, RBC-SOD dropped 69% and the glutathione peroxidase, GSH-Px dropped 35%.) This translates into a small miracle, nothing that any medicine or gene therapy is capable of even coming close to duplicating. Wow! A 500% increase in beta-carotene! That nutrient is what Harvard researchers (that I've cited in *Total Wellness*) turned cancer genes back into normal genes with. Each one of these improvements is a powerful indicator of parts of anti aging success, while taken together they are awesome.

Why not see how you can improve the whole foods in your diet to give you more food power? The key with food is simple. Just eat anything recently living, like a raw fruit or vegetable. And they have more than double (actually 2½ times) the anti-oxidant power (free-radical-fighting) ability when they are organic (Smith). Also in this category are unroasted seeds and nuts plus soaked or sprouted grains and beans. Why, they still have so much life force in them that you can place any organic whole grain like brown rice, or any bean or seed in water and in a few days it will spout. They have so much energy in them that they can create an entire new plant. That's the kind of energy you want in your body. Put bleached white rice or wheat flour or a boxed cereal in water and they will rot.

I've watched some families shop and eat. **They live on dead processed foods**, either fast foods, take-out, order-out, or home delivery, all ready-made. These foods were loaded with disease-producing trans fatty acids (hydrogenated oils), sugars, artificial chemicals like the fake sugar aspartame (that triggers headaches, food addiction and metabolizes into formaldehyde (a carcinogen) and methanol, and causes vision loss), olestra in "fat-free" foods that sops up your vitamins that are needed to properly metabolize cholesterol, addicting MSG, pesticides that can trigger high cholesterol, additives (that trigger hyperactivity and learning disorders, depression, and more), and were generally stripped of nutritional value. Hot dogs, pizza slices made with cheap trans fatty acid vegetable oil, gooey doughnuts with more trans fats, pre-made sandwiches of nitrate-laced cold cuts with large amounts of trans fatty acid sources like mayonnaise, chips, pretzels, plus large Cokes (eight tablespoons of sugar!) dominated the scene. This diet nearly guarantees they will eventually have high cholesterol, early heart attacks and an avalanche of a multitude of other ailments. The closest to living food were some highly waxed apples!

In contrast to dead food, whole recently living foods contain, for example, quercetin, one of the richest phytochemicals in whole foods. **Quercetin actually stops LDL (the "bad" cholesterol) from being oxidized to the cholesterol form that clogs arterial walls**. This and other flavonoids also relax the smooth muscle and decrease coagulability, meaning they make heart attack less likely (Regelson).

176

Processed foods that come out of a factory in a bag, box, a can, jar, or wrapper and have a list of chemical additives have been subjected to manufacturing processes that drop the original nutritional value by as much as 80%. Eating as close to nature as possible can boost the immune system's bug-fighting ability immensely. But I know changing dietary habits is one of the most difficult things to do. So let's see how you could simply just improve breakfast and lunch, two out of three meals.

Whole Foods Diet

Breakfast could be the birdseed cereal (the "birdseed cereal" travels very well in your suitcase, just add your favorite fruit or vegetable juice, yogurt, kefir or nut milk or just water and fruits. It consists of equal parts of soaked (overnight) raw buckwheat groats, sunflower seeds and almonds, or your choice of grains, seeds and nuts. (**Natural Lifestyle** catalog can provide the ingredients, 1-800-752-2775), or a fresh fruit plate, or just freshly squeezed fruit or vegetable juice, or if you need more substantial food or are a carnivore have eggs and/or, smoked wild salmon with sliced sweet onion on whole grain toast.

If you are not a breakfast person, try having just a glass of freshly prepared carrot juice. Remember Harvard researchers have shown high doses of beta-carotene transformed (reprogrammed) the p53 cancer gene back to normal. No chemotherapeutic drug in the world can accomplish this miracle. This is one reason why the program in *Wellness Against All Odds* has more than quadrupled some end-stage cancer survivals (references in *TW*).

Lunch could be a huge salad with unlimited raw vegetables of your choice. Don't forget great additions like avocado, almond slivers or walnuts, freshly grated cheeses, apple or pear slices, pine nuts (pignoli), grated cabbage, sautéed mushrooms or sunflower seeds. Use your imagination. If you need more protein, add some hard boiled eggs, sardines, or canned Alaskan wild salmon that has not been fed pink dye so that it looks artificially fresh (**Seafood Direct**, 1-800-732-1836) or left-over sliced organic chicken or meat from dinner. If you are a carnivore who needs more meat, cook a big roast and slice it off as you go through the week so you can avoid the chemical-laden (nitrates, dyes, preservatives, sugars, potato starch fillers) deli meats.

Your dressing should be a top-quality organic cold pressed oil of your choice, fresh lemon juice or rice wine or balsamic vinegars, plenty of fresh herbs like cilantro or basil, and/or minced fresh garlic with a little maple syrup if you need sweetening. Again, use your imagination, but make sure that ingredients are top-quality. This can easily be prepared the night before (keep your dressing in a separate little jar) for carrying to work. Bring along 2-4 great fruits for dessert and your glass-bottled alkaline water. This makes a great start for a more healthful change toward a raw whole foods diet that has even been used to reverse cancers, after everything else has failed (more details in *Total Wellness* 1999-present). For the more adventuresome, check *Macro Mellow* for whole-grain salads and many more recipes and creative ideas.

If you are on the road and salads are too messy for your lunchtime, bring along humus made at home from your own delicious organic spiced beans (*Macro Mellow* contains recipes galore) or buy it ready-made from the local health food or grocery store. A zip lock baggy keeps a variety of vegetable sticks very fresh. Julienne some carrots, celery, scallions, zucchini, cauliflower, radishes, anise, red cabbage leaves; these are just a few of the many healthful vegetables for your humus dip. Bring along a hunk of organic cheddar cheese or hard-boiled eggs, or a hunk of roast if you like, and some great raw cashews, raisins or tangerine for dessert.

Dinner can be any assortment of vegetables and whole grains. When you make your big salad however, don't forget to add lots of fresh herbs and spices like fresh basil, cilantro, arugula, parsley, dill, tarragon, or whatever you prefer. Just be sure it's alive! Grow herbs on you windowsill. Being high in anti-oxidants, fresh herbs have wonderful healing properties. And don't forget to get the whole family involved. Oftentimes men are much more creative than women because they don't have to cook every day, and who knows what creative genius lies beneath the surface of one of the younger members of the family. Adding fish, fowl or meats is perfectly fine and in fact, necessary for most people. And a glass of red wine contains even more anti-oxidants and polyphenols that keep cholesterol from becoming oxidized, the process that makes it cling to the arterial wall.

Snack with fruits and/or nuts or a small selection of cheeses or sunflower seeds. Or use crudities (raw vegetables) and a dip like humus. Humus can be made from a variety of beans while vegetables blended can be made into tasty dips.

Macrobiotics deserves a word here, because Dr. Dean Ornish in *the Journal of the American Medical Association* reversed angina and other coronary artery disease symptoms with it. Even though you may never choose to eat the macrobiotic way, there's a great deal to be gained by reading first *You Are What You Ate* followed by *The Cure is in the Kitchen,* then *Macro Mellow.* First you'll learn how people who had mere days to live with metastatic cancers not only completely healed themselves but went on to live for decades (I also suggest you learn about this now, so that you are more prepared when you or a loved one need it. It is no longer a question of "if" we'll get cancer, but "when". References are in *TW*). Equally important, learning about macrobiotics teaches you aspects of whole foods selection, preparation and cooking that you won't encounter elsewhere, and explores better choices for foods that you never questioned the quality of, like your choice of salt and sea vegetables. More importantly it will open up a vista of new foods that you can incorporate into your meal plans for much better health. For remember the basis of healthful eating is G, G, & B: **grains, greens, and beans, seeds and weeds, roots, and fruits.**

Additional Tips

Eating like this for just one month will convince you of the power of food. Getting off dead, devitalized, factory processed foods and substituting whole foods that were recently alive (and have not been mangled and cooked to death in some aluminum factory vat) will energize your whole system. First of all, you will have easy non-smelly bowel movements shortly, since all that fiber is not only good for cleansing the bowel, but helps heal the gut's immune system and is strongly anti-carcinogenic. (Be prepared to go through an extra-smelly detox period, however if your gut is super toxic, as many are. I embarrassingly smelled like a dead rat for weeks when I was detoxing with macro years ago. And you may have a period of huge bowel movements, disproportionately larger than what you ate. This is good. It is the bowel cleansing itself of old concretions, layered on like an old rusty drainage pipe.)

Studies show **that vegetables are also rich sources of natural salicylates**. You know that aspirin is salicylic acid, commonly prescribed so that you won't have a heart attack. But the truth is aspirin doubles your stroke risk. However, it turns out that **vegetarians have serum concentrations of salicylic acid as high as those of people ingesting 75 mg of aspirin a day,** the amount in half of a baby aspirin (Blaylock). Maybe the doctor of the future will just say, **"Take two carrots and call me in the morning"**. Clearly it's one more reason to be having a diet high in vegetables.

If you cannot handle the fruits because of Candida, isn't it about time for you to get rid of your Candida? Start with *No More Heartburn* then go to *Detoxify or Die*. If you still can't figure it out, correct your **Cardio/ION Panel** (schedule a phone consultation with myself if you need help interpreting it) then do the heavy-metal detox protocols in *The High Blood Pressure Hoax*. For hidden mercury and other metals make it impossible for many folks to heal their Candida until the heavy metals have been gotten rid of. Or if your gut is too sensitive for all this fiber, likewise, heal it. *No*

More Heartburn tells you how to heal the whole intestinal track from mouth to rectum. After all, time is of the essence and is wasting. Get on with your healing.

And don't be hoodwinked by the about-face of fast food restaurants as they brag about carrying improved fast food salads. Their new crispy chicken bacon ranch salad with dressing has more fat (51 grams) and calories (661) and just as much cholesterol as a hamburger combo, which has 34 grams of fat and 590 calories (Leung). At $4, this is not a bargain. Also avoid salads with iceberg lettuce since it has hardly any nutritional value, and likewise avoid salads with canned tuna, which is high in mercury. The irony is that bringing your own food is not only infinitely more healthful, but it's cheaper. So regardless of where you are asked for lunch, if you're not certain of the quality of the food, why not bring your own or suggest a brownbag lunch while enjoying the fresh air in the park? It's a no-brainer to improved health. If we guard our breakfasts and lunches to make them as health boosting as possible, how bad can dinner be?

They Forgot the Whole Grains!

Belated as they are, recommendations for increasing fruits and vegetables have finally been widely promoted. But true to form, they've missed the boat once more, because **whole grains are actually much higher in antioxidants than fruits and vegetables**. It's just that the concept of whole grains is even harder to get across to the average person than the 6-9 fruits and vegetables a day that is currently being recommended. But brown rice, millet, quinoa, buckwheat, barley, oats and other **whole grains have more than twice the antioxidant activity of fruits and vegetables**.

Furthermore, folks who have **diets containing daily whole grains have 26% less heart disease**, 36% fewer strokes, **and a 43% lower cancer rate**. In another study of 88 folks with high blood pressure, 73% of those who had two meals of whole grains a day dropped their blood pressure medications in half in addition to dropping their cholesterol and blood sugars (Pins, Jones). So learn how to make whole-grain cold salads that travel well and are delicious, like the barley/walnut/tamari/veggie salad in *Macro Mellow*. For remember, whole grains have twice the antioxidant capacity as do fresh fruits and vegetables.

Cereal Killers in Your Pantry?

If you have boxed breakfast cereals in your pantry, two to one they are silently eroding your health. Think about it. One of the most important meals of the day is relegated to companies that load cereals with hydrogenated oils that contain damaging trans fatty acids (Lord). Boxed breakfast cereals also contain sugars that rob you of minerals, plus additives and dyes that needlessly overwork your detoxification system. And high fructose corn syrup (or just labeled "corn syrup" or "corn sugar") is not only in boxed breakfast cereals, but also in fruit juices and breakfast sausage meats that contributes **heavily to the inability of the body to lose weight.** Clearly, when a food is "fortified" that should be a warning that so much has been removed through the work of processing that the addition of a handful of synthetic cheap nutrients is mandated. After all, nature doesn't need to be fortified.

As well, boxed grocery store cereals often contain bleached and pulverized grains that have been dead for months and stripped of their vitamin E (proven to cut heart attack and cancer rates by more than a third). Folks who have sailed their own boats to Europe told me they have to throw out the boxes and put all their cereals in plastic containers before boarding, because the bugs eat the boxes, BUT not the cereal! Bugs know better than to eat dead chemical laden grains that have been through a factory.

Like a serial killer, these boxed cereals, which make up one-third of many Americans' diets, stealthily help create disease and death.

Dr. Lorraine Day, former chief orthopedic surgeon at San Francisco General Hospital, years ago developed breast cancer. She graciously gave me photographs and laboratory reports so that I could show slides of these when I was lecturing to physicians at Oxford University. In the lecture ("The scientific basis for reversing end-stage cancer") I showed how her breast cancer went from grape size to grapefruit size in one month, and how 2 major medical centers had confirmed the biopsy reports as metastatic infiltrating ductal adenocarcinoma.

Yet this leading surgeon did not have surgery and did not have chemotherapy. Instead she did a whole foods diet with hourly carrot juicing and more (drday.com or 1-800-574-2437). You can read about a natural non-prescription program in *Wellness Against All Odds* (1-800-846-6687) that describes diet, enzymes, enemas, juicing and more that has been proven to more than quadruple survival when all else has failed. If a non-prescription program is powerful enough to more than quadruple survival in cancer patients for whom everything that medicine has to offer has failed, just think how easily it can rejuvenate your cholesterol pathways.

Ready for a Healthful "Mac Attack"?

By now you are probably looking for healthful oil for cooking and eating. Macadamia nut oil has great health effects with only 3% pro-inflammatory omega-6 oils compared with 25% of omega-6 for genetically modified (GMO) canola oil and 60% for GMO soybean oil. Try to avoid these latter two. **Macadamia nut oil** is cold-pressed and **does not develop trans fatty acids like canola oil, shortening, grocery store vegetable oils and margarines when cooked.** Since it can tolerate twice the temperature that olive oil can without smoking (200 degrees Fahrenheit vs. 410 degrees Fahrenheit for macadamia nut oil), it is *wonderful for frying and baking*. As well, it *is high in natural antioxidants*, which gives it a *long shelf life*.

The *Archives of Internal Medicine* (June 24, 2002) showed that men who ate **nuts at least twice a week lowered their risk of heart attack by 47% and reduced the risk of general coronary heart disease by 30%**, because of these good nut oils. In fact there are over 20 clinical studies proving the benefits of nuts on cholesterol reduction (Fraser, Albert). And since macadamia nut oil is derived from plants, it has **no cholesterol.**

It is 55% oleic acid (the main fat in healthful olive oil), 15% palmitoleic, 7% palmitic, and 2% or less of lauric, myristic, stearic, linoleic, linolenic, arachidic, eicosenoic, and behenic (for those of you who carefully read your fatty acid reports and wonder where you're going to get those other missing oils). Compared with healthful olive oil that is 70% *monosaturated*, **MacNut Oil** is 85%, while the GMO canola oil is 61% and safflower is 20%, leaving the other common oils even lower. At the same time it has very low amounts of less healthful polyunsaturated and saturated oils. Also for folks who are allergic to certain oils like peanut, this is the only oil that is manufactured in the facility, so there is *no risk of cross contamination*. **No solvents or chemicals are used** and the trees are typically sprayed just once per season, if at all. In this imperfect world, it is simultaneously one of the most delicious and nutritious oils available.

MacNut Oil (realfoodgrocery com, 1-877-673-2536) is available in glass, of course, not health-damaging plastics that you will learn about. Here is your chance to have a sinfully delicious yet healthful "Mac attack".

The Innocent Egg is <u>Eggsactly</u> What the Doctor Ordered

The egg has become the fall guy for cholesterol and folks have passionately avoided eggs since they found they contain cholesterol. But to avoid organic free-range chicken eggs is to miss out on one of nature's many bargains. First, eggs are one of the greatest sources of phosphatidylcholine (PC), the "meat" in your cell membrane "sandwich" and the heart of your oil change.

Not only is the egg a source of much-needed PC and cholesterol, but many potent carotenoids like lutein to prevent macular degeneration, the leading cause of blindness. By bypassing the egg, you miss a great source of natural phosphatidylcholine, crucial to every cell in the body, controller of depression, chronic fatigue, and brain fog, for starters. And recall that PC is another "wheelbarrow" which carts cholesterol overload off from arteries, out of the body and into bile.

A study of **96 adults who ate 12 eggs a week showed no difference in cholesterol compared with those who consumed no eggs** (Morgan). The ability of the body to properly metabolize the needed cholesterol in the egg lies in how replete the nutrient status is. Phytochemicals like indole-3-carbinol from broccoli, cabbage and cauliflower, and diets high in fresh fruits and vegetables, are what contribute to proper metabolism of cholesterol. Just recall the famous *New England Journal of Medicine* article on the very **healthy 88 year old man who ate 25 eggs a day for 15 years**, took no medications, and had nothing wrong with him (Kern).

Yes, diet is important, but the diet that lowers cholesterol is a far cry from the diet recommended by most cardiologists, which actually hurry heart disease along. They recommend plastic foods like margarines in place of butter, plus fake eggs, and corn oils (trans fats), none of which have been proven to prevent arteriosclerosis. In fact, the trans fatty acids of margarine and hydrogenated grocery oils like corn oil actually cause arteriosclerosis as well as raise the bad LDL cholesterol and triglycerides!

Not only have current researchers re-evaluated the data of years to discover that over half the people dying of a heart attack never had **high cholesterol**, but that **it is not consistently associated with coronary heart disease** (McNamara). Furthermore, it made no difference if folks consumed less than one egg a week versus more than one a day. (Kritchevsky). Even a decade ago in a landmark article in the *New England Journal of Medicine* it was admitted that trans fatty acids were an underestimated major cause of arteriosclerosis. The egg is one of nature's gifts, while fractionated factory foods like fake eggs are never an answer to health.

Don't fall for the fake fractionated processed foods that so many dietitians at hospitals recommend that can hide trans fatty acids and other undesirable additives. These dieticians actually hurry heart disease along with recommendations of "plastic foods" like margarines (in place of butter), fake eggs, and corn oil (hydrogenated trans fats!).

Sugar Contributes to High Cholesterol

There are a number of ways that sugar contributes to high cholesterol: (1) The foods sugar is found in are usually processed, which means they have lost on average 80% of nutrients, which you will learn contribute to high cholesterol. (2) High sugar consumption means you are probably not getting other high quality foods that fight abnormal cholesterol metabolism, (3) high sugar foods are usually accompanied by trans fatty acids or, high fructose corn syrup, both of which trigger arteriosclerosis, and (4) sugar causes renal (kidney) wasting of magnesium, a mineral you learned in Chapter II that is needed for proper metabolism of cholesterol. And last but not least, (5) sugar triggers high insulin, and folks on the **higher end of normal for insulin have triple the risk of heart attack** (Pyorala).

Sugar is clearly a risk factor for early heart death, yet its **effects are reversible with simple vitamins C and E**, for example (Title). As well, sugar (cookies, candies, sodas and other junk foods) increases CRP levels (Sesso). And the **fake sugars are no better**, since they can **elevate cholesterol and make you hungrier** than natural sugars. Aspartame (Nutrasweet, Equal), on nearly every restaurant table, is 10% methanol (can cause blindness) and turns into formaldehyde (a known carcinogen). Reports right out of the government's leading environmental journal, *Environmental Health Perspectives* (2007) gave the evidence that is still ignored (*TW* 2007). No wonder it increases headaches and many other symptoms, and in fact in 1994 it represented more than 75% of all the non-drug complaints made to the FDA (Levy).

There is so much more that you need to learn, but has been spelled out already. For example, hidden food allergies can drive food cravings for junk foods (see *The E.I. Syndrome* to learn how to diagnose and treat your food allergies). Sweeten your drinks, dressings and meals with natural sugars, like maple syrup, honey, guava, yinnie rice syrup, molasses, organic sugar, or stevia.

Food Heals Where Medicine Fails

Before we leave this section on food, I just want to be sure you understand the power of food, and that God designed food to heal the body. Any time you get stuck in your future life, having been told by all of your physicians that there is nothing more that can be done, don't believe it. Here is my gift of hope to you. Just refer back to this case history:

Cancer is Just a Label

Janet was the perfect mother of two teenage sons, worked out three times a week, and balanced being a full-time registered nurse who held a couple of part-time teaching jobs in addition to being a full-time manager of a department at the local hospital. When she had constant clearing of her throat and a dull ache in her chest for a couple of weeks, she saw her family doctor who did X-rays. What he found was to forever change her life. She had stage IV metastatic lung cancer. It was unbelievable that a young woman all of 45 who never smoked could have not only three cancers in her left lung and seven cancers in the right lung, but 3 cancers in the liver, another in the pancreas and one the size of a baseball in the abdomen. The first oncologist gave her 3-6 weeks to live, while the second one suggested that if she did some chemotherapy she might live 3-6 months.

She jumped at the opportunity to quadruple her life span, so she took the first dose of chemo. The reaction of her body to it was so horrible that she dropped from 118 pounds to 72 pounds within three weeks after one dose. She had literally lost a third of her body in just a couple of weeks. Now she was screwed. There was nothing left. Here she was with two sons and **over a dozen wildly metastasized and inoperable cancers for which medicine had absolutely nothing to offer.** Just two months after her diagnosis she was reduced to 72 pounds, bald, her fingernails were blue and her skin color was gray, plus she was on oxygen and she had to rely on hospice workers to help her to the bathroom. She had already signed do-not-resuscitate papers. She was totally prepared to die. And doctors feared if she took another dose of chemotherapy and lost any more weight, she would be dead sooner.

As a last resort, she started the macrobiotic diet. After two meals her vomiting stopped. And after one week on the diet she got rid of her pain medications. And **10 months after her diagnosis her CAT scans showed that the tumors were all gone**. As she got stronger and healthier over the months, all sorts of other minor maladies that had plagued her for years melted away as well: migraines, joint pains, insomnia and more.

Today twelve years after her hopelessly terminal diagnosis, she looks more radiant and prettier, and cooks for 40 people. Her case has been presented on Fox News and at NIH (U.S. government's National Institutes of Health), and in fact is one of the best-documented cases they have ever seen. In summary, **in 1995 this registered nurse was diagnosed with 10 small cell adenocarcinomas of the lung, with metastases to the liver, pancreas, abdomen and lymph nodes. There was absolutely no hope.**

There was nothing that medicine could offer; yet she is totally well today 12 years later. For more details, including how to avoid common reasons for failure, see the *Total Wellness* December 2006 issue (prestigepublishing.com or 1-800-846-6687). All the dietary directions are explained in the Macro Trilogy: begin with *You Are What You Ate,* then proceed to *The Cure is in the Kitchen,* and last *Macro Mellow).* The point is that **when medicine has nothing more to offer, even if you're riddled with cancer and have only days to live, you can still heal yourself.** You only have one body to use during this lifetime, and you, not any physician, totally control how well this gift of a body serves you. Food is key.

Drink Your Cholesterol Down

Researchers at major medical schools around the world have proven the cholesterol-lowering effects of green tea (Dulloo). In studies of green tea, they dropped cholesterol 11%, LDL cholesterol 16%, and raised HDL in 12 weeks (Maron). In fact, studies showed that **1-4 habitual cups of green tea a day can reduce the chance of heart problems by 24%!** Or if preferred, why not make a daily huge pitcher of **Green tea** and jazz it up with mint, lemon or maple syrup (if you need) and store it in the refrigerator for a healthful summer cooler. One of my favorite green teas is **Sencha Premium Organic Green tea.**

And if you want a colorful sweet drink for fun, think about pomegranate juice. Most fruit juices consist of fruits that were harvested after the "pretty" ones were sold whole. The leftovers, fallen from the tree, can be moldy and soiled. They are therefore cooked or sterilized which kills their vitamin content. Then a smattering of synthetic nutrients is added back to "fortify" the product while they sweeten it with high fructose corn sugar, a potent trigger for obesity and other body malfunctions.

But pomegranate has the highest antioxidant power of any since it has actually reversed plaque (Tuttle, Aviram) as it slows down arteriosclerosis (Fuhrman, Kaplan). You can jazz it up with limes and sparkling mineral water. However good quality **Pomegranate Juice**, specifying it is high in **punicalgins, inhibits LDL oxidation** (the process that makes cholesterol stick to vessel walls) as it lowers cholesterol synthesis (Kaplan, Huang, Fuhrman). Get **Pomegranate Juice** from your local health food store.

Or if you want something totally inexpensive which is also good for cleansing the gut, how about grating ginger root and squeezing the juice into water, a fruit juice or even salad dressing. Grating about a walnut sized piece is sufficient (you don't have to bother peeling it, just wash it off) and then squeeze it with your fingers or through cheesecloth or a tea strainer. **Ginger juice reduces cholesterol and inhibits the oxidation of cholesterol,** which is the process that makes it stick to arterial walls (Lam, Fuhrman). You can add fresh lemon juice, maple syrup, etc., use your imagination.

Alkalinize or Die

As the body becomes sicker, it becomes more acidic. Think of diabetic acidosis or overwhelming infection or serious trauma from an accident. Even well-honed athletes when they push their bodies too far can develop acidosis, as lactic acid builds up in muscles causing exhaustion and cramping. Any imbalance in the body chemistry can lead to acidosis, even high cholesterol.

Unfortunately regular tap water and the majority of bottled waters are highly acidic, usually with a pH of around 5.1. The body prefers a pH of around 7.4 in the alkaline range for maximum performance. And folks who drink fizzy or carbonated drinks are even in more danger, because the carbon dioxide forms carbonic acid making the water even more acidic. When the body runs out of buffer to neutralize this acidity, it steels calcium from the bones. But this leads to osteoporosis, and makes the body more vulnerable for any disease, since it wastes the body's buffering system and uses up energy trying to neutralize the acidity. As well, diets high in sugars and processed foods lead to further acidity and weaken the body's overworked reserves even more.

Scientists have known for decades that cholesterol is only damaging when it is oxidized by free radicals. These free radicals (that come from metabolizing the unavoidable barrage of chemicals in our air, food, and water) are naked electrons that wildly steal electrons to mate with from cholesterol molecules. This results in an oxidized cholesterol molecule (oxidized LDL), which now is missing an electron itself. So it grabs onto the endothelial lining of the blood vessel, looking for its own electrons. It is oxidized cholesterol, not regular cholesterol, that attaches itself to the blood vessel wall creating cholesterol plaque which eventually plugs off the artery and leads to stroke or heart attack. High doses of antioxidants (that you'll learn about in Chapter VI) are also an important part of the cure to slow this damage by sopping up these free radicals like a sponge.

Likewise, free radicals in our blood burn holes in the lining of blood vessel walls. This makes the body send out an urgent call for its cholesterol Band-Aid to patch up the holes before we bleed to death. Hence, we have two free radical mechanisms to destroy arterial health and trigger early heart attacks: (1) the oxidized LDL cholesterol, and (2) the free radical destruction of the blood vessel lining. And once more the **amount of antioxidant protection we have makes the difference between early aging, early disease or not.** And as you just learned, a diet high in whole foods, many raw, is a great free radical-fighter as well as an alkalinizer.

Wouldn't it be wonderful if we had something else really simple that could alkalinize the body, in other words get us out of this disease-producing acidity quicker and into the alkaline zone? And wouldn't it be even more wonderful if this also served as a free radical sponge, sopping up even more disease-producing free radicals? Well now you can accomplish both feats with one healthful remedy that has even additional benefits (Shirahata).

Healing With Water

In *Detoxify or Die* I showed you how the Alkaline Water Machine (High Tech Health, 1-800-794-5355) is superior to reverse osmosis for removing unwanted chemicals from tap water. As well, through a patented electrolysis of water, the **Alkaline Water Machine** can provide any degree of alkalinization of your drinking water that you want with the push of a button. And it also supplies free radical fighters or antioxidants as strong as the ones your body makes. Since you have to drink water anyway, it might as well be the best quality, alkaline (Shirahata, Price, Ledingham, Plaskett, Groff). And since you need a water filter and you would benefit from alkalinizing water as well as more anti-oxidants, why not combine the two? Call High Tech Health and get information about installing this in your kitchen, pantry, laundry room, or wherever it would be handy.

Common Queries
(References in *Total Wellness* 1999-2006)

Q. In the grocery store is a butter substitute called Smart Balance. It says it improves your cholesterol ratio, has no trans fatty acids and is not hydrogenated. What do you think?

A. The ingredients list soy and canola oils, which are both genetically engineered. Non-organic soy is usually contaminated with the potent herbicide, Roundup, since it has been genetically engineered to be resistant to poisoning by Roundup (Monsanto owns both the patent for the roundup-resistant soybean seed and the herbicide Roundup). As well, they list vitamin E as d,l-a-tocopheryl, which means it is the synthetic vitamin E, known to counter or negate the good effects of natural vitamin E. Plus cooking canola oil can result in trans fats. Would I use it? Never. Regular butter for spreads, cold-pressed unfiltered organic seed or grain or nut oils (sesame, sunflower, corn, safflower, almond, walnut, macadamia, etc.) for salads; extra virgin olive oil or MacNut Oil for salads and cooking are still your best bets.

Q. What about just eating more fish to get the omega-3 oils?

A. Take any healthful food and you will be amazed at how much man has ruined it. As one example from our monthly newsletter, **farmed fish have been implanted with a gene** that turns on their growth hormone. How did they get this gene into the fish? They **used a virus as the carrier or vector**. What virus that did they use? The **rous sarcoma virus, a virus known to cause cancer** in chickens (more information in *Total Wellness 2001*). As well, these genetically engineered "farmed" fish have elevated levels of omega-6 oils instead of omega-3, because they have been fed another product of genetic engineering, soybean pellets (also loaded with Roundup pesticide residue) as fish food. This negates the omega-3 reason for eating the fish! In other studies, the level of **PCBs is ten times higher in farmed fish**. And when they irradiate fish for transport, this destroys a number of the vitamins. And this is just a small example of how giant agri-business massacres one innocent "healthful" food.

Q. What about microwaving foods?

A. Microwaved food virtually eliminates all the antioxidants from a food, **destroying 95% of the nutrients**! (Randerson). Steaming is the best cooking method and leaves antioxidants practically untouched, while pressure cooking and boiling are halfway between the two, but *nothing destroys antioxidants like microwaves*. Some cooking is better than none, however, for folks with poor digestive systems (until they learn how to heal the gut via *No More Heartburn*). So if you want to avoid prematurely aging, give your microwave away.

Q. I hear people now recommending olive oil over butter as being more healthful. They say olive oil and pasta are what make the Mediterranean diet so healthful.

A. Fat is fat. Adding 3 tablespoons of olive oil to pasta or salad is equivalent to adding three scoops of ice cream (Ornish, 1997). And pasta is nothing but bleached dead white flour serving as a vehicle for fat. But there are a multitude of aspects of the Mediterranean and French diets that do contribute to a lowered heart attack rate:

• They shun American processed foods containing trans fatty acids that cause high cholesterol and damage heart cell function in a number of ways (see *Detoxify or Die).*
• They cook with **fresh herbs**, not some old dried up, dead, irradiated weed bottled for grocery store shelves. Herbs have enormous anti-oxidant power, but only if used fresh, consistently raw (or minimally cooked), and in quantity.
• They shun dangerous foods like those "guilt-free" snack chips and pretzels containing Olestra, which blocks absorption of fat-soluble vitamins like A, C, E, CoQ10, lipoic, B-carotene, PC, EPA/DHA, and more.
• They take time to chew, eat, and digest in pleasant surroundings without TV violence.
• They frequent local markets with fresh local produce, not picked green, pesticided and shipped from South America or China, and they are often on first name basis with their baker, butcher, and fish and produce mongers, and there is a responsibility for wholesomeness. For example, breads are bought daily, not loaded with trans fatty acids (disguised as partially hydrogenated oils) and preservatives to last all week.
• They balance meals with lots of herbs, vegetables, bean dishes and whole foods cooking. The grand scale super markets and the myriad of packaged foods is not the norm. **They basically eat from the farm, while we eat from the factory.**

Q. I still don't have a clear idea about trans fatty acids and their role in causing high cholesterol and heart disease. A short version please?

A. Picture these two types of diets and then tell me which person more than doubles his chance of having a heart attack.

Diet #1
Breakfast is cereal with skim milk; lunch is a green salad and tuna sandwich; and dinner is another salad and pizza, and snack is pretzels or ice cream.

Diet #2
Breakfast is scrambled eggs and sprouted whole grain bread with butter, lunch is homemade bean/vegetable soup, and dinner is a juicy grilled steak with broccoli cheese sauce and oven-baked sweet potato "fries", and snack is almonds.

Most folks would choose diet #1 as the heart attack prevention diet, because they have been brainwashed to think that eggs, butter, juicy steaks, nuts and cheese are what cause elevated cholesterol and heart attacks. WRONG. They only cause high cholesterol if you are missing some of the minerals, vitamins and fatty acids that properly metabolize your cholesterol. And they only cause high cholesterol if you have another cause of abnormal cell chemistry, for example, the accumulation of trans fatty acids, or toxins that you will learn about like plasticizers, Teflon, and more.

The famed Dr. Walter Willett, of the Dept. of Nutrition and Epidemiology at Harvard School of Public Health in Boston has set the record straight with multiple publications. Yet appreciation of his evidence is still overshadowed by the food industry and its clever marketing and powerful lobbying.

The trans fatty acids are in most grocery store oils, disguised as margarines, commercial salad dressings, commercial breads, fried foods, fast foods, breakfast cereals, pretzels, potato chips and other snacks, and foods containing vegetable oil, hydrogenated oils, and soybean oils. These **trans fatty acids lower the HDL (high-density lipoprotein) cholesterol, in other words the "good" cholesterol. They also elevate triglycerides** that also predispose to early coronary death. In the diet #1, trans fats are hidden in the boxed cereal, salad dressings and croutons, mayonnaise of the sandwich, pizza, pretzels, and ice cream. It's your standard trans fat special. Pizza is especially laden with trans fats, as most places cut their olive oil with (hydrogenated) vegetable oil, making it a trans fat vehicle. Ask to see the oils that are used, and see if you can find a pizzeria that uses only pure olive oil.

Folks tanking up on trans fats each day who eat lots of salads like this diet (two salads a day) think they are eating great. But they may never lower their cholesterol as long as they are damaging the very chemistry that governs it with hidden trans fats. And since the average doc doesn't even measure the trans fats in their blood tests, ignorance appears to be bliss.

Over half the people who have a heart attack do not even have high cholesterol. But they do have trans fatty acids, low HDL's, elevated triglycerides, or elevated fibrinogen, lipoprotein(a) or hs-CRP, or any of the other abnormalities in the **Cardio/ION Panel** that measure the damage done. Bottom-line: **if you only get your cholesterol measured, you're being cheated, and if it won't come down naturally, look first at the trans fats.**

Q. I know when I eat the whole foods diet I feel great. But I live in the boonies and getting whole grains, nuts and other organic foods is out of the question. I don't have time to go to the city an hour and a half away and scout up some health food store. My nearest store is a 7-11!

A. Don't worry. You are not alone. You and I know that the bottom line is **whoever cooks your food is a more important determinant of your overall health than who your doctor is.** Studies prove that organic foods have on average twice the nutrition of conventionally contaminated foods and a quarter of the pesticides. On the flip side, it is estimated now that at least 80% of foods in the grocery store contain foods that have been genetically modified and over 95 % contain pesticides.

That's why I place a simple order for whole grains, beans, seeds, nuts, flours, condiments and much more three or four times a year from **Natural Lifestyle** (natural-lifestyle.com or 1-800-752-2775). I don't know about you, but as the world gets bigger and more impersonal, I find there are fewer and fewer people that I trust. I find I like businesses who put their pictures, their family, an even their names in their catalogs. Just as I would never go to a physician or dentist who is not proud enough of his reputation to put his name on the door, but instead calls himself "Family Dentistry" or "Gastroenterology Associates", I do not trust my food to just anyone, especially a faceless corporation.

Natural Lifestyle on the other hand, is a family-owned business. Tom Athos puts his entire reputation on the line every time he sends us a product. In a world turned topsy-turvy, this is where I put my money and trust. And the beauty of it all is that we don't have to live in a huge polluted city with great health food stores like Boston or San Francisco, because we can have this brought to our doorsteps, whenever and wherever we want.

Q. You don't stress soy. Why?

A. Nix on soy. I am no fan of soy, since 80% of it is genetically engineered and loaded with roundup pesticide residues. As well, being loaded with estrogen mimics we have no business feeding it to infant males as the first experimental generation. In previous *TW* issues I've shown how it has decreased mental function in adults. Now researchers have found that low concentrations act like fertilizer for cancer and stimulate cancer cell growth (Allred, Ju). I would not recommend soy products for anyone, but especially for women with a family history or other increased risks for breast cancer. If you are in doubt you might want to check out the references.

Another soy ploy: it damages the immune system. In the *Proceedings of the National Academy of Sciences* (May 28, 2002) university researchers show that genistein shrinks the cell thymus and reduces the number of immune cells (Harder). Why is this important? Because 25% of infant formulas are soy-based, providing 10 times more genistein than an adult would get with an abnormally high soy diet. Soy formulas are the sole nutrition for over 750,000 U.S. infants each year. I've documented for you in past *TW* issues how **soy has been linked to elevated risk of uterine and breast cancer, and dwindling brainpower.** And it's no secret now that learning disability and behavior problems are epidemic, in fact government studies say that **one in six children born today has a neuro-behavioral problem.** Now it looks like we can add shrinking of the immune system with spawning of allergies and recurrent infections to the list. On the flip side, learning how to cook healthful bean dishes weekly is health boosting. Start with the *Macro Mellow* cookbook.

Q. What about using flax oil for high cholesterol?

A. You are right in that flax (linolenic acid) is the precursor in the body to the two oils found in cod liver oil, EPA (eicosapentaenoic acid) and DHA (docosapentaenoic acid). And so this can correct high cholesterol in folks if it is their relevant deficiency (Prasad). But many folks lack the necessary co-factors, like simple magnesium, to pull it off, or as you will learn in Chapter VII, they are so poisoned by plasticizers that they cannot make the conversion. For the plasticizers (in every human including newborns and animals in the wild) actually poison the chemistry that converts flax to more healthful fatty acids, EPA and DHA. We know this from published research results as well as seeing it repeatedly in folks who have had their fatty acids assayed. If you are sick enough, why take the chance? Go for the cod.

Q. Foods that are enriched should be good for us, right?

A. Absolutely not. When a food is "enriched", it's because manufacturers have destroyed so much nutrition that they are legally bound to put a little bit back. Since they can never one-up Nature and they want to accomplish this as cheaply as possible, you usually get a smattering of the poorest quality of synthetic nutrients in the lowest dose possible and not the whole package of harmonizing nutrients as Nature designed it in the original food. For example, the RDA for vitamin E is less than 15 IU, but the studies that cut heart disease nearly in half used an average of 800 IU. If a company puts vitamin E in a food, it is usually synthetic and actually fights the natural E you get from your food. If they use 15 IU, then the package can state it provides over 100% of your daily need. An absolute ruse. But most folks believe it because they leave their health to the "experts".

Diet Superior to Medications

Clearly, as studies verify, folks can lower their cholesterol and CRP (an indicator of inflammation which is one of the molecular causes of high cholesterol) just as well with diet as they can with the dangerous statin drugs that do not repair anything. Nor do statins correct an underlying cause of high cholesterol as diet can. And this is right out of the high profile *Journal of the American Medical Association* (Jenkins). This **study showed that diet or a statin drug equally lowered the LDL cholesterol and CRP, both 30%.** And these folks did not do as good a whole foods diet as we have discussed nor an oil change, much less all the other healing goodies you will learn about. What will it take to supersede the mindset that high cholesterol is a deficiency of expensive, side effect-ridden statin drugs that do not fix what is broken, but merely sentence the unknowledgeable to a lifetime of drugs? In other studies, diet made no difference at all for many reasons (too many processed foods were allowed, no oil change was done, and general ignorance of the other things you will learn about).

Meanwhile, **when you don't fix what is the underlying cause, you set yourself up for an avalanche of symptoms,** the least of which is cancer. And indeed right out of the same journal, *JAMA*, we saw the increased incidence of cancer in folks who silently persist in having elevated free radicals and merely take drugs (Newman). So let's move on to Chapter V to find out about another dangerous hidden cause that is completely fixable, that can be permanently cured and negate a lifetime of drugs.

Busy Executive Summary

High cholesterol doesn't simply mean you need a toxic drug guaranteed to cause other symptoms. It is a God-given warning that something more serious is going on. To take a cholesterol-lowering drug is like seeing the red oil light in your car go on and smashing it with a hammer. High cholesterol usually means free radicals are on the rampage and that trans fatty acids (disguised as polyunsaturated, hydrogenated, partially hydrogenated oil, or just "oil") have invaded and damaged your cell membranes. The whole foods diet and an oil change may be all you need. Animals in the wild don't have high cholesterol as they eat whole foods. But pets fed from the dinner table do get "human" diseases. You must do an oil change by getting rid of the trans fats and restore your membrane sandwich with cod liver oil and the highest quality phosphatidylcholine, for starters. If you are still stuck with high cholesterol, let's go to the next chapter.

Sources for this Chapter's Recommendations

- Organic, non-GMO grains, beans, seeds, nuts, teas, cookware, prepared foods, and so much more. There is no excuse for not eating healthfully, no matter where you live. Get the catalog: natural-lifestyle.com, 1-800-752-2775
- PhosChol, nutrasal.com, 1-800-777-1886
- Alkaline Water Machine, hightechhealth.com, 1-800-794-5355
- IndolPlex and Calcium-D Glucarate, integrativeinc.com, 1-800-917-3690
- Cardio/ION, metametrix.com, 1-800-221-4640

- Cod Liver Oil, carlsonlabs.com, 1-800-323-4141
- Green tea infuser, natural-lifestyle.com, 1-800-752-2775
- Sencha Premium Organic Green tea, indigo-tea.com, 1-866-248-3516
- Macadamia Nut Oil, realfoodgrocery com, 1-877-673-2536
- Books on whole foods diets, The Price-Pottenger Nutrition Foundation, ppnf.org, 1-800-366-3748
- Dr. Ohhira's 12+ Probiotic, realfoodgrocery.com, 1-877-673-2536, or 1-877-VIT-AMEN
- GPLC, ALCA, jarrow.com, or 877-VIT-AMEN, or 1-800-634-1380
- Pomegranate Juice, your local health food store

References:

McWhinney VGA, Lombardo YB, Chicco AG, Effects of dietary polyunsaturated **n-3 fatty** acids on **dyslipidemia** and **insulin resistance** in rodents and humans. A review, *J Nutr Biochem*, 17: 1-13, 2006

Levy TE, *Optimal Nutrition for Optimal Health*, Keats Publishing, a division of McGraw-Hill, NY, 2001

Blaylock CJ, et al, Salicylic acid concentrations in the serum of subjects not taking aspirin: comparison of salicylic acid concentration in the serum of vegetarians, non-vegetarians and patients taking low-dose aspirin, *J Clin Pathol*, 54: 553-55, 2001

Sesso HD, et al, *J Am Med Assoc*, 290: 2945-2951, 2003)

Pyoralas M, et al, Hyperinsulinemia predicted coronary heart disease risk in healthy middle-aged men: the 22-year follow-up results of the Helsinki Policemen Study, *Circulation*, 98; 5:398-404, 1998

Title LM, et al, Oral glucose loading acutely attenuates endothelium-dependent vasodilation in healthy adults without diabetes: an effect prevented by vitamins C and E, *J Am Coll Cardiol*, 36; 7:2185-91, Dec 2000

Newman TB, Hulley SB, **Carcinogenicity of lipid lowering drugs, *J Am Med Assoc***, 55-60, 1993

Dulloo AG, et al, Efficacy of a green tea extract rich in catechins polyphenols and caffeine in increasing 24-h energy expenditure and fat oxidation in humans, *Am J Clin Nutr*, 70: 1040-1045, 1999

Parker-Pope T, Health advice that's tough to swallow: Nine helpings of fruits and veggies a day, *Wall St J*, D1, April 29, 2003

Pins JJ, et al, Do whole-grain oat cereals reduce the need for antihypertensive medications and improve blood pressure control? *J Fam Pract* 51: 353-359, 2002

Jones JM, Reicks M, Marquart L, et al, The importance of promoting a whole grain foods message. *J Am Coll Nutr*, 21; 4:293-297, 2002

Shirahata S, Kabayama Sm Nakano M, Katakura Y, et al, Electrolized-reduced water scavenges active oxygen species and protects DNA from oxidative damage, *Biochem Biophys Res Commun*, 234:269-274, 1997

Ravnskov U, *The Cholesterol Myths, Exposing the Fallacy That Saturated Fat and Cholesterol Cause Heart Disease*, New Trends Publ., Wash. DC, 2000 (877-707-1776 and thincs.org)

Ornish D, Low-fat diets, *New Engl J Med*, 338; 2: 127, 1997

Alper CA, Mattes RD, Peanut consumption improves indices of cardiovascular disease risk in healthy adults, *J Am Coll Nutr*, 22; 2:133-141, 2003

Prasad K, Dietary flax seed in prevention of hypercholesterolemic atherosclerosis. *Atherosclerosis*, 132:69-76, 1997

Graham K, *Food Irradiation. A Canadian Folly*, 1992, Paper Birch Publishing 83 Wilkinson Crescent, Portage la Prairie, Manitoba, Canada, R1N 1A7

Leung S, Experts differ on healthiness of "fast" salads, *Wall St J*, B 1, May 8, 2003

Flint J, Johnson & Johnson is pushing Tylenol product to younger set. Publicist Groupe campaign includes deal with Disney to air some spots on ESPN, *Wall St J*, B 13, May 6, 2003

Anderson JW, Short-chain fatty acids and lipid metabolism. In: Cummings JH, et al, eds. *Physiological and Clinical Aspects of Short-Chain Fatty Acids*, NY: Cambridge University Press 509-523, 1995

Parker-Pope T, Heart disease hits the preschool set. Chicken-nugget boom leads to concerns about kids' health, *Wall St J*, D1, D4, Mar 18, 2003

Winslow R, New research shows warning signs begin in early childhood, *Wall St J*, D1, D4, Mar 18, 2003

Bruce B, Spiller GA, Klevay LM, Gallagher SK, A diet high in whole and unrefined foods favorably alters lipids, antioxidant defenses, and colon function, J *Amer Coll Nutr*, 19; 1:61-67, 2000

Allred CE, et al, Soy diets containing varying amounts of genistein stimulate growth of estrogen-dependent (MCF-7) tumors in a dose-dependent manner, *Ca Res* 61: 5045-50, 2001

Allred CE, et al, Dietary genistein stimulates growth of estrogen-dependent breast cancer tumors similar to that observed with genistein, *Carcinogenesis* 22; 10: 1667-73, 2001

Ju YH, et al, Physiological concentrations of dietary genistein dose-dependently stimulates growth of estrogen-dependent human breast cancer (MCF-7) tumors implanted in athymic nude mice, *J Nutr*, 131: 2957-62, 2001

Harder B, Look Ma, Too much soy, *Sci News*, 161:325, May 25, 2002

Moore S, Cholesterol revisited: Prime mover or a factor in the progression of atherosclerosis?, *Ann Roy Coll Phys Surg Canada*, 32:198-204, 1999

Oliver MF, Might treatment of hypercholesterolaemia increase non-cardiac mortality? *Lancet*, 1: 1087-89, 1991

Oliver MF, **Reducing cholesterol does not reduce mortality**, *J Am Coll Cardiol*, 12:814-17, 1988

Oliver MF, Doubts about preventing coronary heart disease. Multiple interventions in middle-aged men may do more harm than good. *Brit Med J*, 304:393-4, 1992

Hulley SB, Walsh JMB, Newman TB, Health policy on blood cholesterol. Time to change directions, *Circulation,* 86:1026-29, 1992

Smith GD, Pekkanen J, Should there be a moratorium on the use of cholesterol lowering drugs, *Brit Med J,* 304:431-34, 1992

Editorial, Atherosclerosis and auto-oxidation of cholesterol, *Lancet* 1:964-5, 1980.

Steinberg D, et al, Beyond cholesterol. Modifications of low-density lipoprotein that increases its atherogenicity, *N Engl J Med,* 320:915-24, 1989

Randerson J, Microwaved cooking zaps nutrients, *New Scientist* October 25, pg 14, 2003

Jenkins DJA, Kendall CWC, Marchie A, et al, Effects of dietary portfolio of cholesterol-lowering foods vs lovastatin on serum lipids and C-reactive protein, *J Am Med Assoc,* 290:502-510, 2003

Pinckney ER, Pinckney C, *The Cholesterol Controversy,* Sherbourne Press LA, 1973

Smith RL, Pinckney ER, *The Cholesterol Controversy,* Warren H. Green Inc., St. Louis MO, 1991

Maron DJ, Lu GP, Cai NS, et al, Cholesterol-lowering effect of a thea-flavin-enriched green tea extract, *Arch Intern Med,* 163:1448-53, 2003

Corinna MA, Mattes RD, Peanut consumption improves indices of cardiovascular disease risk in healthy adults, *J Am Coll Nutr,* 22; 2:133-41, 2003

Hu FB, et al, Dietary fat and risk of coronary heart disease in women, *New Engl J Med,* 337:1491-99, 1997

Oomen CM, et al, Association between trans fatty acid intake and risk of coronary heart disease in the Zutphen Elderly Study: a prospective population-based study, *Lancet* 357:746-51, 2001

Lemaitre RN, et al, Cell membrane trans fatty acids and the risk of primary cardiac arrest, *Circulation* 105: 697-701, 2002

Hu FB, et al, Fish and omega-3 fatty acid intake and risk of coronary heart disease in women, *J Am Med Assoc,* 287:1815-21, 2002

Wang C, et al, N-3 fatty acids from fish oil or fish oil supplements, but not [alpha]-linolenic acids, benefit cardiovascular disease outcomes in primary- and secondary-prevention studies: a systematic review, *Am J Clin Nutr,* 84:5-17, 2006

Teitelbaum JE, Walker WA, Review: the role of omega-3 fatty acids in intestinal inflammation, *J Nutr Biochem,* 12, 1. 21-32, January 2001

Jenski LJ, Strudevant LK, et al, Omega-3 fatty acid modification of membrane structure and function. Dietary manipulation of tumor cell susceptibility to cell- and complement-mediated lysis, Nutr *Cancer,* 19: 135-146, 1993

Albert CM, Hennekens CH, O'Donnell CJ, et al, Fish consumption and risk of sudden cardiac death, *J Am Med Assoc,* 279: 23-28, 1998

Soria A, Chicco A, Lombardo YB, et al, Dietary fish oil reverses epididymal tissue adiposity, cell hypertrophy and insulin resistance in dyslipemic sucrose fed rat model, *Nutr Biochem*, 13: 209-2 18, 2002

Haglund O, Wallin R, Saldeen T, et al, Effects of a new fluid fish oil concentrate, ESKIMO-3 on triglycerides, cholesterol, fibrinogen and blood pressure, *J Intern Med*, 227; 347-53, 1990

Haglund O, Luostarinien R, Wallin R, Saldeen T, Effects of fish oil on triglycerides, cholesterol, lipoprotein(a), atherogenic index, and fibrinogen. Influence of degree of purification of the oil, *Nutr Res*, 12:1419-30, 1992

Enig MG, *Trans Fatty Acids in the Food supply: A Comprehencsive Report Covering 60 Years of Research*, Enig Associates, Inc., Silver Spring MD, 1993

Koletzko B, Trans fatty acids may impair biosynthesis of long-chain polyunsaturates and growth in man, *Acta Pediatrica*, 81:302-06, 1992

Mensinck RP, Katan MB, Effect of dietary trans fatty acids on high density and low-density lipoprotein cholesterol levels in healthy subjects, *N Engl J Med*, 323:439-45, 1990

Simopoulos AP, Omega-3 fatty acids and inflammation and autoimmune diseases, *J Am Coll Nutr*, 12; 6: 495-505, 2002

Augustsson K, Michaud DS, Rimm EB, Leitzmann MF, Stampfer MJ, Willett WC, Giovannucci EM, A prospective study of intake of fish and marine fatty acids and prostate cancer, *Ca Epid Biomark Prevent*, 12; 1: 64-67, Jan. 2003

Laidlow M, Holub BJ, Effects of supplementation with fish oil-derived n-3 fatty acids and gamma-linolenic acid on circulating plasma lipids and fatty acid profiles in women, *Am J Clin Nutr*, 77; 1: 37-42, Jan 2003

Abboud L, The truth about trans fats: coming to a label near you. FDA orders disclosure of more details on packages; a new excuse to eat Cheetos, *Wall St J*, D1, July 10, 2003

Lord RS, Bralley JA, Polyunsaturated fatty acid-induced antioxidant insufficiency, *Integrat Med*, 1; 138-43, Dec 2002/Jan 2003

Gundermann KJ, ed., *The "Essential" Phospholipids as a Membrane Therapeutic*, Polish Section of European Society of Biochemical Pharmacology, Institute of Pharmacology and Toxicology, Medical Academy, Szczecin, 1993

Archakov AI, Gundermann KJ, *Phosphatidylcholine (Polyenephosphatidyl-choline/PPC): Effects on Cell Membranes and Transport of Cholesterol*, PPC Workshop, Cologne, May 2-3, 1988, Verlag, Bingen/Rhein, 1989

Peeters, H, ed., *Phosphatidyl-choline, Biochemical and Clinical Aspects of Essential Phospholipids*, Springer-Verlag, NY, 1976

Schlettler G, *Phospholipids, Biochemistry, Experimentation, Clinical Application*, Georg Thieme Verlag, Stuttgart, 1972

Wojcicki JT, Dutkiewicz J, Kadlubowska D, et al, Essential phospholipids (EPL) modify immunological functions and reduce experimental atherosclerosis in rabbits, *Atherosclerosis* 93:7-16, 1992

204

Howard AN, Patelski E, Gresham GA, et al, Phospholipids in experimental atherosclerosis, in Schlettler G, *Phospholipids, Biochemistry, Experimentation, Clinical Application*, Georg Thieme Verlag, Stuttgart, 1972

Vroulis G, Smith RC, Misra Ch, et al, Reduction of cholesterol risk factors by lecithin in patients with Alzheimer's disease, *Am J Psychiat,* 139; 12:1633-34, 1982

Avogaro P, Bittolo-Bon G, Cazzolato G, A role for phospahtidyl choline in reducing the damage of oxydized low density lipoproteins, in Archakov AI, Gundermann KJ, *Phosphatidylcholine (Polyenephosphatidyl-choline/PPC): Effects on Cell Membranes and Transport of Cholesterol*, PPC Workshop, Cologne, May 2-3, 1988, Verlag, Bingen/Rhein, 1989

Ornish D, Intensive lifestyle changes for reversal of coronary heart disease, *J Am Med Assoc*, 280: 2001-07, 1998

Kooyenga DK, Geller M, Bierenbaum ML, et al, Palm oil antioxidant effects in patients with hyper-lipidaemia and carotid stenosis: 2-year experience, *Asia Pacific J Clin Nutr,* 6; 1:72-75, 1997

LaPointe A, et al, Effects of dietary factors on oxidation of low-density lipoproteins particles, *J Nutr Biochem,* 17:645-58, 2006

Toshima S, et al, Circulating oxidized low-density lipoproteins levels. A biochemical risk marker for coronary heart disease, *Arterioscler Thromb Vasc Biol,* 20: 2243-47, 2000

Wang TTY, et al, Estrogen receptor alpha as a target for indole-3-carbinol, *J Nutr biochem,* 17:759-64, 2006

Pereira MA, et al, Dietary fiber and risk of coronary heart disease, *Arch Intern Med,* 164:370-76, 2004

Anderson JW, et al, Whole grain foods and heart disease risk, *J Am Coll Nutr,* 19:291s-99s, 2000

Price JM, *Coronaries/Cholesterol Chlorine*, Jove Books, Berkeley Publishing, NY, 1969

Ledingham JGG, Warrell DA, *Concise Oxford Textbook of Medicine*, Oxford: Oxford University Press, 2000

Plaskett LG, On the essentiality of dietary carbohydrate, *J Nutr Environ Med* 13; 3:161-68, Sept 2003

Groff JL, Gropper SS, Hunt SM, *Advanced Nutrition and Human Metabolism*, P. 138, West Publishing, 1995

Plaskett LG, *The Wherewithal to Detoxify*, Tiverton: Nutrigold, 2001

Lombardo YB, Chicco AG, Effects of dietary polyunsaturated n-three fatty acids on dyslipidemia and insulin resistance in rodents and humans. A review, *J Nutr Biochem,* 17: 1-13, 2006

Willett, WC, Will high-carbohydrate/low-fat diets reduce the risk of coronary heart disease?, *Soc Exper Biol Med,* 187-190, 2000

Hu FB, Mason JE, Willett WC, Types of dietary fat and risk of coronary heart disease: A critical review, *J Am Coll Nutr,* 20; 1:5-19, 2001

Peskin BS, *The Hidden Story Of Cancer*, pgs 255-259, Pinnacle Press, Houston, Texas, 2006

www.BanTransFats.com exposes the legalized lying loophole of the FDA

Sinclair HM, Deficiency of essential fatty acid and atherosclerosis, *Lancet* April 7, 1956

Waddington, Kuhn, Felton, Felton CV, et al, Dietary polyunsaturated fatty acids and compositions of human aortic plaque, *Lancet,* 344:1195-96, 1994

Waddingon E, et al, Identification and quantification of unique fatty acid and oxidative products in human atherosclerotic plaque using high-performance liquid chromatography, *Ann Biochem,* 292:234-44, 2001

Kuhn H, et al, Structural elucidation of oxygenated lipids in human atherosclerotic lesions, *Eicosanoids,* 5: 17-22, 1992

Estruch R, et al, Effects of a Mediterranean-style diet on cardiovascular risk factors, *Ann Int Med,* 4; 145; 1:1-118, Jul 2006

Kern F, Normal plasma cholesterol in an 88-year-old man who eats 25 eggs a day–mechanism of adaptation, *N Engl J Med,* 324:896-899, 1991

Morgan JM, et al, Effect of dietary (egg) cholesterol on serum cholesterol in free-living adults, *J Appl Nutr,* 45; 3,4:73-84, 1993

McNamara DJ, The impact of egg limitations on coronary heart disease risk: Do the numbers add up?, *J Amer Coll Nutr,* 19;5:540S-548S, Oct 2000

Kritchevsky SB, Kritchevsky D, Egg consumption and coronary heart disease: An epidemiologic overview, *J Amer Coll Nutr,* 19; 5:549S-555S. Oct 2000

Altman R, et al, Phospholipids associated with vitamin C in experimental atherosclerosis, *Arzneimittelforschung,* 30; 4:627-30, 1980

Dobiasova M, Lecithin: cholesterol acyltransferase and the regulation of endogenous cholesterol transport, *Adv Lipid Res,* 20:107-194, 1983

Chen C, et al, Effect of peroxyl radicals on lecithin/cholesterol acyltransferase activity in human plasma, *Lipids,* 30; 7:627-31, 1995

Polichetti E, et al, Dietary polyenylphosphatidylcholine decreases cholesterolemia in hypercholesterolemia, rabbits: role of hepato-biliary axis, *Life Sci,* 67; 21:2563-76, 2000

Polichetti E, et al, Cholesterol-lowering effect of soyabean lecithin in normal lipidemic rats by stimulation of biliary lipid secretion, *Brit J Nutr,* 75; 3:471-78, 1996

Mastellone IE, et al, Dietary soybean phosphatidylcholines lower lipidemia: Mechanisms at the levels of intestine, endothelial cell, and hepato-biliary axis, *J Nutr Biochem,* 11; 9:461-66, 2000

Adams C, et al, The effect of saturated and polyunsaturated lecithins on the resorption of 4-14C-cholesterol from subcutaneous implants, *J Pathol Bacteriol,* 94; 1:73-76, 1967

Adams C, et al, Modification of aortic atheroma and fatty liver in unsaturated and polyunsaturated lecithins, *J Pathol Bacteriol,* 94; 1:77-87, 1967

Bielicki J, et al, Copper and gas-phase cigarette smoke, inhibit plasma lecithin: cholesterol acyltransferase activity by different mechanisms, *J Lipid Res*, 32; 2:322-31, 1995

Leuschner F, Wagener HH, Neumann B, The anti-hyperlidemic and anti-atherogenic effect of 'essential' phospholipids: A pharmacologic trial, *Arzneimittelforschung*, 2:9a: 1743-72, 1976

Duan JM, Karmazyn M, Protection of the reperfused ischemic isolated rat heart by phosphatidylcholine, *J Cardiovasc Pharmacol*, 15; 1:163-71, Jan 1990

Duan JM, Moffat MP, Protective effects of phosphatidylcholine against mechanisms of ischemia and reperfusion-induced arrhythmia in isolated guinea pig ventricular tissues, *Naunyn Schmiedebergs Arch Pharmacol*, 342; 3:342-8, Sept 1990

Anonymous monograph, Phosphatidylcholine, *Altern Med Rev*, 7; 2: 150-154, 2002

Foster JS, Kane PC, Speight N, *The Detoxx Book*, 1-866-293-3945, fax: 856-825-2143

Mensink RP, Katan MB, Effect of dietary trans fatty acids on high-density and low-density lipoprotein cholesterol levels in healthy subjects, *N Engl J Med*, 323:439-445, 1990

Lichtenstein AH, Ausman LM, Schaefer EJ, Effects of different forms of dietary hydrogenated fats on serum lipoprotein cholesterol levels, *N Engl J Med*, 34:1933-40, 1999

Estruch R, et al, Effects of a Mediterranean-style diet on cardiovascular risk factors, *Ann Int Med*, 4; 145; 1:1-118, Jul 2006

Lombardo YB, Chicco AG, Effects of dietary polyunsaturated n-three fatty acids on dyslipidemia and insulin resistance in rodents and humans. A review, *J Nutr Biochem*, 17: 1-13, 2006

Willett, WC, Will high-carbohydrate/low-fat diets reduce the risk of coronary heart disease?, *Soc Exper Biol Med*, 187-190, 2000

Hu FB, Mason JE, Willett WC, Types of dietary fat and risk of coronary heart disease: A critical review, *J Am Coll Nutr*, 20; 1:5-19, 2001

Plotnick GD, et al, Effect of antioxidant vitamins on the transient impairment of endothelium-dependent brachial artery vasoactivity following a single high-fat meal, *J Am Med Assoc*, 278; 20: 1682-86, Nov. 26, 1997

Assoc. Press, Heart Association sets trans-fat limit, *Wall St J*, D4, June 20, 2006

Pond WG, Mersmann HJ, Ontogeny and Dietary Modulation of 3-Hydroxy-3-Methylglutaryl-CoA Reductase Activities in Neonatal Pigs, *J Animal Sci*, 74: 2203-10, 1996

Enig MG, *Know Your Fats: The Complete Primer for Understanding the Nutrition of Fats, Oils, and Cholesterol*, Bethesda Press, 12501 Prosperity Dr., Ste 340, Silver Spring MD 20904-1 689, fax: 301-680-8100, Web: bethesdapress.com, 2000

Enig MG, Atal S, Keeney, et al, Isomeric trans fatty acids in the U.S. diet, *J Am Coll Nutr*, 9: 471-86, 1990

Blackburn GL, et al, A re-evaluation of coconut oil's effect on serum cholesterol and atherogenesis, *J Philippine Med Assoc*, 65: 144-52, 1989

Eaton MDL, et al, Preliminary examination of contaminant loadings in farmed salmon, wild salmon and commercial salmon feed, *Chemosphere,* 46:1053-74, 2002

Iacobs M, et al, Investigation of polychlorinated dibenzo-p-dioxins, dibenzo-p-furans and selected coplanar biphenyls in Scottish farmed Atlantic salmon, *Chemosphere,* 47:183-90 1, 2002

Jacobson TA, Secondary Prevention of coronary artery disease with Omega-3 fatty acids, *Am J Cardiol,* 98 [supple]: 60i-70i, 2006

Reiffel JA, McDonald A, Anti-arrhythmia, effects of Omega-3 fatty acids, *Am J Cardiol,* 98 [supple]: 50i-60i, 2006

Olthof MR, et al, Choline supplemented as phosphatidylcholine decreases fasting and postmethionine-loading plasma homocysteine concentrations in healthy men, *Am J Clin Nutr,* 82: 111-17, 2005

Kaplan M, et al, Pomegranate juice supplementation to arteriosclerotic mice reduces macrophage lipid peroxidation, cellular cholesterol accumulation and development of atherosclerosis, *J Nutr,* 131; 8: 2082-89, Aug 2001

Huang TH, et al, Pomegranate flower improves cardiac lipid metabolism in a diabetic rat model: role of lowering circulating lipids, *Brit J Pharmacol,* 145; 6:767-74, July 2004

Fuhrman B, et al, Pomegranate juice inhibits oxidized LDL uptake and cholesterol biosynthesis in macrophages, *J Nutr Biochem,* 16; 570-76, Sept 2005

Aviram M, et al, Pomegranate juice consumption for three years by patients with carotid artery stenosis reduces common carotid intima-media thickness, blood pressure and LDL oxidation, *Clin Nutr,* 23; 3:423-33, June 2004

Tuttle D, Pomegranate reverses atherosclerosis and slows the progression of prostate cancer, *Life Extension,* 13; 2:72-77, Feb 2007

Arockia P, et al, Carnitine as a free radical scavenger in aging, *Exp Gerontol,* 36:1713-26, 2001

Dayanandan A, et al, Protective role of L-carnitine on liver and heart lipid peroxidation in atherosclerotic rats, *J Nutr Biochem,* 12:254-50 7, 2001

Sayed-Ahmed MM, et al, L-Carnitine prevents the progression of atherosclerotic lesions in hypercholesterolemia rabbits, *Pharm Res,* 44: 235-42, 2001

Gomez-Amores L, et al, Antioxidant activity of proprionyl,-L-carnitine in liver and heart of spontaneously hypertensive rats, 78:1945-52, 2006

Fraser GE, et al, A possible protective effect of nut consumption on risk of coronary heart disease, The Adventist Heart Study, *Arch Int Med,* 152:1416-24, 1992

Albert CM, et al, Nut consumption and decreased risk of sudden cardiac death in the Physicians' Health Study, *Arch Int Med,* 162:1382-87, 2002

Kooyenga DK, Geller M, Bierenbaum ML, et al, Palm oil antioxidant effects in patients with hyperlipidemia and carotid stenosis: 2-year experience, *Asia Pacific J Clin Nutr,* 6; 1:72-75, 1997

Ornish D, Scherwitz LW, Brand RJ, et al, Intensive lifestyle changes for reversal of coronary heart disease, *J Am Med Assoc,* 280:2001-2007, 1998

Lam RYY, et al, Antioxidant actions of phenolic compounds found in dietary plants on low-density lipoproteins and erythrocytes in vitro, *J Am Coll Nutr,* 26; 3:233-42, 2007

Fuhrman B, et al, Ginger extract consumption reduces plasma cholesterol, inhibits LDL oxidation and attenuates development of arteriosclerosis in atherosclerotic, apolipoprotein E-deficient mice, *J Nutr,* 130:1224-31, 2000

Jacoba R, et al, Effect of L-carnitine on the limitation in infarct size in one-month post-myocardial infarction cases: A multicenter, randomized, parallel, placebo-controlled trial, *Clin Drug Investig,* 11; 2: 90-96, 1996

Defelice Sl, *The Carnitine Defense*, rodalebooks.com, 1999

Chapter V

You Can "Catch" a Heart Attack:
The Infection Connection

It should be clear to you now that real scientists know that choles-terol is not the cause of coronary artery disease. When you exam-ine arteriosclerotic arteries under a microscope they show inflam-mation and clotting (van der Wal, Ross). That means the body is reacting to something and trying to get rid of it. One of the things that can trigger this inflammatory reaction is infection. Just as your body tries to get rid of a splinter or sliver by getting "in-fected" or inflamed, so do the coronary arteries.

It has been abundantly proven now for decades that arteriosclero-sis, coronary artery disease, cholesterol plaque or whatever you want to call it, begins as an inflammatory process. In other words, just as inflammation occurs around a splinter, no matter where there is inflammation it is merely the body's last-ditch attempt to clean up a mess that was started by some agent. And coronary ar-tery disease is no exception. **Hidden infection is one of the main causes of coronary artery inflammation.** The most common sources for bugs that cause heart disease are:

- Gut
- Teeth
- Sinuses
- Chest cold bacteria

Let's look at the chief ones. In terms of the gut, the symptoms may be nothing, or it can merely be heartburn, acid indigestion, irritable bowel, gas and bloating or alternating diarrhea and constipation. In terms of the teeth, the symptoms may be nothing or an occa-sional tooth that is just irritated transiently but simmers down. And then there are numerous viruses and bacteria that can remain dormant in the system for years until the immune system finally takes a nosedive and now the organism silently attacks the coronary arteries. Or there is molecular mimicry. For some bugs have long been banished from the body, but while they were there, the body learned to make antibodies against them to ward them off. So far, so good. The hooker is that sometimes the antigenic recognition sites on the bug look similar to sites on our own cells. So now these antibodies that we made to fight the bug attack our very cells by **mistaken identity or molecular mimicry**. Strep throat leading to rheumatic heart disease is a simple time-honored example. **An autoimmune inflammation can be born at any time**. The immune system takes a nosedive when finally the total nutrient deficiencies and toxicities reach a critical point. Let's take a look at how silent bugs in the gut can eat away at the coronary arteries.

Heartburn Leads to a Heart Attack

Heartburn or indigestion, they seem innocent enough, but watch out! Taking medications to quiet the symptoms can lead to accelerated aging, cancer, a heart attack, and high cholesterol. The problem lies in not knowing what the real cause of your heartburn is. For in the vast majority of folks, a common stomach bug causes it, *Helicobacter pylori*, called H. pylori for short. This bug is so common that it has been shown to lurk silently in the stomachs of two out of three people. It can be there and cause absolutely no symptoms. Or it can cause heartburn and indigestion of any degree (sometimes being mistaken for a hiatus hernia or GERD), or an ulcer that can eventually rupture, leaving you hemorrhaging to death.

But worse is the fact that when you use common non-prescription drugs that turn off or sop up acid (antacids and acid inhibitors), you have lost one of nature's main tools for killing bugs. And when not killed because of lack of stomach acid (poisoned by heartburn drugs), *H. pylori* can go on to cause cancer of the stomach. In fact it is such a potent cause that the prevalence of cancer of the stomach has risen over eight-fold in the last 20 years as these stomach drugs have become more popular. Remember a few years back, many were prescription that are now available over-the-counter, like Prilosec (funny how a medicine requires a prescription until its patent runs out, then it magically is safe enough to no longer require one). Turning off your natural stomach acid secretion is counterproductive (God designed it to kill bugs), and studies show that folks unknowledgeable enough to take **medications for their heartburn (prescription or over the counter) have a cancer risk of not 8 times but 43 times normal!**

But bleeding to death from an ulcer or getting fatal stomach cancer is not the end of the line. ***H. pylori* can silently rot out the lining of your stomach causing atrophic gastritis.** Now you no longer absorb your nutrients and are on a fast downhill course of **accelerated aging** and start developing all sorts of symptoms that no one can cure. This bug has even been incriminated in glaucoma (Kountouras).

Cholesterol is Nature's Band-Aid

But H. pylori can do something even worse. It is taken up in white blood cells where it rides piggyback through the blood stream to coronary artery walls (Mendell). Here the enzymes that the bug secretes drill holes in the lining of coronary arteries. Our body defenses send in cholesterol to patch up these microscopic holes so we don't bleed to death. In time when enough of the cholesterol band-aid has been piled on, it can plug the artery. If it is the coronary artery that is plugged, a heart attack results. Because the excess cholesterol is directed to such a tiny area, you may not even have elevated blood cholesterol that any doc can measure. Hence, another part of the reason for the statistic is that half the folks who die of a heart attack never even had high cholesterol.

H. pylori is surprising the medical community by being a major cause of arteriosclerosis, when all along cholesterol was

touted as the main cause. Instead, as you are learning, cholesterol is merely an innocent bystander, which is actually protecting us from bleeding to death when *H. pylori* and other hidden bugs have eaten holes in our arteries. No wonder folks still get heart attacks even though they have diligently followed a low cholesterol diet or taken cholesterol-lowering medications. **By lowering cholesterol with drugs we have only been shooting the messenger.**

So what can you do? Your doctor can order a blood test at any local lab that will show if you have *H. pylori*. Since many other bugs like Herpes, Cytomegalovirus, Chlamydia, and others from flus, colds, silently infected teeth roots, and more can also cause arteriosclerosis, it seems like a good idea to go after the bugs. The problem is antibiotics often miss their mark, since they are dispersed to the entire body and therefore are not concentrated enough to penetrate a specific area.

In addition, bugs develop resistance to antibiotics and when taken for a while then can cause the leaky gut syndrome that snowballs into fibromyalgia, chronic fatigue, autoimmune diseases, and allergies (see *No More Heartburn* for the diagnosis, causes and cures of all these). Meanwhile, **taking an antacid or any medication that turns off stomach acid makes H. pylori grow even more wildly, because stomach acid is meant to kill bugs.** So you begin to see again how counterproductive it is to take any medications, because they merely poison enzymes so that your symptom turns off, but they don't identify and get rid of the underlying cause. Therefore you have only one way to go: **with drugs the sick get sicker quicker.**

Clearly, **you can literally go from heartburn to a heart attack**. Fortunately there are several non-prescription items that can nip *H. pylori, Candida* (a common yeast), and other unwanted bugs in the bud. One is the special form of aged garlic you have learned about in Chapters II and IV. Sounds too easy, doesn't it? But don't be fooled by nature's simplicity. This proprietary form of aged garlic has withstood the test of time and has over 300 research papers behind its anti-bacterial, anti-fungal, and anti-viral properties. And not only does **Kyolic Liquid** kill bugs like *H. pylori*, but it lowers the cholesterol in some folks, lowers blood pressure, makes the blood less likely to clot, lowers homocysteine (the amino acid that is a stronger risk factor for heart attack than having high cholesterol), and raises one of the body's cells that kill bugs and cancer cells, the natural killer or NK cells (Liu, and see all related Kyolic references in Chapters II and IV).

As one of nature's anti-oxidants, **Kyolic** also protects LDL from becoming oxidized and turning it into the bad guy (that hungry electron-seeking beast) that glues itself to arterial linings, eventually plugging them up (Ide). So what could be more perfect than a safe, natural substance that not only kills the bug, plus fights cancer and arteriosclerosis, all rolled into one? No medication does all that, but **Kyolic** does (by Wakunaga, the same company that makes the **Kyolic Formula 107 Red Yeast Rice** that you learned about in Chapter II that is so effective in lowering cholesterol). The beauty of **Kyolic Liquid** is that (1) not only does it lower cholesterol, but also (2) it kills *H. pylori* and (3) acts as an antioxidant protecting the coronary vessel walls. Furthermore, (4) it lowers platelet aggregation or the ability of blood to adversely clot (Liu, Ide, Steiner, Orekhov, Warshafsky, Rahman, Munday, Yeh).

Another powerful tool to kill H. pylori and heal ulcers and heartburn is **Mastic Gum** (Jarrow) 500 mg 1 or 2 twice a day. This also has been used to kill even resistant strains of H. pylori, as well as accelerate healing and regeneration of damaged tissue (Huwez, Marone, Al-Habbal). *H. pylori* currently is diagnosed by PCR (polymerized chain reaction) blood tests and then 3 potent antibiotics are prescribed. You can imagine the amount of fungal Candida overgrowth that this will generate, which then leads to leaky gut syndrome and autoimmune disease! I sure would want to evaluate natural products with no side effects a long time before I would ever consider such a nasty and expensive treatment.

So start to think about the possible causes and consequences of not getting to the bottom of the true underlying cause, the next time you feel indigestion. If either of these shotgun approaches, together or alone, simmers down your gut and your cholesterol, you have hit the jackpot. But if your gut is still flared up and cholesterol is not moving, you may need to become much more of an expert in the cause and cure of your gut symptoms before your cholesterol will ever budge. Read *No More Heartburn* and you'll learn about many more simple cures, like Pepto-Bismol® that can kill H. pylori, too. It all depends on how far you have to go for your particular body. Whatever you have to do, it is worth it. Many diseases are never cured until the gut is first healed, for **the road to health is paved with good intestines.**

Tar and Feather Docs Who Prescribe the Purple Pill

And in case you think that your heartburn will be "cured" by your doctor's prescription, consider this: Newspapers, magazines and TV commercials are loaded with ads for "the purple pill", Nexium®. But I want to show you how **prescribing Nexium is a warning sign of an inadequate physician.** You already learned that the cholesterol-lowering drug Lipitor is the largest selling blockbuster drug currently in the world. But the first blockbuster drug in the history of the world was Prilosec, a prescription acid inhibitor that made over $26 billion. You need to know that when the patent expires on a drug, the huge profits for the company that had exclusivity stop rolling in, since now it is generic and can be made by lots of people who can competitively bring the price down, often 5- to 10-fold. Hence, Prilosec is now as little as 40¢ a capsule versus the former prescription at nearly $4.

So what did the makers of Prilosec do? They attached a small chemical side chain to their old Prilosec molecule, thereby creating a "brand new drug" which was called Nexium, and was again patentable so they were able to continue to charge obscene prices. The problem is this new creation, Nexium, makes more work for the body because in order for the body to use Nexium, it must first use up precious body nutrients in order to rip off the useless attached sidearm. This leaves the original product Prilosec that works to turn off acid. But don't forget that Prilosec is now OTC (over-the-counter), and often eight times cheaper than the prescription Nexium, depending on where you buy it.

So I ask you: what knowledgeable doctor would prescribe a drug that is (1) eight times more expensive than it needs to be, and that (2) makes the body go through extra metabolic work which wastes healing nutrients? **No self-respecting physician prescribing Nexium could possibly be aware of this double disadvantage and still prescribe it for any one.** I believe it has to be done out of total biochemical and pharmacologic ignorance. That means his prescribing practices are directed by drug company advertising, as frequent *Wall Street Journal* articles remind us, and that **he never even looked up the chemical structure of what he is licensed to prescribe** for your body. Meanwhile there are many inexpensive cures for heartburn (see *No More Heartburn*) that the average person will never be aware of. For many people they are at a standstill and can never get better from whatever disease they have merely because they did not begin by making the gut healthy. **Since the gut houses half the immune system and half the detoxification system for the entire body, the gut has to be entirely healed before you can get to second base with any disease, and high cholesterol is no exception.**

The Tooth Connection to Heart Disease

When somebody gets pneumonia, it's usually blamed on some exposure. Or if their diabetes goes haywire, it's blamed on their genetics or diet. Or when they have a heart attack it's blamed on their diet or family history. We can always find some excuse for just about every disease. But many diseases begin right inside the victim's mouth. For those crevices between the gums and the teeth harbor an army of bugs that have easy access into every nook and cranny of the body. You know now that much disease begins in the gut. But most forget that the gut begins in the mouth.

Many systemic medical problems, including coronary artery disease, with or without high cholesterol, start from bugs harbored in tooth crevices, called gum disease or **periodontal disease**, and high cholesterol and coronary artery disease are no exception (Iacopino). These bugs can just cause bad breath, occasional bleeding of gums, an occasionally tender tooth, or no symptoms at all until you have a heart attack. But mouth bugs clearly can get into the circulation and invade coronary artery cells (Dorn). Most importantly, **mouth bugs have been found in coronary artery plaque** (Haraszthy), and harboring them clearly raises your heart attack rate (Matilla).

For example, the risk of **early heart problems is 300% higher with one or more oral bacteria** and in another study, the heart attack death rate is 2 1/2 times greater in patients with bacteria in the crevices between teeth and gums. In other studies **having periodontal infection also markedly increased the risk of death from coronary heart disease.** And **always look for periodontal disease when you find an elevated fibrinogen or hsCRP,** since you recall from Chapter III how much more serious risk is present when one or more of these parameters are elevated. In fact, the greater the number of abnormal parameters there are on your **Cardio/ION Panel**, the greater the risk of a heart attack and/or early death.

I've discovered a great periodontal package, designed and distributed by a dentist that is complete, logical, safe and efficacious. The best toothpaste by far that I have found is PerioPaste, designed by Dr. James Harrison, DDS, which is a natural toothpaste containing organic herbs, vitamins and oils while avoiding the toxins like fluoride and other preservatives that are so ubiquitous in standard commercial toothpastes. It's great for sensitive teeth, dry mouth and contains even folic acid, CoQ10 and Aloe Vera, all very good for helping to heal inflamed gum tissues. After a gentle scrub of the teeth now you are ready to clean out the dangerous bacteria-filled crypts between gums and teeth.

Next you want PerioScript, a concentrated solution of herbs and nutrients that is preservative-free and organic. Following the directions put some into the Hydro Floss, an oral irrigator that comes with two separate sizes of jet tips for really getting to the root of the problem. Dr. Harrison is a dentist who is a member of the International Academy of Oral Medicine and Toxicology. You may want to check their website for a possible biological dentist in your area who is aware of mercury and other dangers commonly ignored by conventional dentists (iaomt.org). For example, mercury in "silver" fillings makes bacteria in the mouth and intestines resistant to antibiotics. If your dentist fights you on the mercury issue and is unaware of these facts, it may be time to switch (there's much more on this including the convincing scientific backup in *Detoxify or Die* and Chapter VII here).

Bare minimum you want to use daily (1) **PerioPaste**, (2) the **Hydro Floss** irrigator, and (3) **PerioScript**. It is imperative to clean out those crypts between the teeth and gums twice daily to keep them as free from heart-destroying bacteria as possible. Clearly mouth bacteria lurking in periodontal crevices are a major risk for heart disease (Scannapieco, Beck, Dorn, Matilla).

The Chlamydia Calamity

A species of bacteria that commonly causes colds, sinus infections, bronchitis, asthma or pneumonia is called *Chlamydia pneumoniae*. Unfortunately when you search chlamydia in the medical literature, one usually ends up with one of the other two species of chlamydia that either causes blindness in tropical areas or another one that causes venereal disease. We are not concerned with these two.

Chlamydia is an odd bug because once you have gotten it, and it's very common, it can live silently in the body for decades without causing any problem. Unfortunately in many people it causes a silent infection with inflammation inside the coronary arteries. In fact, **in 79% of folks with carotid plaque there are antibodies against chlamydia as opposed to only 4% of those without plaque** (Muhlestrin). And although many other cardiologists have reported this as well, many cardiologists still do not routinely check it even though this has been known for decades (Linnan-maki, Bachmaier).

Interestingly studies giving people six months of tetracycline-type antibiotics did not help them. But others who used single three-day courses of antibiotic a month had a drop in antibody titers (Gupta). And of course none of these cardiology-based researchers knew a thing about assaying all the nutrients and getting the toxins out that you'll learn about here to make sure that the body's immune system is maximally capable of fighting infection.

Therefore my plan of choice would be to (1) measure the **Chlamydia antibodies by PCR** at any commercial medical lab to establish that there is indeed infection, and (2) measure and correct the vitamin, mineral, fatty acid, amino acid and organic acid abnormalities and abnormal cardiovascular risk factors via the **Cardio/ION Panel** (MetaMetrix Lab). Also very important is the fact that within this test are parameters that will tell you how successful you have been in defeating the inflammation. An elevated **fibrinogen and a high sensitivity CRP as well as lipid peroxides** are among the many important indicators of serious inflammation that are included in this test. (3) Then use expensive azithromycin 500 mg twice a day (on an empty stomach) for 3-5 days 1-2 times a month for 6 months. Follow this by probiotics like **Dr. Ohhira's 12 Plus** or **Abx Support**, either 2 twice a day for 10 days at the end of the 10 days of antibiotics each time. (4) Then repeat the antibody titers. If they are still up then you most likely need to get rid of the toxins that you will learn about in Chapter VII, and important updates will be coming in *TW* 2008 and subsequent issues, as we are actively researching this.

Protect Against Meat That is Getting Buggier

Where do all these bugs that can cause high cholesterol come from? As one example, the Food and Drug Administration is worried about the rise of antibiotic-resistant bugs that are cropping up in meat. The reason we have so many "super bugs" in meat is that cattle, pigs, and chickens (and now farmed fish) are fed antibiotics routinely, to make them grow faster so they can get to market sooner. The problem is this use of antibiotics (prophylactically, when there is no infection) kills off normal bacteria and generates the emergence of bugs that resist the average antibiotic. But don't hold your breath for reform, because these changes take a long time, and bucking the $4 billion annual market for animal drugs, dominated by powerful pharmaceutical firms is a daunting task.

Meanwhile according to the U.S. Centers for Disease Control and Prevention (*Wall Street Journal*, D7, April 16, 2003), there are 76 million food borne human illnesses annually in the U.S. There are **over 325,000 hospitalizations for food poisoning each year and over 5,200 deaths in the U.S. each year just from food poisoning** (that are recognized, reported and included in the statistics). This is not a light issue.

Freeze Your Meats

You might think the biggest user of antibiotics would be people. But not so, for **80% of the antibiotics produced in the United States are fed to healthy, not sick, livestock.** This fosters antibiotic-resistant strains of bacteria and other "super-bug" infectious agents, which silently grow in the tissues of the animals and then

220

are passed on to us when we eat them. For example, after the FDA approved a particular antibiotic (fluoroquinolones, like Cipro) for poultry production in 1995, bacteria like Campylobacter became resistant to that antibiotic. Worse, as a result, *Campylobacter jejuni* **increased tenfold in humans in the United States.** But this bacterium did not increase tenfold in Australia, because Aussies smartly refused to approve the antibiotic for use in their animal farming. This is but one small example of **how antibiotic use in animals has then dangerously transferred to a 10-fold antibiotic resistance for humans.**

But the problem gets even worse because a study from Johns Hopkins Medical School showed that once the FDA finally banned this particular antibiotic from being used routinely in chicken farming, all it had amounted to was "too little, too late". They found that banning the antibiotic for animal prophylaxis after it had been used so recklessly didn't accomplish anything for the marked increase in antibiotic-resistant bugs in humans that had already resulted in increased Campylobacter (H. pylori). Once the horse is out of the barn the damage appears to be irreconcilable. For this new onslaught of bugs in humans was now fluoroquinolone-resistant (antibiotics like Cipro). This is epidemic of antibiotic-resistant bugs in humans is one major contributor to the overall **hospital-acquired infections that kill over hundred thousand people each year in the United States and add over $27 billion to the nation's already bloated health tab** (Osby). In one study 34 of every thousand patients in the hospital were infected with methacillin-resistant Staphylococcus (MRSA) and it is increasing. This can be fatal, especially in infants, the elderly and immunocompromised, not to mention the silently nutrient deficient.

In addition, in another study **85% of the feed ingredients for poultry, cattle, and farmed fish contained bacteria that were resistant to one or more antibiotics.** As well, some of the most potent cancer-causing toxins from moldy feed are able to survive in animals and be passed on to humans. Then to top it off, industrial processing and incineration of plastics have put large amounts of PCBs and dioxins into the atmosphere and into the soil and plants. Animals bio-accumulate or concentrate these most potent cancer-causing chemicals in their fat and pass these on to us.

We've already seen how breaking the laws of nature and feeding animals to animals who don't normally search out and eat that type of animal has led to prions creating mad cow disease and other fatal brain degenerating diseases (Creutzfeld-Jakob). Recycling not only dead animal products, but also putting animal waste into animal feed has become a means of cutting feed costs. For example, dead hog parts are ground into poultry feed. But in all my years on the farm, I never saw a chicken chase down a pig for her dinner!

As well, processed oils and garbage from restaurants containing trans fatty acids are used for feeds which then actually change the chemistry of the animal meat and, of course, our chemistry when we eat it. I remember 35 years ago standing on a hillside with my neighbor dairy farmer who could name every one of his cows in a 60-head herd from half a mile away. Now, thousands of those cows are raised in an area of the same size but never see a fresh pasture or blade of grass, receiving only chemicalized feed.

It seems like every month there is a report of some new catastrophe of food poisoning. What's your best protection? First of all **freeze all of your meats and poultry** for a few days before thawing and cooking. This at least can kill the bacteria from the emerging onslaught of antibiotic-resistant bugs. For all of the other toxins, Chapter VII will guide you. It's no longer an option. We have to detoxify in order to cure our present ills, and then to stay healthy. It's a totally different world and we are the first experimental generation of an unprecedented and unstudied onslaught of toxins. If you wait for someone to fix it or for some official proclamation of what you should do, it will be too late.

Friendly Gut Bugs Fight Bad Bugs
While They Lower Your Cholesterol

Probiotics are necessary after every antibiotic prescription. Antibiotics invariably upset the balance of good bugs versus bad bugs in the intestines, so you always want to replenish the good bugs with probiotics. Millions of doses of antibiotics are prescribed each year. They may kill the bug you are targeting, but they leave their damage behind. Eight years ago the prestigious *Journal of the American Medical Association* showed that **when doctors fail to prescribe probiotics for patients after antibiotics, their patients have a five-fold increased risk of getting other infections**. And why shouldn't they? For overgrowth of bugs resistant to the antibiotic then cause leaky gut (the cause and cure are described in *No More Heartburn*) which makes for ready access of the nasty putrefied intestinal organisms right into the bloodstream, brain, kidney, liver, coronary blood vessels and every other organ. This ushers in autoimmune diseases, fibromyalgia, depression, polymyalgia rheumatica, chronic fatigue, colitis and much more.

Even worse, this *JAMA* article showed that **when doctors fail to prescribe probiotics after antibiotics, there's a threefold increase in the chance of death**. This is a *300% increase in death because of failure to recommend something that doesn't require a prescription*, is totally harmless and without side effects. But it is not on the hospital formulary because it does not require a prescription. **This is serious negligence of a drug-ruled profession**. We're talking about people's lives. Yet there are rarely probiotics on hospital formularies, and studies confirm the yogurts that are served are dead in terms of Lactobacillus or Bifidus. Do we need a law that doctors have to Rx probiotics?

The lucky patients who do not die can get overgrowth of *Clostridium difficile* in the gut after antibiotics. This bacterium causes a mysteriously intractable life-threatening diarrhea and colitis. Yet the probiotic *Saccharomyces boullardii* produces an enzyme that degrades the Clostridia's toxin. And if the patient takes it right after an antibiotic, he never gets the Clostridium anyway. Of course, probiotics have many other uses like preventing traveler's diarrhea, Candida vaginitis after antibiotics, and naturally improving the health of the whole gut which houses over half the immune system and half the detox system for the entire body. **Probiotics also increase the main antibody for protecting the gut, secretory IgA. This then leads to improved immunity against all sorts of infections** and even against bio-terrorism organisms. For probiotics like Lactobacillus bind to intestinal cells and inhibit the attachment and cell invasion of nasty bugs. **God-given probiotics actually prevent folks from dying from the inside out.**

The **gut has ten times more bacteria than there are cells in the human body** (Gill). Our "good" intestinal bugs do more than just "rot" our food to break it down into absorbable portions. They also rev up the detoxification of the gut lining and power up the gut's immune system. And, **probiotics also help control abnormal cholesterol and LDL** (Anderson, Dambekodi, Sanders). The solution is to periodically restore the good bugs in the gut beginning with a probiotic that supplies multiple beneficial organisms. There are many to chose from. For multiple strains of Lactobacillus I like **Dr. Ohhira's 12 Plus** (realfoodgrocery.com or 1-877-262-7843), and for Saccharomyces and Bifidus plus Lactobacillus, I like **ABx Support** (protherainc.com or 1-888-488-2488).   Use either one of these, 1-4 capsules twice a day between meals for at least a couple of weeks to restore the good flora.

There are many good brands of probiotics, but many inferior as well. For example, some producers will shake up the Petri dish to generate higher colony counts for the label. So to safeguard yourself, **a good test of a probiotic is to take a one-time triple dose**. If you feel like the Pillsbury doughboy with bloat for a few hours, that is a great sign that it is alive and growing in your gut. Also, another test of a good probiotic is after taking a large dose for three or four days your stools should finally smell sweet like baby poop and not like gross adult stools where "a little gas" could empty a shopping mall. Remember, that foul smelling stools cause leaky guts that then actually leak putrefying toxins into the bloodstream, ushering in autoimmune diseases, chronic fatigue, mysterious muscle and joint aches and/or itching or burning skin, fibromyalgia, and more. These gut toxins also use up detox nutrients that could have been used to protect your LDL cholesterol from being oxidized and gluing itself to your arterial wall. Once the gut is healthy, then a high-fiber diet has an easier time of lowering your cholesterol, naturally and safely. Confirmed once again: The road to health is paved with good intestines (No More Heartburn gives all of the directions for diagnosing and healing the leaky gut).

And by the way, don't be intimidated by doctors who are unknowledgeable about the contents of this book and consequently try to make you feel inferior. Stick to your guns until you get yourself well. As an example of **how important the infection connection is for arteriosclerosis**, it was written about over a hundred years ago in mainstream medical journals, plus in 1929 in the Journal of the American Medical Association and has been written about ever since (Ophuls, Frothingham). I could fill a book just on the references alone. I find it disgusting that it continues to be ignored. Why is it ignored?

So How Do We Keep Our Blood Clean?

Step One: The Detox Cocktail

A lot easier than the macrobiotic diet, which is a great detoxifier, is the daily detox cocktail. Since cholesterol is metabolized by our detoxification pathway (cytochromes P-450 via 7-alpha-hydroxylation), the **Detox Cocktail** not only **lowers cholesterol, but also boosts your daily blood and gut detoxification** (Levy). As well, the quicker you empty out the gallbladder plus the more you rev up liver detoxification, the more cholesterol the body can get rid of. That is why combining it with the **Detox Enema**, as described in *Wellness Against All Odds,* also helps to fight infection and lower cholesterol (Danielsson).

The detox cocktail's ingredients could each fill a book with their benefits to the body. In terms of hypercholesterolemia, the vitamin C keeps our arteries clean and protected and "cholesterol-resistant" (Krumdieck, Rath), while the glutathione relaxes, cleanses and heals the blood vessel lining (Prasad). Yet even though these findings were in the *Journal of the American College of Cardiology*, where are the cardiologists who should be recommending something as simple, easy, inexpensive, safe, non-prescription, and protective as the detox cocktail?

Detox Cocktail
Your detoxification booster, the **Detox Cocktail**, contains bare minimum:

- **Klaire Ultrafine Vitamin C Pure Ascorbic Acid Powder** (1-5 grams, depending on individual gut tolerance)
- **R-Lipoic Acid** (300-600 mg)
- **Recancostat** (400-800 mg, a special form of glutathione proven to be orally absorbed and that recycles or regenerates itself via an anthocyanidin) in a big glass of water (details, verifying scientific references, sources and much more are fully covered in *Detoxify or Die*).

Studies show the synergistic effect of these detox nutrients is powerful in aborting not only infections and high cholesterol, but the symptoms of the sick building syndrome, traveler's diarrhea, flus, migraines, inhibiting cancerous gene mutation after a chemical exposure, and much more. Don't forget from Chapter II how vitamin C actually helps lower cholesterol as well as revs up detoxification of our daily chemicals. Resist letting its simplicity fool you. **We should all do the detox cocktail every day forever.** You can double its power with the detox enema, described in *Wellness Against All Odds.* I hesitate to mention it because so many have an aversion to enemas. But in all fairness, I must because so many folks over the years have raved about the results for their health once they got over the psychological barrier and did it. Anyway, it is there for folks who need another easy step toward wellness.

For those who prefer, there are liposomal forms of vitamin C and glutathione to the rescue. Lyposome technology basically is an improved way of getting medications or nutrients inside cells. This is accomplished by wrapping the nutrient in a little microscopic bubble of another nutrient, phosphatidyl choline (that you learned about in the last chapter). Since phosphatidylcholine (PC) is an integral part of the cell membrane, hiding nutrients inside of a tiny microscopic nanometer bubble of PC allows it to be carried into the cell in Trojan horse fashion.

We now have available **Lypo-Spheric Vitamin C** in airtight packets containing 3000 mg of the Essential Phospholipids wrapped around 1000 mg of vitamin C. These essential phospholipids are derived from non-GMO soy and are non-hydrogenated. The dose can be whatever you need, from 1-5 packets spread out through the day, or more (it's great for emergency situations, like aborting infections).

When you use it, be sure to put a quarter cup of filtered water into a cup before you open the package, and then squeeze the contents into the cup. Don't put the lyposomal product in the cup without water for it to float on. Do not try to stir it, because it will not dissolve. It is meant to stay in this form until it gets across the gut lining. So just swig it down. You can use 1 3 packcts of **Lypo-Spheric Vitamin C** 1-3 times a day, as much as you need to bring down your cholesterol and free radical markers, lipid peroxides (available from 1-877-VIT-AMEN).

For liposomal glutathione, there is either **Essential GSH** (1-877-VIT-AMEN with a benzoate preservative) or **LipoCeutical Glutathione** (gshnow.com or 1-650-323-3238 with a glycerol preservative). You might want to reserve these liposomal forms for special cases because of cost and taste, but keep them in mind for possibly improved absorption or cases where you need fast intracellular rescuing with a detox cocktail boost, as in a heart attack. There will be more information in *TW*.

Step Two

In terms of making the immune system stronger to fight off infections, two things are crucial and they will be covered in the next two chapters: having good nutritional levels and getting the toxins out. In previous books and the *TW* newsletters we have detailed many items that are non-prescription that help to boost the immune system's strength and fight off infection. We've given the 800 numbers and web sites of the suppliers plus the scientific backup. If you want one simple recommendation, I would suggest a couple of large squirts of **Kyolic Liquid** down your throat four to six times a day. It has an enormous volume of evidence behind it, most important of which is that it slows down the progression of coronary artery disease by multiple mechanisms. It's an anticoagulant, anti-inflammatory, antioxidant, kills Candida, kills *H. pylori*, lowers cholesterol, reduces hypercoagulability and blood pressure, and much more (Milner, Budoff, Liu, Ide, Rogers). How can you go wrong?

In the Myths Chapter III, I told you about the D.O.C. Ultrafast Heartscan and the coronary calcium score. I want to repeat this because it's so important. **If your calcium score is over 400, you have a 50% chance of a heart attack within the next year** (Davis). **The annual rate of increase in the coronary calcifications score is 39% per year** if you are untreated (Budoff). This means you should have a heart attack in minimum 3 years. Mere progression of your calcium score more than 15% per year is associated with a 13-fold greater risk of having a heart attack each year (Raggi, Budoff). But you can cut this risk down two thirds, because **a huge swig of Kyolic Liquid twice a day is like a triple**

damper on the progression of your coronary artery disease. How can you afford not to do it?

Likewise if you are on a statin drug and an aspirin, your plaque volume increases 129% (+/- 102%) per year. But if you add Kyolic, it drops dramatically to a volume increase of 45% (+/- 57%) per year. Bear in mind that the large +/- variation is because there is a huge variability among individuals, especially in regard to their other contributing factors (each person's diet, nutrients, toxins, knowledge, reading commitment and implementation, etc.).

Clearly, the healing of all ailments must begin with a healthy, clean gut. To keep the gut clean, I would recommend five days every month a huge tablespoon of **Organic Green Barley Grass** in a large glass of water. You can even do it several times a day if you have particularly foul smelling stools. Chlorophyll is one of nature's best gut detoxifiers.

Yeasts to the Rescue?

There are so many ways to enhance the power of the immune system to fight this daily onslaught of infectious organisms, that we'll just take a quick look at one category, beta-glucans (since enhancing the immune system could take a whole book by itself, there has been and will continue to be more in *TW* on this subject).

'
First let me caution you that if you have fallen for any of the biological response modifiers so flagrantly advertised on TV and in magazines, forget it. They are more dangerous than steroids, as they are a concentrate of one of the most potent parts. Hidden under such names as Enbrel, Remicade and Humira (with new ones emerging continually), they are TNF or **tumor necrosis factor inhibitors**. By poisoning one of God's factors made in our blood to fight cancer, they actually **raise your risk of cancer and infection,** as their black box warnings indicate. They are prescribed for arthritis, psoriasis, colitis, and other inflammatory conditions. If

you have already taken some of these dangerous drugs and poisoned your tumor necrosis factor, you need to boost it back up. And you should want to boost it anyway, since we are all vulnerable to the bugs you just learned about.

How can you do that? You can boost the potency of the immune system by super-charging the white blood cells (macrophages) with yeasts! Yes, yeasts have good benefits. One of the cell wall components of yeast is beta glucan. And if properly prepared, can repair or boost the immune system without undesirable yeast allergy effects.

God designed the body in unfathomably clever ways that we will never fully appreciate. One way that the immune system is boosted to keep us fighting off daily invasions is by stimulating (turning on) receptor (docking) sites on the outside surface of white blood cells. When yeast fragments fit into these docking sites, they trigger the white blood cells of our immune system to make more cytokines, proteins that fight infection, like TNF (tumor necrosis factor). In order to turn on these receptors on white cells, there has to be a steady exposure to antigens or substances to trigger this. What better way than with the many fungi we are unavoidably exposed to? For fungi are necessary parts of life. They turn everything "from ashes to ashes", for if it were not for fungi degrading dead plants and animal life, we would be up to our eyeballs in refuse and there would be no life on earth.

One manufacturer uses beta-glucan from the cell wall of the bread yeast, *Saccharomyces,* to boost our infection fighting macrophages. But they first sonicate (bounce sound waves off the yeast) to bring it to a small enough molecular size to fit into the B-glucan receptors on the surface of the white cell in order to turn them on. I have not seen comparable research by any other company that makes B-glucan, nor has anyone compared the effects of competing brands which derive their beta-glucans from different sources or use different manufacturing techniques. The jury is still out on which is superior. But voluminous studies from Harvard, The Medical School of Tulane and others prove for sure that these fragments from yeasts and plants can super-charge the immune system and in particular prime the white blood cells to fight infection more powerfully than usual. Let's look at 3 types.

NSC-100 Extra Strength Formula is 10 mg of micro-particulate beta glucan from a proprietary method for making the small 1-2 μ size beta glucan. Why is this important? It is the same size as the beta glucan receptors on white blood cells (called macrophages) for fighting off infection. You'll find lots of other brands of beta-glucan with much higher doses, but they may not be useful if they clump together in the acidic environment of the stomach and pass right through the digestive tract without getting absorbed. And they may be too big to fit into the white blood cell docking sites to turn on infection-fighting cytokines if they did get in.

You may want to boost your immune system with a trial of **NSC-100 Extra Strength Formula**, 1-2, twice a day, if you have, for example, resistant Candida, a troublesome tooth (in which case I would definitely add the **Lumen** (that you will learn about in Chapter VII, since it has incomparable infection-fighting ability to rescue without antibiotics, extraction or root canal, more details are found in *TW* 2007). You might also want to keep **NSC-100 Extra Strength Formula** on hand for the flu season, especially since you now know that seemingly innocuous infections like Chlamydia can masquerade as colds and bronchitis. And once it gains entry into the vascular system, it may hide there for years before wreaking coronary havoc. Don't forget that the majority of our environmental chemicals have a hidden side effect of also damaging or at least weakening the immune system. **NSC-100 Extra Strength Formula** is one tool to consider keeping in your non-drug emergency drug box to boost the immune system, making it more efficient at thwarting inflammation and stronger at fighting off infection.

Alternatively, one (of many) studies by Harvard Medical School researchers showed mice were protected against lethal peritonitis from E. coli or Staphylococcus using a different manufacturing source of beta glucan, now sold as **Life Source Basics**. In other studies it even had strong protective effects against agents of bioterrorism agents like anthrax, and they have sponsored a vast amount of research, spawning patents as well. Use 1-3 capsules per day for immune system boosting and compare.

Because beta-glucan is such a powerful immune stimulant, I give you a third and highly purified form, and yet again backed by studies and referenced. **Beta-1, 3-D Glucan** can be used as 1-2 capsules two to three times a day for starters. As I say, no one has compared all 3 of these different forms side by side to determine which gives the best immune stimulation; so once more we are the experimental generation. There is one study but it omits the NSC type in its comparison. The one that came out on top was the last form mentioned, **Beta-1, 3-D Glucan** (Vetvicka). The science behind the beta-glucan neutraceuticals (which sport a variety of manufacturing differences in the market) is too convincing to ignore as an immune system booster. Clearly the best proof of which product is best for you is in the absence of infection or dropping of some barometer of infection, like your hsCRP or fibrinogen.

Using the Lab to Bail You Out

One very serious sign of a bad gut with hidden toxins is an elevated fibrinogen (Patel). You should hope that the infection is in the gut, because that is a lot easier to heal than if you have to search for the needle in the haystack, looking for an infected tooth, sinus, bone, lung abscess, or vasculitis (infection in the blood vessels, like the coronaries) from Chlamydia, as examples. If there are also elevated lipid peroxides, hsCRP, or evidence of gene damage as with an elevated 8-OhdG, these are bad signs. But if they are accompanied by elevated organic acids that suggest evidence of bad bugs in the gut, you are in luck, for it helps narrow your search and point you in the direction to reverse these bad warning signs. All of these tests and more are in your **Cardio/ION**.

The various organic acids provide oodles of clues. As an example, elevated D-arabinitol suggests infection with yeast, usually Candida. Dihydroxyphenylpropionate suggests Clostridia. Elevated **tricarballyate** suggest a bacterium that also acts like a claw and **chelates out your magnesium**, making it difficult to maintain healthful levels until the bug is killed. **Indican indicates bugs** in the upper small intestine **that can damage pancreatic function** and other digestive juices. There is much more to be learned from these gut organic acids. All of the above tests and more are included in your, yes, you guessed it, **Cardio/ION** (MetaMetrix). Are you beginning to appreciate why I call it a crystal ball test?

Use any of the above products and clean out the gut. If you are not successful, you may need to actually identify the exact bugs in the gut to know how to get rid of them. I like the best stool study for identifying live bugs and so easy to do at home, the **Comprehensive Stool with Purged Parasites** (CSPP, Doctors' Data). I like to combine it with the next test for tough cases.

If the gut issue is not solved, the **GI fx** test (MetaMetrix) is unique among gut tests. With most tests you collect stool and it is shipped to the lab, being bounced around and exposed to various temperature changes. This causes some bacteria to grow more rapidly than others and seed themselves, giving fictitiously higher colony counts for some, while smothering out the growth of others, resulting in an erroneous estimation of the prevalence of each bug. This yields higher counts for some bugs than there actually were in your gut, and lower or no counts at all for the bugs that were stifled or smothered by the fast growers.

To avoid this misinterpretation, for the **GI fx** test you put your stool right away into formaldehyde, thereby killing everything. When it reaches the lab, the DNA of organisms is measured, not a possibly fictitious colony count. This gives a much more accurate representation of the bugs that are present in your stool and in which amounts. And you will be able to identify bugs that with other stool culture techniques were smothered by faster growing types and therefore never seen. Just have your doctor, chiropractor or naturopath order the **GI fx** test, and/or CSPP above, collect your stool at home, and call FedEx for easy return.

And one more point. If you have Candida, for example, that is resistant to treatment, be sure to check the protocols in *No More Heartburn* (it covers the entire gut). Furthermore, if any bug is still resistant, heavy metals like mercury can make bugs resistant to any eradication attempts (Summers). Follow the protocols in *The High Blood Pressure Hoax* to get rid of the heavy metals. Chapter VII here will get you started.

The bottom line is that if you have coronary artery disease and someone has merely started you on a statin and never looked at your gut and other sources of infection, especially if you have further evidence of hidden infection like an elevated hsCRP, fibrinogen, lipid peroxides, or gut-related organic acids, you have not had a complete evaluation and have been grossly short-changed.

Busy Executive Summary

Infection is a common cause of arteriosclerosis. Start with the detox cocktail and other adjuncts to keep the blood cleaner. Diagnosis includes blood antibodies and stool tests. But above all, don't ignore the gut, especially if there are any symptoms, since some folks will never heal what they have, cholesterol elevation, coronary artery disease, or anything else, until the gut is first healed. Housing half the immune system and half the detox system for the entire body, a sick gut can hold back progress indefinitely.

Sources for this Chapter's Recommendations

- PerioPaste, Hydro Floss, PerioScript, docharrison.com, 1-800-650-9060
- Kyolic Liquid, wakunaga.com, 1-800-421-2998
- Organic Green Barley Grass, livingfoodsusa.com, 785-856-0701
- Mastic Gum, jarrow.com, or 1-877-VIT-AMEN
- Dr. Ohhira's 12 Plus, realfoodgrocery.com, or 1-877-262-7843, or 1-877-VIT-AMEN
- ABx Support, protherainc.com, 1-888-488-2488
- GI fx, Cardio/ION, metametrix.com, 1-800-221-4640
- Comprehensive Stool with Purged Parasites, doctorsdata.com, 1-800-323-2784
- Klaire Ultrafine Pure Ascorbic Acid Powder, protherainc.com, 1-888-488-2488
- Recancostat, integrativeinc.com, 1-800-917-3690
- R-Lipoic Acid, intensivenutrition.com, 1-800-333-7414
- Lypo-Spheric Vitamin C, livonlabs.com, 1-866-682-6193, or 1-877-VIT-AMEN
- Essential GSH, 1-877-VIT-AMEN
- LipoCeutical Glutathione, gshnow.com, 650-323-3238
- NSC-100 Extra Strength Formula, nsc24.com, 1-888-541-3997
- Life Source Basics, lifesourcebasics.com, 1-877-346-6863
- Beta-1, 3-D Glucan, transferpoint.com, 1-877-407-3999

References:

Prasad A, Andrews NP, Padder FA, et al, Glutathione reverses endothelial dysfunction and improves nitric oxide bioavailability, *J Am Cardiol*, 34: 507-14, 1999

Krumdieck C, et al, Ascorbate-cholesterol-lecithin interactions: factors of potential importance in the pathogenesis of atherosclerosis, *Am J Clin Nutr*, 27: 866-876, Aug 1974

Rath M, Pauling L, Hypothesis: lipoprotein(a), is a surrogate for ascorbate, *Proc Natl Acad Sci USA*, 87: 6204-07, August 1990

Kugiyama K, et al, Intracoronary infusion of reduced glutathione improved endothelial vasomotor response to acetylcholine in human coronary circulation, *Circulation*, 97: 2299-2301, 1998

Usal A, et al, **Decreased glutathione levels in acute myocardial infarction**, *Jpn Heart J*, 37: 1 77-1 82, 1996

Heuser C, Vojdani A, Enhancement of natural killer cell activity and T and B cell function by buffered vitamin C (ultra potent-C), in patients exposed to toxic chemicals: the role of protein kinase-C, *Immunopharmacol Immunotoxicol*, 19:291, 1997

Lenton KJ, Therriault H, Wagner JR, et al, Glutathione and ascorbate are negatively correlated with oxidative DNA damage in human lymphocytes, *Carcinogenesis*, 20; 4: 607-613, 1999

Meister A, Glutathione-ascorbic acid antioxidant system in animals, *J Biol Chem* 269: 9397-9400, 1994

Gupta P, Kar A, Role of ascorbic acid in cadmium-induced thyroid dysfunction and lipid peroxidation, *J Appl Tox*, 18: 317-320, 1998

Ophuls W, Arteriosclerosis and cardiovascular disease: And their relation to infectious diseases, *J Am Med Assoc*, 76:700-7 01, 1921

Frothingham C, Relation between acute infectious diseases and arterial lesions, *Arch Intern Med*, 8: 153-162, 1911

Ross R, Atherosclerosis-----and inflammatory disease, *New Engl J Med*, 340:115-126, 1999

van der Wal AC, et al, Site of intimal rupture or erosion of thrombosed coronary atherosclerotic plaques is characterized by an inflammatory process irrespective of the dominant plaque morphology, *Circul*, 89:306-44, 1994

McWhinney VGA, Pond WG, Mersmann HJ, Ontogeny and Dietary Modulation of 3-Hydroxy-3-Methylglutaryl-CoA Reductase Activities in Neonatal Pigs, *J Animal Sci*, 74: 2203-10, 1996

Kountouras J, Mylopoulos N, Venizelos J, et al, Eradication of *Helicobacter pylori* may be beneficial in the management of chronic open-angle glaucoma, *Arch Intern Med*, 162: 1237-1244, 2002

Steinberg K, Arthasarathy S, Witztum JL, et al, Beyond cholesterol: Modification of low-density lipoprotein that increase its atherogenicity, *N Eng. J Med*, 320:915-24, 1989

Cox DA, Cophen ML, Effects of oxidized low-density lipoprotein on vascular contraction and relaxation: Clinical and pharmacological implications in atherosclerosis, *Pharmacol Rev*, 48:3-19, 1996

Meyer M, Is this the drug for you? Doctors say millions more should take cholesterol drugs -- but are there risks?, *AARP Bulletin*, 20-21, Nov. 2002

McKay B, Caution is prescribed for antibiotics. U.S. agency moves to urge doctors and patients to use treatments in moderation, *Wall Street Journal*, D11, Sept. 17, 2003

Williams JE, *Viral Immunity*, Hampton Roads Publ., (1-800-7665-8009) Charlottesville VA, 2002

Patel P, Carrington D, Strachean DP, Leatham E, Goggin P, Northfield TC, Mendall MA, **Fibrinogen: a link between chronic infection and coronary heart disease**, *Lancet*, 343; 1634-5, June 25, 1994

Kusters JG, Kuipers EJ, Helicobacter and atherosclerosis, *Am Heart J,* 1999 Nov, 138(5 pt 2): S523-7

Mendell MA, Goggin PM, Moineaux N, et al, Relation of Helicobacter pylori infection and coronary heart disease, *Brit Heart J,* 71:437-39, 1994

Mendall MA, Goggin PM, Molineaux N, et al, Childhood living conditions and *Helicobacter pylori* seropositivity in adult life, *Lancet,* 339:896-7, 1992

Danesh J, Koreth J, Roskell D, et al, Is Helicobacter pylori a factor in coronary atherosclerosis? *J Clin Microbiol,* 1999 May, 37; 5:1651

Rogers SA, *No More Heartburn*, 2000, prestigepublishing.com or 1-800-846-6687

Elmer GW, Surawicz CM, McFarland LV, Biotherapeutic agents, a neglected modality for the treatment and prevention of selected intestinal and vaginal infections, *J Am Med Assoc,* 275: 870-876, 1996

Salminen E, Elomaa I, Salminen S, et al, Preservation of intestinal integrity during radiotherapy using live *Lactobacillus acidophilus* cultures, *Clin Radiol,* 39: 435-437, 1988

Hensley S, Side effect concerns grow for drugs to treat rheumatoid arthritis, D1, *Wall Street Journal,* May 17, 2006

Hamilton DP, New treatments for rheumatoid arthritis, *Wall St J,* Jun 20, 2006, D1, D4

Bao B, Prasad AS, Beck FWJ, Godmere M, Zinc modulates mRNA levels of cytokines, *Am J Physiol Endocrinol Metab*, 285:1095-1102, 2003

Periodontal References:
Beck, et al, Periodontal disease and cardiovascular disease, *J Perio*, 67; 1:1123-37, 1996

Dorn, et al, Invasion of human coronary artery cells by periodontal pathogens, *Infect Immun,* 67; 11:5792-98, 1999

Matilla, et al, Dental infection and the risk of new coronary events: Prospective study of patients with documented coronary artery disease, *Clin Infect Dis,* 20; 3:588-92, 1995

Edlund, et al, Resistance of the normal human microflora to mercury and anti-microbials after exposure to mercury from dental amalgam fillings, *Clin Infect Dis*, 22; 6:944-50, 1996

Summers A, et al, Mercury released from dental "silver" fillings provokes an increase in mercury- and antibiotic-resistant bacteria in oral and intestinal floras of primates, *Antimicrob Agents Chemother*, 37; 4:825-34, 1993

Joshipura KJ, Poor oral health and coronary heart disease, *J Dent Res*, 75; 9"1631-6, 1996

Iacopino, et al, Pathophysiological relationships between periodontitis and systemic disease: Recent concepts involving serum lipids, *J Periodont,* 71; 8:1375-84, 2000

Haraszthy, et al, Identification of periodontal pathogens in atheromatous plaques, *J Periodontol,* 71; 10:1554-60, 1999

Matilla, et al, Dental infections as a risk factor for acute myocardial infarction, *Eur Heart J,* 14; supp; K: 51-3, 1993

Scannapieco F, et al, Association of periodontal infections with atherosclerotic and pulmonary diseases, *J Perio Res*, 34; 7:340-45, 1999

Demmer RT, et al, Periodontal infections and cardiovascular disease: the heart of the matter, *J Am Dental Assoc*, 137 supp; 14S-20S, Oct 2006

Noack B, et al, Periodontal infections contribute to elevated C-reactive protein level, *J Periodontal,* 72; 9:1221-27, Sep 2001

Chlamydia References:
Vojdani A, A look at infectious agents as a possible causative factor in cardiovascular disease: part II, *Lab Med,* 4; 34: 5-9, April 2003

Bachmaier K, et al, Chlamydia infections and heart disease linked through antigenic mimicry, *Sci,* 5406; 283: 1335-39, Feb 26, 1999

Linnanmaki E, et al, Chlamydia pneumoniae---Specific Circulating Immune Complexes in Patients with Chronic Coronary Heart Disease, *Circulation,* 87:1130-30 4, 1993

Muhlestrin JB, et al, Increased incidence of Chlamydia species within the coronary arteries of patients with symptomatic atherosclerotic versus other forms of cardiovascular disease, *J Am Coll Cardiol*, 27:1555-61, 1996

Gupta S, et al, The effect of azithromycin in post-myocardial infarction patients with elevated Chlamydia pneumoniae antibody titers, *J Am Coll Cardiol,* 29:209 a, 1997

Gupta S, et al, Elevated Chlamydia pneumoniae antibodies, cardiovascular events, and azithromycin in male survivors of myocardial infarction, *Circulation*, 96:404-07, 1997

Gurfinkel E, ifich G, et al, for the ROXIS study group. Randomized trial of roxithromycin in non-Q-wave coronary syndromes, *Lancet,* 350:444-407, 1997

Buggy Meat References:
Sapkota AR, et al, What do we feed to food-production animals? A review of animal feed ingredients and their potential impacts on human health, *Environ Health Persp*, 115; 5: 663-70, 2007

Price LB, et al, The persistence of fluoroquinolones-resistant Campylobacter in poultry production, *Environ Health Persp*, 150:1035-39, 2007

Osby L, Serious infection won't be tracked by hospitals, Dangerous Staph cases don't yet need to be reported by health facilities, 1C, *The Greenville News,* Greenville South Carolina, July 1, 2007

Antibiotic-resistant Staph more common B5, *Wall Street J*, June 25, 2007

Probiotic References:
Anderson JW, Gilliland DE, Effect of fermented milk (yogurt) containing Lactobacillus acidophilus L1 on serum cholesterol in hypercholesterolemic humans, *J Am Coll Nutr*, 1;18:43-50, 1999

Dambekidi PC, Gilliland SE, Incorporation of cholesterol into the cellular membrane of Bifidbacterium longum, *J Dairy Sci*, 81:1818-24, 1998

Sanders ME, Considerations for use of probiotic bacterial to modulate human health, *J Nutr,* 130; 384s-90s, 2000

Gill HS, Guarner F, Probiotics and human health: a clinical perspective, *Post grad Med J,* 80:516-26, 2004

Beta-Glucan References:
Blaylock, R, Yeast B1, 3-glucan and its use against anthrax infection and in the treatment of cancer, *J Am Neutraceut Assoc,* 5;2, Spring 2002

Onderdonk AB, et al., Anti-infective effect of poly-B1-6-glucotriosyl-B1-3-glucopyranose glucan in vivo, *Infect Immun,* 1642-47, Apr. 1992

Berner MD, Sura ME, Alves BN, Hunter KW, IFN-y primes macrophages for enhanced TNF-a expression in response to stimulatory and non-stimulatory amounts of microparticulate B-glucan, *Immunol Lett,* 98:115-22, 2005

Hunter KW, Gault RA, Berner MD, Preparation of micro-particulate B-glucan from *Saccharomyces cerevisiae* for use in immune potentiation, *Lett Appl Microbiol,* 35-4:267-71, Oct 2002

Lee DY, Ji IH, Kim CW, et al, High-level TNF-secretion and macrophage activity with soluble B-glucans from *Saccharomyces cerevisiaae, Biosci Biotechnol Biochem,* 66:233-8, 2002

Hoffman OA, Olson EJ, Limper AH, Fungal B-glucans modulate macrophage release of tumor necrosis factor in response to bacterial lipopolysaccharide, *Immunol Lett,* 37:19-25, 1993

Vetvicka V, et al, An Evaluation of the immunological activites of commercially available B1, 3-glucans, *J Am Neutraceut Assoc,* 10; 1:25-31, 2007

Kyolic References:
See End of Chapters II and IV

239

Chapter VI

The Nutrient Connection

The *Journal of the American Medical Association* **urges docs to learn about, ask about, and prescribe nutrients for chronic diseases.**

I continually hear, " My doctor insists there is not enough evidence for using vitamins yet. How can I convince him?"

My answer could fill volumes (and has), but let's see what we can convince him with for starters. It is pretty sad how the pharmaceutical industry has controlled medicine. As an example, the February 2002 *Journal of the American Medical Association* showed that for the vast majority of physicians making up the rules or recipes that physicians are supposed to follow for every disease (called the practice guidelines of medicine), **87% of these "experts" were found to be financially connected to the pharmaceutical industry.** No wonder every symptom turns out to be a deficiency of the latest drug. No wonder finding the underlying cause and cure is frowned upon. That's bad for the drug industry's bottom line. And no wonder the media is frequently reporting on the worthlessness of some nutrient when the shoddy "science" is funded by the pharmaceutical industry. Not only have I shown you some of the evidence, but the past editor of *The New England Journal of Medicine*, heads of medical school departments, congressman and others have much more carefully documented this control of medicine (Angell, Cohen, Epstein, Haley, Breggin, Glenmullen, Moore, Richards, *TW*).

In defense of nutrients, plenty of research shows that not only can **many diseases be prevented, but also they can be cured by nutrients**. And since we are the first generation of man to ever eat so many processed foods lower in nutrients and grown on depleted soils, **nutrient deficiencies are epidemic**. In addition, **this is the** first generation of man to ever be exposed to so many chemi-**cals** in our everyday lives. **The work of detoxifying these chemicals also uses up nutrients.** I've reference all of this heavily in past books and newsletters showing that taking supplemental nutrients is absolutely essential for health in this era.

I like to quote from a paper from the prestigious University of California at Berkeley, Dept. of Biochemistry and Molecular Biology. "High levels of vitamins have been used to successfully treat many human genetic diseases." (My gosh! You mean we can stop blaming our genes?) " The **therapeutic vitamin regimens work by** increasing intercellular coenzyme concentrations, stimulating a defective enzyme and thereby **alleviating the primary defect and curing the disease**."

Furthermore, "**diseases involving dysfunctional enzymes can be remedied by <u>high levels of the vitamin</u> component of the enzyme**" (Liu). Translation: some people, by nature of their individual biochemistry, **need much higher levels of nutrients than others in order to correct their** (genetic and/or acquired) **deficiencies. Standard or RDA levels will not do the trick.** And don't forget the "norms" for blood tests are not the values for best health. They are population norms, meaning this is where the ranges for most folks fall, folks who eat junk food, who know little about health, and are unknowingly the "walking wounded" or an accident waiting to happen. These are the folks who two-thirds of which are overweight, a quarter of whom have hypertension, arthritis, fatigue, heart disease, high cholesterol, or other diseases. But they just hire a drug-prescriber and go on their merry ways.

This article beautifully shows physicians how **vitamins are absolutely essential for turning off diseases.** It is only through ignorance of the molecular biochemistry that a physician would fail to assay for or prescribe nutrients. And what monumental savings in medical costs and lives are possible! But nutrients can only be prescribed if docs stop being sold the idea that every symptom is a deficiency of some drug. Instead they could learn the real medicine (nutritional and environmental molecular biochemistry) of healing.

In other equally recent papers in the *Journal of the American Medical Association,* it was clearly outlined how **"suboptimal intake of some vitamins, above levels causing classic vitamin deficiencies, is a risk factor for chronic diseases and common in the general population"**. Translation? <u>It is common for folks with chronic diseases to need nutrient doses higher than the doses classically used to alleviate deficiency symptoms.</u> In other words, just because 50 mg of vitamin C might cure someone's scurvy has no bearing on the fact that you may need 2000 mg to keep cholesterol from oxidizing and clinging to your arterial walls. Furthermore, this JAMA paper went on to emphatically state, **"Physicians should make specific effort to learn about their patients' use of vitamins to ensure that they are taking the vitamins they should,"** (Fletcher).

The authors go on to reaffirm that **"Many physicians may be unaware... or unsure which vitamins they should recommend for their patients. Inadequate intake of several vitamins has been linked to chronic diseases, including <u>coronary heart disease,</u> cancer, and osteoporosis.** The vitamins are organic compounds that cannot be synthesized by humans and therefore **must be ingested** to prevent metabolic disorders." In case any physician readers did not get the message, they went on further: **"Physicians need to be informed about available preparations and prepared to counsel their patients"** (Fairfield). I don't know how much planer it can be, and right out of the journals that are quoted every week for reporting on some new drug that drives the stock market. **Clearly, it's inferior medicine to fail to assess and prescribe nutrients for all symptoms.**

And these two papers were only talking about vitamins, ignoring minerals, fatty acids, amino acids, and orphan nutrients. And how can anyone evaluate your nutrient status without blood tests? **They do not check your cholesterol without a blood test, or your diabetes without a blood test. They don't check your liver or kidney function without a blood test. How come they are suddenly clairvoyant and don't need to look at your vitamins, minerals and fatty acids? Nutrients are the very backbone of health that separate us from disease.**

Even **cardiac transplant patients who take 500 mg of vitamin C and 400 I. U. of vitamin E each twice a day slow down the progression of arteriosclerosis an incredible *10-fold*.** No medication has this kind of power to delay restenosis (reclotting) of (new) blood vessels, which is the leading cause of death during the first year after cardiac transplant (Stein).

It will be a long time before you hear this news on TV, because it does not make any money for the drug industry. But it certainly points out what we've said all along, that you should be on guided nutritional treatment every day. Why wait until you need a heart transplant to delay aging of your heart's blood vessels?

No, the evidence for nutritional medicine is overwhelming, but the drug industry rules medicine. It would take volumes to show the evidence for turning back the hands of time and reversing blood vessel damage by simple vitamin C (Richartz, Levy, Rogers) or cod liver oil in people with high cholesterol (Chin, Goodfellow). And these examples are in leading cardiology journals! Fortunately, you do not have to be deprived of up-to-date state-of-the-art medicine. You can find physicians who attend courses, read and are fascinated by getting you well through molecular biochemistry, by finding what is broken and fixing it, once and for all. In *TW*, you will find questions you can innocently ask to secretly tell you where the doc you are interviewing stands on the knowledge scale. And in the chapters to follow, I'll give you other guidelines that will enable you to tell the knowledgeable from the rest. Your life depends on these surreptitious physician evaluations. Meanwhile, when will it be malpractice to fail to prescribe vitamins?

Pennies Worth of Nutrients Reverse "Incurable" Conditions

Nutrient deficiencies are epidemic and the rule, not the exception, as I've referenced *ad nauseam* elsewhere. So for the unconvinced, I'd like to give you an idea of the unappreciated power of simple, but knowledgeable nutrient corrections. We've all had the misfortune to witness the humiliating devastation that Alzheimer's brings to the end of life. What would you say the chances of reversing Alzheimer's would be in an 87 year old who has not been unable to care for himself for years? Most all physicians would say," Slim to none". Wrong!

A group of patients in their 70s and 80s was studied because the patients had two things in common: (1) they had an elevated blood test for homocysteine, and (2) they had progressively lost their memories with senile dementia. They couldn't remember simple things, they got lost trying to find their way home, or couldn't even leave home, they were often confused and basically had to have someone else looking after them at all times. They essentially were in the category of "warehoused" humans, needing 24 x 7 custodial care, just like an infant.

The great thing about this study was that their family doctor didn't give up. In medicine usually B12 and folic acid deficiencies are not looked for unless someone has an anemia, specifically a macrocytic anemia (cells become overly large hanging around the bone marrow waiting for the missing nutrients that are not about to come). An interesting part of this whole study was that none of these patients had the typical macrocytic anemia, thus increasing their chances of the deficiencies being missed. But that didn't stop this physician from looking for a curable cause (and actually Harvard's Dr. Lindenbaum warned about this years ago).

Another thing is that most doctors don't look for homocysteine elevations in older people, because they figure they've outlived the norm, so why look at preventive medicine factors. But this doctor was not your average doctor and he looked for elevated homocysteine and found it. It has been known to cause not only early heart attacks and cancers, but also many other problems like brain shrinkage or atrophy as well as Alzheimer's and other types of senile dementias (mind loss).

This physician was also smarter than most because he didn't just settle for a normal B12 or folic acid blood level. Even though the blood levels were normal, he gave these folks a trial of them. Of course, that is one reason why the **Organic Acids** in the **ION Panel** are so important, for they will spot deficiencies that are missed if the blood tests for circulating levels of nutrients are normal. Organic Acids (part of the Cardio/ION) show when you have a functional deficiency of a nutrient. In other words, **it shows if you are one of the folks who need higher levels than normal** for a specific nutrient in order for your body to heal, **even though your blood level for that nutrient may look normal.**

This is very important because docs unknowledgeable in or new to learning about nutritional medicine naively think that a normal blood level, of say a serum or plasma B12, means you don't need any more. But as you will see, **finding that this person needs more than the average in order to heal could mean the difference between living as a warehoused person or as an independent person.** So when these folks did not improve with B12 or folic acid, this physician still did not give up, but went another step further and looked for something else that might be able to improve the chemistry of these folks, and he found it.

N-Acetyl Cysteine or **NAC** is the rate limiting amino acid the body uses to make glutathione, the detoxifier that's in your detox cocktail (that you will learn more about in the next chapter). Glutathione is needed to not only detoxify the body, but also to lower homocysteine as well as to convert B-12 into a useful form to lower homocysteine. In addition, **NAC has actually made the body dump out homocysteine into the urine** and thereby get rid of this toxic amino acid that accelerates aging and brain deterioration (McCaddon, Sachdev, Adair).

The bottom line to this fantastic paper is that it is a perfect, yet simple, example that shows **we should NEVER give up on the elderly just because they have lost their memories or minds.** Some of the folks in this study were **as old as 84 and 87 and they got better.** They got their minds back, many were **able to live independently again with no supervision** or caretaker, and some even **got their drivers' licenses back!** These are folks that medicine had basically discarded into the nursing home dump. Medicine tends to give up when it comes to the elderly and is sloppy in neglecting to look at nutrient deficiencies in general, but instead starts throwing a lot of expensive prescription drugs into a body chemistry that is already deficient. That's when you kill folks off quicker with the more drugs you pile on, especially when they are older and more depleted. This brings on an avalanche of mysterious symptoms before they die.

If you or someone you love has started going downhill with brain rot, at least do a trial of the sublingual B12 in the form of **Methylcobalamin 5mg** and **Folixor 5m**, one each a day dissolved under the tongue, as well as 1-2 **NAC** 500 mg or 800 mg glutathione in the form of **Liposomal GSH** or **LipoCeutical Glutathione** or **Recancostat** (see Chapter III and more in this chapter for the other nutrients). You have a lot of options to choose from. And if you remember nothing else from this, remember to **never give up on any condition until you've properly looked at all the chemistry, or more precisely, someone who knows enough body chemistry has been consulted.**

These folks in their last decades were given their minds, freedom, independence, dignity and lives back with just pennies of nutrients a day (McCaddon, Sachdev, Maurath, Adair, Lietha). But current medicine directives would have thrown them away. They would have been warehoused in a nursing home forever, waiting to die. All of the clues for this vital brain-restoring information and more are in your **Cardio/ION Panel**. And this article with all its references was originally in our monthly newsletter of 18 years, *Total Wellness*, to give you an example of the priceless life-saving, practical and referenced information you get for a dollar a week. You can't afford to be without it.

Meanwhile, I hope you get the bottom line: **Never give up until a true biochemical assessment and expert interpretation have been done**. You will amaze yourself with the healing power that God designed, yet current medicine is totally in the dark with.

Vitamins C & E Reverse the Effect of a High Fat Meal

Worried when you eat "wrong" that you could trigger a heart attack? You should be, for a high fat meal raises your risk of a heart attack within the next few hours. Scientists needed a standard easily accessible high fat meal to do their study on. They chose one available to millions, containing 900 calories with 50 grams of fat and 225 mg cholesterol. They chose a McDonald's Egg McMuffin, Sausage McMuffin, and 2 hash browns.

Compared with the group that took no vitamins, another group took a mere **1000 mg of vitamin C and 800 I.U. of vitamin E** before the meal. The amazing results? By taking only vitamins C and E, folks **cut their heart attack rate by 28%** (measured as vascular constriction) (Plotnick). Now that is nutrient power. Think what you can do with even more nutrients that are balanced and tailored to the individual. In Chapter II, I showed you the power of vitamins C and E in regulating cholesterol. Just make sure that you now put this information to use and take these (extra) doses after a high fat meal.

Merely 2 Vitamins Save Lives in ICU

Every once in a while I see another article that gets plastered over the media showing that we don't need nutrients or antioxidants. But the evidence is so overwhelmingly just the opposite that I think it should border on malpractice to fail to give nutrients (more evidence in June 2003 *TW*). The only reason it's not malpractice is because **the definition of malpractice is based on what everybody else is doing, not on what the scientific evidence shows we should be doing.** Some system, huh? And you thought it was based on science! No, it's based on finance and control.

But let's get you even more armed with some irrefutable evidence to get you prepared for the day when you might need it. For starters, in a leading cardiology journal, studies show that the ability to form blood clots leading to a heart attack or stroke is greater in patients who already have had heart attacks or strokes. Patients who have known hypertension or coronary artery calcifications and plaque are at much greater risk of earlier heart attacks and strokes. Yet inexpensive *vitamin C actually reversed the blood vessel abnormalities that would cause another heart attack and stroke.* This makes a lot more sense than an aspirin which cannot reverse all of these vascular changes, and as I showed the evidence for in Chapter II, is based on the erroneous interpretation of one drug-funded study, using a magnesium-containing aspirin (as a buffer). Furthermore, you recall that aspirin doubles your risk of stroke and causes leaky gut, which then goes on to cause auto-immune diseases like arthritis, fibromyalgia, multiple sclerosis, lupus, as just a few examples, plus poor absorption of nutrients, joint deterioration, and much more.

In an even more important study of 595 people in ICU (intensive care unit of the hospital) who had had accidents and surgery, they were randomized into two groups. One group was merely given vitamin E and vitamin C along with the standard care versus the other group that was given the standard care but no nutrients (as are most ICU patients to this day). The **folks who had the pennies of nutrients were remarkably healthier, and got out of the hospital quicker**. **They had fewer deaths, less organ failure** like dying from acute respiratory distress syndrome, which is common in this scenario, and they had a shorter ICU length of stay, which means less money and less chance of dying from infection, arrhythmias and other complications. **We're talking pennies worth of therapy, not rocket science that makes a difference between thousands of dollars, not to mention the increased chance of dying.**

This monumental paper from the _Annals of Surgery_ should just by itself be enough evidence that **it should be considered malpractice to neglect to prescribe at least vitamins C and E to every patient in the intensive care unit**. First of all, it cut the chance of dying from lung failure from 40% to 19%. Without the 2 vitamins there was a triple chance of organ death like death of the lung, heart, brain, kidney or liver. And once one of these organs dies, the patient is pretty much certain to die shortly, and all because two inexpensive vitamins were not prescribed. There was a startling **57% decrease in organ death just from prescribing two inexpensive vitamins.**

Put another way, **the overall chance of dying in ICU dropped in half, from 81% to 43% by giving two inexpensive vitamins.** No drug does this. This in itself should be enough evidence for insurance companies and hospital formularies to insist that nutrients be given to patients sick enough to be in ICU, especially if it's from accidents and other forms of trauma as well as post-surgery, like these 595 patients were. Yet nutrients of this caliber are not even in most hospital pharmacies, not available for doctors to order, and patients are not allowed to bring nutrients from home (although I know many who attribute their successful healing to smuggled nutrients from home).

If that were not enough reason, there are multiple papers showing that folks admitted to ICU already have markedly reduced antioxidants, including low levels of vitamins E and C. Furthermore, other studies show that *the more depleted of antioxidants the patient is, the greater his chance of organ death.* Another important feature of this article from a leading surgery journal showed that **antioxidants work best when they are administered as early as possible,** not waiting until signs of organ death and infection show up. Even if the insurance companies were not interested in saving lives, they should at least be interested in saving money, for the costs were lower as well, since patients got out of the ICU earlier and did not require expensive organ failure dialysis and other heroic measures. I could give you many more examples, but you get the message. This type of research has been coming on for over a decade and yet still has not taken off, for many financial reasons. (Did you ever look at the prices of drugs given to you in the hospital?) But let's not let you or your loved ones become victims of inexcusable ignorance. **Remember the current definition of malpractice is not that a physician is doing bad medicine, but that he is not doing what all the other physicians are doing.**

Where are the cardiologists, internists, family practitioners, surgeons, consultants, ICU specialists, emergency room physicians, and other practitioners who should be doing nutritional medicine? Please show them the references if someone you love is admitted, so they will be put on notice to be sure to at least include these nutrients. Because the hospital probably does not even have these in the formulary, you might be allowed to bring in your own, which would most likely be of superior quality anyway. Unfortunately those unschooled in nutritional biochemistry would have no way of appreciating the superior quality of your choices. Meanwhile, I hope this reminds you to do your daily **Detox Cocktail** along with **E-Gems Elite**.

What About Other Parts of Vitamin E

Remember in Chapter II how you learned about the other half of vitamin E, the four tocotrienols? They are much stronger HMG COA reductase inhibitors than the statin drugs and they lower cholesterol by not poisoning the gene like the statins do (Parker). New information is constantly emerging and it turns out that the **delta tocotrienols are the strongest for reducing cholesterol** (Song, Chao, Naito). And they have strong anti-clotting and plaque-inhibiting action. You can now get delta tocotrienols as **Delta-Fraction Tocotrienols** (Allergy Research Group), containing 45 mg of delta tocotrienols and 5 mg of the gamma. You can use 1-2 twice a day to compliment your three-part vitamin E program in Chapter II.

Neglected Nutrients Contribute to Heart Disease

We could devote a whole book just to the vitamins, so let me just give you a brief overview of the enormous problem (and some easy solutions). When I was in grade school in the early 50s, I remember first learning about vitamin D that it was important for our teeth and bones. Sadly the recommendation at that time was 400 international units a day and it still remains the same over half a century later in spite of enormous evidence to the contrary. In that were not enough of a travesty, that the official agencies have not kept up with science and modified the daily recommendation, there are many worse problems.

There is a hidden epidemic of folks, regardless of age, finances or country with deficiencies of nearly every nutrient, and vitamin D is no exception. As a brilliant Boston researcher has proven, **vitamin D deficiency is a silent epidemic affecting as much as half the population in the United States,** the land of plenty, and fortified foods (Holick). For starters, vitamin D is extremely important for many other diseases including multiple sclerosis, autoimmune diseases, cancers and yes; you guessed it, for preventing cardiovascular disease. And vitamin D is essential for preventing diabetes, high triglycerides, hypertension, and other risks that elevate your chance of early heart death (Martins, also see *The High Blood Pressure Hoax* for more).

It is also crucial as part of a package for melting away of coronary artery plaque or stalling its progression (Watson, Zittermann). Vitamin D keeps calcium metabolism from going awry. It puts calcium in bone and not in arteries. It turns out the average daily amount should be more like 4000 I.U. not 400. Along with vitamin K, **vitamin D helps keep unwanted calcifications and plaque out of arteries** (Rogers). Luckily a vitamin D level is part of your **Cardio/ION Panel**, one more reason why it is an indispensable part of diagnosis, healing and cure (Vieth, Holick, van der Mei, Hollis, Zitterman). I suggest at least one a day of **Vitamin D3 2000 mg** (Carlson).

Vitamin <u>K</u> to <u>K</u>ick and <u>K</u>eep Cholesterol Off the Vessel Wall

The big myth about cholesterol is that it is supposed to glue itself on to the blood vessel wall and calcify. This is why we call the number one cause of death "hardening of the arteries" or arteriosclerosis. But once more, God has designed our nutrients and foods to harmonize, to support the beautifully orchestrated chemistry of the body. For many folks, the use of vitamin K is only known in terms of helping blood clot. But this notion is also 50 years out of date. **We need vitamin K so that osteocalcin can transport calcium from the blood and vessel walls, and bind it to bone.** If vitamin K is deficient, this calcium instead goes to the body's toxic waste site, the inflamed arterial wall to become another Band-Aid. **Instead of piling calcium into the bones, when vitamin K2 is deficient the body piles the leftover calcium onto the arterial wall.** This is one reason why the recommendation of over 1000 mg of calcium daily to prevent osteoporosis is so ridiculous. It actually accelerates aging and arteriosclerosis, especially if no one has measured the levels of vitamin D first, the intracellular minerals, and also prescribed vitamin K.

How potent a protection is vitamin K? **Folks who have higher levels of vitamin K2 have a 57% reduction in heart disease** (Geleijnse). And for folks with higher levels of vitamin K on board they also have **68% less arteriosclerosis in the main artery of the body, the aorta** (Geleijnse). For **vitamin K** controls calcium regulation and specifically **inhibits arterial vascular calcifications** (Vermeer, Shearer, Schugers). In addition, **vitamin K decreases circulating cholesterol** (Kawashima).

And as usual, commonly prescribed medicines, like the common blood thinner Coumadin, that are supposed to help you live longer actually do the reverse. Blood thinners like coumadin (warfarin) speed up arteriosclerosis because they inhibit vitamin K (Schugars). In *TW* we have gone through the evidence that proves vitamin K safely prevents this and is safe to use with warfarin or Coumadin (Spronk). If that were not bad enough, **Coumadin also causes osteoporosis.** There's also more information in *The High Blood Pressure Hoax*. Meanwhile, **since vitamin K lowers cholesterol and keeps calcium out of plaque,** my recommendation would be **5 mg Vitamin K2** daily. Vitamins K2 and D3 are especially important if you are on blood thinners like Coumadin, which promotes calcium dumping into the arteries versus bones where it belongs (*TW*).

Fibrinogen's Secrets

Fibrinogen is a blood indicator that you must have checked. But why is it often neglected? Again, the cure is nutrients, not a billion dollar drug. To give you an idea of how much more important it is than high cholesterol, **if you've already had a heart attack, having elevated fibrinogen shows you who is <u>most likely to die within less than four years</u>** (Coppola). So if you have already had a heart attack and you're not having your fibrinogen measured, you sure are being very cheated, because it's totally reversible, once you know to go after it. Many other studies show, for example, that a **fibrinogen over 300 mg/dL indicates that you are at very high risk for an early heart attack**, stroke, and other vascular diseases. Of course the standard laboratory reference range for fibrinogen goes up to 423, but that's no surprise since most cut-offs for dangerous levels are too high, while on the flip side the lower cut-off for minimal levels for nutrient sufficiency are notoriously too low.

Unfortunately, **elevated fibrinogen can also be a warning sign of a cancer** that is brewing. And certainly if you have already had a cancer and the fibrinogen is elevated I would be very concerned. You see, cancer cells use sialoglycoproteins and fibrinogen to coat themselves, making their antigenic recognition sites invisible to the immune system cells. You recall from April 2007 *TW* how various enzymes dissolve off this coating so that now the immune system can "see" cancer cells and gobble them up (see the protocols in *Wellness Against All Odds*). Meanwhile, every doctor caring for a cancer patient should obviously measure fibrinogen (as well as all the other parameters in the **Cardio/ ION Panel**).

You might wonder why your cardiologist hasn't checked the fibrinogen level, and I do, too. Even in the *Journal of the American Medical Association* they showed that for every 100 mg/dL increase in fibrinogen over the norm there's a 2.4 fold greater likelihood of getting coronary heart disease (Danesh). Thus, fibrinogen joins the ranks of homocysteine in making **elevated fibrinogen more dangerous than the commonly checked cholesterol.** But because there are pricey drugs for cholesterol, it receives more attention. **One of the many other causes of elevated fibrinogen, besides coronary plaque, infection or cancer, which you'll learn about in the next chapter, includes common diesel exhaust.**

Taming Fibrinogen

So how do you lower your fibrinogen if you have this dangerous indicator of hidden infection, cancer or eventual clots? It won't surprise you that many of the nutrients that you take for other reasons have a potent effect on taming fibrinogen, depending upon your individual deficiencies and toxicities, in other words, your personal total load. Since fibrinogen is part of an inflammatory response of the body to protect itself and needing an oil change produces inflammation, **Cod Liver Oil** is crucial in many people to lower fibrinogen (Calder). Why doesn't it work in everyone? Many reasons:

- Not everyone has a deficiency of EPA and DHA fatty acids.
- Most were never analyzed to begin with to see how much and which oil forms they needed. In other words, they were not biochemically balanced.
- Anyone deficient in EPA and DHA is deficient in many other things that were also not assayed much less corrected in those studies. PC is a great example.
- And worse, they may have a serious cancer or infection making it impossible to lower fibrinogen until that underlying cause is corrected. **You must find the cause.**

What about negative studies on cod liver oil? Many studies look at one or two nutrients and try use them solo like a drug. Ridiculous! **Since cod liver oil helps correct inflammation, makes blood less able to clot, repairs cell membranes and protects against cardiac arrhythmia, it's a pretty important nutrient to correct, especially for folks who can't afford an assay, but have already had a heart attack.** We find it so commonly deficient and at such low levels that it really is a testament to the design of the body how low a level folks can endure and still be functioning. Refer back to Chapter IV for your complete oil change.

Next to consider for lowering and elevated fibrinogen would be an old friend you learned about in Chapter II, **Niacin-Time.** Vitamin B3, or niacin, is not only a vasodilator, energy booster, detox helper, and cholesterol fighter, but lowers fibrinogen (Philipp, Johansson). Next, vitamin C in doses above 2000 mg also lowers fibrinogen (Bordia). Use **Ultrafine Pure Ascorbic Acid** (Klaire, ProThera) ½-2 tsp 2-4 times a day as tolerated without diarrhea. Don't be surprised if you don't tolerate it after a few weeks or months, for as your need for it goes down, so often does your tolerance. For example, some can take 3-10 gm of vitamin C (1 gm = 1,000 mg) for flu with no loose stools, and barely tolerate 2 gm when the flu is over. Lots of other things I've told you about already have a positive bearing on fibrinogen, like aged garlic (Rahman) as exclusively found in **Kyolic Liquid Cardiovascular**, vitamin E's alpha tocopherol (Azzi) as in **E Gems Elite**, and much more that we'll eventually cover here and in future *TW* (and there are many other solutions to fibrinogen in past *TW*). Isn't it beautiful how nutrients you have already learned about have multiple other benefits you never dreamed of?

In the meantime this one component, fibrinogen, of the **Cardio/ION** is so important that I firmly believe everyone should have it measured. And if you have any suspicion that all is not well, like a past history of heart surgery or cancer, I would definitely get your fibrinogen measured because it is such a critical barometer of silent trouble brewing that needs immediate attention. Even if you are well, if this comes out elevated, **an elevated fibrinogen is an imperative sign that you had better find the underlying cause**, especially if you cannot nullify it with nutrients. It is too much of a gift to be ignored, and a much greater harbinger of serious trouble than high cholesterol.

The cardiologist who does not check fibrinogen as a standard will embarrassingly find that it has been recommended for over a decade. If not for you, he should order one for himself, for it can warn even if he has never had heart disease (Palmieri).

There will be much updating on this important subject in future *TW* issues. For now, you have seen a miniscule sample from the enormous evidence for the beneficial effects of a few vitamins, so now let's look at some minerals.

Think Zinc to Zap Inflammation
That Underlies Arteriosclerosis, Arthritis and Cancer

As you will learn in the next chapter, we have so successfully polluted the world that plasticizers are the number one pollutant in all humans and even in animals in the wild in pristine areas of the globe. Because industrial smokestacks and incinerators have spewed phthalates to the soils and waters over the globe, they are in all humans and animals. But humans lead the way in ingesting and stockpiling unprecedented amounts, because we go out of our way to get even higher levels of plasticizers. We are the only species whose foods are packaged in plastic. This leaches right into the food, as Tufts Medical School researchers proved. Once in the person, **plasticizers poison** the very chemistry (**peroxisomes**, little organelles that govern genes inside our cells) that **governs how cholesterol is metabolized.** But more on this subject later.

Plasticizers do something else equally damaging to cholesterol metabolism. They **create a silent zinc deficiency** (Peters, *TW*). What is so important about zinc? It is in over 200 enzymes, many of which control cholesterol metabolism and better yet, the inflammation chemistry that makes or breaks our blood vessel and heart health. **Zinc governs homocysteine** which you recall is much more dangerous than high cholesterol (via impaired conversion of B6 to its useable form).

Zinc also **runs the desaturase enzymes that metabolize fatty acids for every cell membrane, which in turn determine every disease**, including heart and blood vessel health. As one example, without enough zinc in the desaturase enzymes, you cannot convert the fatty acid EPA to DHA. Fortunately you get both in your cod liver oil in the oil change you learned about in Chapter IV. Why is DHA so important? Besides being crucial in the brain for intelligence, **DHA lowers cholesterol.**

(*For physicians* who want more, **DHA re-programs 504 genes (while zinc alone programs 33 genes), DHA depresses the P21** gene (turns off one of the cancer genes), DHA controls inflammation via Cox-II pathways (the place your pain meds work), DHA **activates PPAR that control cholesterol metabolism (the PPAR genes are damaged by plasticizers, but zinc doubles the PPAR),** and DHA increases cytochrome C (which is needed to metabolize cholesterol, makes cancer cells commit suicide, and more). You see how when we cannot make enough DHA because plasticizers have poisoned our zinc, we get a myriad of diseases.)

Zinc deficiency also controls your genes that determine which diseases you get (via DNA polymerase), it makes stomach acid which is needed to absorb minerals that fight cholesterol abnormalities (via carbonic anhydrase enzyme), converts beta-carotene into two molecules of vitamin A, accelerates wound healing, runs the bone and liver enzymes alkaline phosphatase and LDH plus insulin. Can you appreciate how you invite every disease with just one mineral deficiency? So how on earth can a physician heal you if he is working blindly and doesn't measure your minerals like zinc? And he needs to interpret them in view of the fact that the "norm" often includes folks who may have inferior nutrition (they subsist on fast foods), but are considered "normally healthy" merely because they don't as yet have a disease label. And he needs to balance your deficient nutrients with other nutrients, including those not measured yet. And recall minerals must be measured *inside* the cell!

As an example, some folks, they may never correct their homocysteine, or any other cardiovascular risk factors, because no matter how many nutrients are recommended, no one has assayed to find that they don't have enough zinc to convert vitamin B6 into its active form. And likewise without sufficient zinc they cannot metabolize the omega-3 fatty acids that make the "bread" of the membrane sandwich. And without zinc, we cannot turn down the flames of inflammation. **Inflammation is not a Celebrex deficiency, but it can be a zinc deficiency** (Fong, Raederstorff). We certainly see zinc deficiency commonly on the **Cardio/ION Panels**. And you might want to bear in mind that for years the intracellular zinc "norm was 6-11, but in 2007 it magically became 3.6-8.0 ppm packed cells. That is because as the population gets progressively and silently more deficient, the "norm" goes lower. Therefore, this too, must be compensated for when interpreting this sophisticated blood work. For depletion of soil zinc by acid rain and repeated growing, depletion of food zinc from processing, depletion of body zinc from the phthalates, prescription medications, and cadmium are just a few examples of the many factors contributing to a zinc deficiency. And zinc is just one of dozens essential minerals in the body.

Organic Acids to the Rescue

Luckily this is where functional assays of zinc repletion come to your rescue. For example, even if your RBC zinc is normal, we need to know if that is enough zinc for *your* body. This is where the vitamin and **organic acids on the Cardio/ION come to your rescue**. If beta carotene is high normal and vitamin A is low normal, even though they are both normal, this suggests a **deficiency of zinc in the enzyme to convert one molecule of beta carotene to two molecules of vitamin A.** Likewise, when specific organic acids are elevated, like kynurenate, quinolinate and others, they suggest a need for more B6. But no matter how much B6 you give, B6 cannot be converted to its active form without the zinc-dependent enzyme, pyridoxal kinase. And for many, B6 not only controls homocysteine but the neurotransmitters of happy mood.

You might start taking **Chelated Zinc** daily. Remember, however, when you need extra zinc you are at risk of creating an imbalance and lowering molybdenum, copper, manganese, vanadium and other minerals. Then if you factor in what drugs folks take, all bets are off. For all drugs deplete nutrients (Pelton). There are no free rides on the drug train. That's why this era of unprecedented chemicals in the human body has made even more necessary the assay of your mineral balance, as in **RBC Minerals,** which are also part of your **Cardio/ION Panel.**

Copper Solves High Homocysteine

Let's look at a common example of having trouble getting an elevated homocysteine down and how to approach it. One reader of the *TW* newsletter wrote in:

Q. "My homocysteine was high, but a B vitamin did not correct it. Now my doctor is stumped as to how to reduce this serious indicator of early heart attack, stroke, Alzheimer's and other diseases of aging."

A. You are right in trusting that there is a biochemical solution. First you may not process your B vitamins normally any more. The organic acids in your **Cardio/ION** will rescue you. If your methylmalonic acid is high normal or above, that shows you need either B12 sublingually (under the tongue) as **Methylcobalamin** 5 mg, or by injection. I suggest a trial of each. If your formiminoglutamate is up, you need sublingual folic acid as **Folixor.** If your B-hydroxyisovalerate is up, you need **Biotin** 5 mg. Remember that **organic acids are metabolic indicators. They are not direct measures of a vitamin level. They are better, because they show if you are one of the folks who need higher levels than "ordinary"**, just as the *Journal of the American Medical Association* spoke of (page 241 of this book). Organic acids measure how the deficiency of a vitamin distorts and arrests specific chemical pathways *in you,* stopping them dead in their tracks. A deficiency of a nutrient raises levels of abnormal metabolites (since the normal progression has been stopped by your deficiency).

If your hippuric acid or 3-methylhippurate is high, you may benefit from **DMG**. That is because toluene and benzene, from say too much auto exhaust, a new car, new carpet, or home or office new paint or renovations is detoxified in the body by hooking a molecule of glycine onto it, forming a hippurate, to drag it out into the bile and dump it into the gut. These metabolites can also come from food preservatives or abnormal bugs in the gut. Nevertheless, elevations of these metabolites are a sign you are using up too much glycine, which is also needed for homocysteine normalization. Glycine 500 mg once or twice a day can help that, and remember there are 920 mg of glycine in each **Carlson Chelated Magnesium,** or you can use **Glycine Powder**.

One nutrient however, that is rarely thought of to correct high homocysteine, even among nutritionally trained physicians, is **Chelated Copper**. One a day can correct it. Copper is important for the enzyme **methionine synthase**, the enzyme needed to pull methyl groups off folic acid precursors and put them on homocysteine to generate methionine (Tamura). An alternative way to correct that is with **Zinc Balance** (Jarrow), containing zinc and copper. Balancing copper with zinc accomplishes two things: (1) it avoids creating a copper-induced zinc deficiency later on, and (2) combining the copper with zinc tends to negate the stomach irritation that is sometimes caused by solo copper nutrients (although I have not seen it with the Carlson Chelated Copper).

Other common deficiencies include **PhosChol** that you learned about in Chapter IV and another methyl donor, **DMG**, dimethyl glycine. But a far more common deficiency, depending on your genetics, is riboflavin or vitamin B2 (McNully). I would also add a **Vitamin B2** one a day and if your homocysteine level is still up get your **Cardio/ION Panel** to determine what other deficiencies are present.

There are many other causes, for example, **many prescription medications raise your homocysteine levels, like blood pressure**

meds (see *The High Blood Pressure Hoax* for more on the causes and cures of high homocysteine, an indicator of early death that is more deadly than high cholesterol, yet totally reversible). After every new medication is introduced (should you have any), you should check (in a few months) to see if it has raised your homocysteine level and is possibly propelling you toward Alzheimer's or early heart disease. You are now too smart to be fooled. You are great to have remembered that when you're stuck, there is always a biochemical explanation. That's the beauty of your **Cardio/ION Panel**. It takes a lot of the guesswork out of diagnostic problems.

Meanwhile, even though a lot of the preceding chemistry may be way over your head, you can use information in this brief section to test your doctor's ability to properly interpret your Cardio/Ion Panel. A simple question like, "Even though my zinc looks normal, what other results on here will tell you it is enough for me personally?" If he doesn't know the beta-carotene to vitamin A ratio and other organics, you can find better.

Chromium to Stop Your Arteries From "Rusting"

Let's look at another mineral that is commonly deficient and tied to proper cholesterol metabolism. In the past days of bumpers and fenders on cars, chromium was used to keep them from rusting. Well, it sort of does that in your blood vessels. By protecting the LDL cholesterol from oxidizing or rusting, **it keeps the main dangerous form of cholesterol, oxidized cholesterol, from depositing on arteries**. And because it is essential in the metabolism of sugars, it also **lowers triglycerides and keeps sugars from causing arteriosclerosis**. And that is not all, for Nature always provides multiple "good" side effects. Chromium **raises the good HDL cholesterol** that acts as a wheelbarrow carrying cholesterol into the liver to make bile, and lowers serum cholesterol.

On the flipside, if you don't have enough chromium you can be plagued by hypoglycemia with mood swings, inability to lose weight, constant cravings, headaches or exhaustion triggered by low sugar. Also chromium is important in some people for **curing their depression** because it reacts with serotonin receptors. And of course, **all diabetics** should have their chromium levels checked and corrected. It is the sign of an antiquated diabetologist who does not insist on checking your chromium levels (and vanadium, manganese, DHA, etc., as you will learn).

Furthermore some people cannot metabolize chromium like others so they need much larger doses, especially **folks who just can't lose weight.** But perhaps it won't surprise you that the powers that be have not yet established whether chromium is even essential yet, so there's no official RDI (referenced daily intake). You can be sure that when it does come along it will, as history repeats itself, be much lower than it should be for decades. A hidden deficiency of chromium is extremely common because, for example, the moment wheat berries are refined into flour, **70% of chromium is lost,** and a typical diet only gives us 25 µg per day, not enough to stave off obesity, arteriosclerosis, hypoglycemia, diabetes, or any degenerative diseases. With all the alcohol and sweets that we have, it may be time to get a little chromium boost. Since sweets and alcohol increase deficiencies, we could probably all use a daily boost for several months of one or two **Chelated Chromium** providing 200 µg of elemental chromium.

Alternatively, you can improve your cholesterol metabolism and antioxidant defenses by adding **Kyo-Chrome** (Wakunaga, the Kyolic people). It contains 200 mg of Kyolic aged garlic extract (which lowers cholesterol, is an anti-oxidant, slows down progression of arterial plaque, etc.), 100 mcg of chromium picolinate and 10 mg of niacin per capsule. Use one to four capsules twice a day. An additional benefit is **garlic is a legitimate aspirin substitute.** This by no means is a complete examination of all the vitamins and minerals, but just a sampling so you get an idea of the voluminous evidence of how miserably we are being mislead and actually cheated by drug-oriented medicine.

Vanadium Saves Lives

Most people including most physicians have never heard of vanadium, but it's one of many crucial trace minerals upon which health hinges. As you have learned here, there are many factors to promote early heart death that are **much stronger risk factors than high cholesterol.** One major factor is **elevated insulin**, which is one of the many important risk factors measured on your **Cardio/ION** panel. Elevated insulin comes about for many reasons. In the next chapter you will learn that plasticizers, the highest pollutant in humans and even in animals in the wild raises insulin while creating insulin resistance. Common conditions in which folks have raised insulin levels include **Metabolic Syndrome or Syndrome X,** as well as **diabetes, hypertension, early heart disease**, and yes, high cholesterol.

You've learned that when insulin receptors on the cell membrane are damaged, insulin comes knocking at the door so you can usher in sugar to make energy. But with **insulin resistance**, the door is locked. So the body sends out even more insulin in attempt to get the needed sugar into the cell. But this extra insulin doesn't do the trick, because as you learned, the cell wall receptors or docking sites for it are damaged. You learned how to repair those in Chapter IV. So let's explore the many reasons that make vanadium another crucial part of the puzzle of insulin resistance that leads to diabetes, hypertension, high cholesterol, arteriosclerosis, early heart death, and even inability to lose weight. In fact **dieting is powerless for reducing weight when vanadium is deficient.**

First though, I must marvel at your indomitable spirit. By now, even though you did not go to medical school, even though you never aspired to have this much biochemical knowledge of the human body, and you have lots of other pressing things in life to at-

tend to, I greatly admire folks like you who take responsibility for their health. Okay, so on to how vanadium helps without getting you too mired in chemistry.

You recall from *TW* how D-ribose in the form of **Corvalen** actually boosts the energy in the heart, ATP. Vanadium plays a role in this as well. In fact, **heart muscle cells are "hand-cuffed" without enough vanadium.** Also many environmental toxins like pesticides in our foods and household items poison ATP (via oxidative phosphorylation) so that energy cannot be made as easily. This is one of the main causes of chronic fatigue, accelerated aging and many diseases. Vanadium counters this. It also decreases the heart vessel-damaging action of too much insulin by increasing the sensitivity of the target organ, like the heart (independent of the cell membrane receptor repair). Also when folks eat too much sugar or they are diabetic, the extra sugar literally fries proteins accelerating arteriosclerosis, heart death and aging. **Vanadium counters this glycosylation** as well while lowering sugar levels in addition to insulin. **It also is the limiting mineral for some folks who can never lose weight or get rid of nagging sugar cravings that are not related to Candida.**

By reducing the damage to heart vessels from extra insulin, sugar and even some environmental chemicals, as well as increasing the energy in the heart and blood vessels, vanadium lowers blood pressure. But its benefits continue: vanadium also improves the chemistry of cholesterol so that it can become more normal. As well, it reduces another cardiovascular risk factor, the triglycerides. And recall, lots of meds like B-blockers for heart arrhythmias and blood pressure raise **triglycerides**. Vanadium could even repair some of the damage from the high fructose corn syrup that permeates the junk food industry. Even though scientists have called it **an insulin mimic, this mineral actually does more than insulin.**

Okay, I promise not to say another word about the chemistry of vanadium, as others have done it better (Noda, Verma, Cohen, Natesampillai, Green). But I hope this has convinced you that you want to at least know your vanadium level and make sure that it is at the top of normal (5th quintile), not anywhere near the middle or the bottom of the reference range which is actually a "population average". The sad fact is the government has not gotten around to establishing that vanadium is even needed, much less an RDA. Sadly, the average daily intake is only 50 µg and we need over 10 times that to protect the heart. You should be sure to include one or two **Vanadium 250 µg Krebs** (douglaslabs.com) into your daily regimen, especially if it's not measured.

Correcting Your Mineral Deficiencies

Here's an easy formula with which many have completely cor-rected their mineral deficiencies (and even totally reversed osteo-porosis) within 3 to 12 months. Glucosamine sulfate, chondroitin, and MSM are important for osteoporosis, but don't kid yourself. They are also important for the integrity of arterial walls to make them more resistant to arteriosclerosis (and resistant to rupture from stroke). For example, the **matrix of the blood vessel wall actually makes heparin, our natural anti-coagulant or clot-buster** (*The High Blood Pressure Hoax* contains more details). You can get all three in one product called **Nutra Support Joint**, two twice a day. As well, boron is very important and you can get this with **SilBoron**, one a day. As you learned, **Vitamin D3 2000 mg** is crucial, 1-2 a day, **Vitamin K2** 5 mg, one a day, and **ACES with Zinc** can give you more antioxidant protection as well as provide you with additional selenium and zinc.

In addition, I've found that many folks need to take their minerals individually, in a chelated form, and **spread them out** with only a couple every few hours to maximize their absorption. You see there are only so many mineral transporters (carrier proteins) the body makes to carry the minerals across the gut wall. That's why many folks will not correct their osteoporosis with a multiple mineral preparation, whereas they will correct with individual minerals that are spread out throughout the day. A typical protocol often includes (in addition to the above) the prescription form of **Magnesium Chloride Solution**, ½ a tsp twice a day, plus one a day each of **Chelated Chromium, Chelated Selenium, Chelated Manganese, Chelated Zinc, Chelated Copper, Iodoral, Vanadium 250 (from vanadium Krebs),** and **Moly B** (chelated molybdenum). And don't forget the **BioSil** (a whole dropper full daily) that you learned about in *Pain Free In 6 Weeks*.

In addition, because minerals run all your enzymes and they are progressively depleted from processed foods and foods grown on chemically fertilized soils, depleted by medications, etc., I also suggest a hefty tablespoonful daily of **IntraMin,** a specially formulated and easily absorbed fulvic acid form of multiple organic trace minerals that are difficult to get elsewhere, especially in a better absorbed form and that help chelate heavy metals (Wershaw, Klocking in next chapter).

These are all especially important if you cannot get your nutrients measured with the **Cardio/ION**. For they represent the most commonly low minerals contributing to arteriosclerosis and other diseases that we have seen over 38 years. Most of all, **remember not to dump them all into your gut at once,** but **space them out** taking a few every few hours, to maximize their absorption. Why so many? Because the soils are more depleted by repeated growing, plus acid rain with cadmium, mercury, aluminum, arsenic, and other heavy metals displace minerals from the soil. Then soils are compromised further with chemical fertilizers and pesticides. The real icing on the cake is the processing of foods. Mineral deficiencies are the norm, not the rare finding.

An easy plan is to put them in old-fashioned ice-cube trays, or little pill bottles (two bottles for every day of the week, you will understand why in the next chapter) every Sunday. Don't worry if you can't get them all in within 24 hours. If you have to take 2-3 days to finish one day's worth, it is still better than what you did before. And frankly, some folks' systems cannot absorb and assimilate any faster. So be it. Does it sound like a lot of work? Not if you learn how to get organized. The alternative is to suffer with the effects of drugs and the inevitable avalanche into a myriad of other seemingly unrelated diseases and miseries. Only you have the power to reverse the ravages of disease. Just correcting the mineral deficiencies and doing the oil change in Chapter IV has turned around much cardiovascular disease.

Magnesium the Mineral That Resurrects Hearts

I showed you how **magnesium works like a statin drug in Chapter II. It does more. Magnesium deficiency is one of the most common causes of heart diseases, yet rarely is correctly checked**, much less corrected. In brief, government studies show that the average American daily diet only provides 40% of what you need, less than half. So clearly nearly everyone is deficient. Furthermore, other things like sweets, processed foods, soda, stress, alcohol, and sweating increase the deficiency even more (Marier). In fact so much magnesium is lost in sweating, that I suspect it is the main cause of death in high profile young athletes.

The nasty part is that the regular blood test done most commonly by physicians for magnesium is grossly inferior, so much so that even the exceedingly conventional 2007, 32nd edition of *The Washington Manual of Medical Therapeutic* warns that the **serum magnesium is a poor indicator and physicians should not use** it (LWW.com). For less than 1% of the body's magnesium resides there. Basically your doc can tell you your serum magnesium level is fine and you can walk right out the door and have a fatal heart attack or cardiac arrhythmia from an improperly diagnosed magnesium deficiency. You need at least the erythrocyte (intracellular RBC or red blood cell) level done for greater accuracy. And even then that is not foolproof, for some folks harbor normal amounts in the RBC, but are deficient in other tissues, like the heart (the magnesium loading test in *Tired or Toxic?* is even more accurate).

Why all the fuss about magnesium? Because magnesium deficiency is the **number one cause of arrhythmias or irregular heart beats that can lead to a heart attack**. It is also a **major cause of sudden heart attack**, especially in folks who do not even have high cholesterol or any plaque. It **causes the same amount of pain and death as if you had coronaries full of cholesterol**. How? But causing the coronaries to go into sudden spasm or cramp, closing down tighter than if they were completely plugged with plaque. **You do not need any plaque in coronary arteries to have a heart attack. Just being magnesium deficient can do the trick.**

The evidence that undiagnosed and untreated magnesium deficiency is a major cause of heart disease is overwhelming (Ma, Gartside, Rayssiguier, Ravn, Altura, Seelig, Rogers), for it causes thickening of the arterial wall spasm, increased clotting, arrhythmias, and high cholesterol just for starters, not to mention sudden cardiac arrest. And, bear in mind **current recommendations for how much magnesium you should take** (remembering as reporters have verified that many "experts" on these boards are connected to the drug industry) **are too low to prevent heart disease** (Cleveland, Gartside, Seelig).

Over a decade ago physicians studied folks who presented to the emergency room with a heart attack. It was clearly shown then in numerous studies, and continues to be, that one of the major differences between folks who walked out of the hospital in a few days versus those carried out in a mortician's bag was how much magnesium they had on board when they entered. And further studies showed that giving magnesium as soon as possible was the next best thing. In fact, an **IV of magnesium cut** the chance of having a life-threatening cardiac **arrhythmia by a walloping 49%**. And there was a **54% drop in the number of deaths in folks given magnesium** (Horner SM, *Circulation,* 86:774-9, 1992).

As I referenced in *The High Blood Pressure Hoax,* **over 61% of people who enter the hospital for surgery are deficient in magnesium,** and that is determined by using the inferior magnesium test! **When they come out the hospital a few days or weeks later 81% are deficient.** Low magnesium doubles your risk for high blood pressure, angina, arrhythmia, and sudden cardiac arrest. And low magnesium raises your cholesterol (Alltur). It is astonishing to me the apparent **disconnect between the great contributions to science and the lack of application to medical practice.** For example, this paper (Alltur BT, et al, Magnesium dietary intake modulates blood lipid levels and atherogenesis, *Proc Nat Acad Sci USA,* 87: 1840-44, 1990) is from a highly respected journal, but 18 years later doctors don't even check RBC magnesium before they place someone on a statin drug for life.

Who in their right mind would ever consider being treated by a physician who does not know their magnesium status? Especially when you learned in Chapter II how a magnesium deficiency causes high cholesterol and that **magnesium acts like a statin** (Rosanoff). Is it standard to check and give magnesium today? Do cardiologists routinely check the correct erythrocyte (RBC or red blood cell) magnesium prophylactically? Do they understand that **magnesium deficiency is epidemic and a major cause of sudden heart attack?** Do they even know that in 2007 the government standard or norm for RBC magnesium plunged from 40-50 to 15-35 ppm packed cells? This reflects our fast food cravings, toxin overloads, and epidemic diseases. (See *Depression Cured At Last* and *Detoxify or Die* for much more on magnesium and voluminous evidence). **There is an enormous "disconnect" and knowledge gap in medicine.**

Best Emergency Form of Magnesium

The most potent form of magnesium available is **Magnesium Chloride Solution, 200 mg/cc**. Have your doctor write a prescription for a 12 oz. bottle, then call the **Windham Pharmacy**, in Windham New York, (windhampharmacy.com) 1-518-734-3033 to fill the prescription. The dose is 1/2 tsp once or preferably twice a day for most folks. There isn't a person I can think of who shouldn't have this emergency magnesium form on hand at home at all times, especially since government studies show the average daily intake of magnesium from food is less than half of what we need each day.

If you can't get your doctor to prescribe this (he ought to at least for himself!), there are excellent forms of magnesium that do not require a prescription that you learned about in Chapter I. You could start with 2-3 twice a day of **Chelated Magnesium** (Carlson) 200 mg /capsule with 920 mg of detox-promoting and homo-cysteine-lowering glycine.

A Glance at the Evidence

A doctor just has to read a couple of medical journals from this year to appreciate that nutritional medicine is superior to drug therapy. In one study, researchers from the Harvard School of Public Health showed that a mere **500 mg of vitamin C and 600 units of vitamin E cut the heart attack rate by 22%** (Cook). **That's cheaper and more healthful for you than Lipitor, which you recall causes a vitamin E deficiency!** Or take another high-profile journal showing that **low vitamin D** levels (which are epidemic) **increase the likelihood of hypertriglyceridemia 50%** and high blood pressure, plus diabetes by 30%, and that vitamin D has a huge bearing on heart failure, inflammatory cardiovascular disease, and coronary plaque (Martins).

In yet another cardiology journal this year they showed once more that **doctors really should be prescribing coenzyme Q10 for all statin patients** (Caso). And then there were three papers showing beyond a doubt that magnesium deficiencies are not only common, but when you correct them you improve not only cholesterol but other important cardiovascular risk factors like diabetes, syndrome X, arrhythmias, elevated CRP, congestive heart failure, and sometimes by as much as 44% improvement (Almoznino-Sarafian, Nielsen, Ford). And some of these diagnoses like heart failure mean that half the patients will be dead in less than five years. These folks can't wait for doctors to get on board. They need this kind of medicine now!

LDL is Not the "Bad" Cholesterol

Cardiologists call the LDL cholesterol the "bad" cholesterol. But this is not true. In fact **LDL has many crucial roles, like carrying vitamin E and other anti-oxidants piggyback** where they are needed in the body (Archakov). But when the balance between free radicals or reactive oxygen species (ROS) and anti-oxidants is distorted and **ROS reign, LDL becomes transformed into the "bad" molecule that glues itself to the arterial wall** (Steinberg, Cox). Because it has lost an electron, this now makes the LDL cholesterol molecule viciously hungry for another electron. So it steels one from the nearest place, the heart artery lining, clinging to its newfound electron for dear life. So **the bad cholesterol is only "bad" if we don't have enough antioxidants,** *for lack of antioxidant vitamins is what makes cholesterol stick like Velcro to the inside of the coronary blood vessel walls.*

One simple antioxidant is CoQ10, as you learned. A simple 1-3 **Q-ODT** under the tongue on your way out the door is one of many nutrients that guards against LDL cholesterol becoming a bad guy (DeRijke). And as you learned in Chapter III, it has other benefits like **reducing the lipoprotein(a) and insulin resistance** (Singh).

Remember when you use nutrients you get multiple benefits. But who has measured your CoQ10 level lately?

Meanwhile on the **Cardio/ION** you can see the precise levels of antioxidant vitamins like A, E, beta-carotene, CoQ10, and organic acids that reflect vitamin C adequacy as well as elevated lipid peroxides, the end result of antioxidant in adequacy. **Your antioxidant level in the blood determines whether or not cholesterol is good or bad.** That's why a *New England Journal of Medicine* study showed that **low LDL cholesterol is meaningless** in terms of being a guarantee of safety or even a decent predictor of your risk of having a heart attack (Ridker). Much more important is the CRP and other inflammatory markers like fibrinogen that you are learning about. But unfortunately medicine still uses the useless LDL to scare or falsely assure folks. And what's worse, cardiologists across the country use an elevated LDL as an excuse to prescribe a statin, even if the victim has a normal cholesterol!!

Needless to say, if you have a doctor who is relying on your LDL, he is years behind. Just remind him that 50% of the people who have a heart attack have normal cholesterol levels and that **76% of the people on statin drugs get coronary artery disease anyway** (Delany).

Whenever you take any drug, it uses up detox nutrients, including antioxidants, that could have and should have been used to heal the body and protect you against aging, degenerative diseases, and cancer. Remember, the statins lower your CoQ10, vitamin E, selenium and more. And recall that getting any of the types of cardiovascular diseases from these deficiencies is only the tip of the iceberg, because **by inhibiting proper cholesterol metabolism in the cell with statins, you also increase the rate of cancer** (Newman, Sacks). So no wonder that *the use of cholesterol-lowering drugs can increase your heart attack and cancer rates while ushering in new diseases.* Drugs make matters infinitely worse by accelerating damage in many ways, one of which is stealing anti-oxidant nutrients. Meanwhile the innocent victim has all the confidence in his expensive medication and the knowledge that his cholesterol level is now down and there is "nothing to worry about".

Cholesterol is the Body's Smoke Detector

Whenever I hear some politician, or worse, physician, talk about winning the war against cholesterol, cancer or some other disease, I'm amazed at their ignorance of the actual causes. They act as though the answer is in just discovering the right drug, gene therapy or surgery and the disease will be magically conquered. But unless they've been living in a cave, most physicians now know that all disease is caused by *free radicals*, or more properly, *reactive oxygen species*, *ROS* which lead to inflammation (Halliwell). When we overwhelm the body's ability to quench or neutralize them, they cause damage that results in symptoms, then disease, and then death. **In health, the body has an ample balance between the forces of destruction, ROS, and the body's arsenal of anti-oxidants to sop them up to put out their fires of destruction. Otherwise, unbalanced ROS burn holes in our cell membranes** (called lipid peroxidation and measured on your Cardio/ION), damage genes that regulate cholesterol, and damage hormones and other proteins that we rely on for total wellness.

But ROS are not all bad. Harnessed in packets inside the white blood cell, they are used to burn up or oxidize nasty bugs in the blood stream like bacteria from food, Candida that sneaked through the leaky gut, or viruses that enter the blood through the lungs. It is only when the balance of ROS (versus our counterbalance of anti-oxidants) swings in favor of the free radicals or ROS, that we begin the downhill course of disease.

What else besides infection can swing this imbalance out of our favor? Common producers of free radicals or reactive oxygen species are environmental chemicals. We inhale over 1000 chemicals every day in the average home environment, and this does not even count the office, factory or traffic and the rest of out of doors. A famous study by the U.S. government's EPA analyzed the exhaled breath of 356 urban residents of New Jersey (see *Tired or Toxic?*). In this breath analysis they found all sorts of chemicals that (through giving birth to armies of free radicals) are notorious for triggering high cholesterol, cancers and every other disease, as you'll learn in the next chapter.

And when ROS get high enough or persist long enough, the ultimate cumulative effect is that they damage genes to create the instructions for a cancer, or they damage an enzyme that is needed to properly metabolize cholesterol, as examples. Finally when our anti-oxidant levels are not high enough to counter this attack, this leaves our arsenal deficient and unable to detoxify the next chemical that comes along. This may provoke a symptom, like a headache or mood swing or muscle ache from the undetoxified chemical. You see how the **domino effect of disease** gets you on a roll with ROS.

Once these naked, wildly destructive electrons are on the loose, they also eat holes in arteries that then attract nature's cholesterol band-aid. But as you've learned, instead of seeing the **cholesterol as a messenger of ROS overload**, or a call to arms to find the underlying cause and fix it, we kill the messenger with drugs that also guarantee an avalanche of symptoms. We can go on to get hypertension, heart failure, cancer, nutrient deficiencies and other serious consequences. For the popular prescription statin drugs not only dampen cholesterol manufacture, they stop the manufacture of our essential internal vitamin-like CoQ10, create deficiencies of selenium and vitamin E, and neutralize the blood thinning activity of Plavix, as examples you have already mastered.

Furthermore, you now know that cholesterol itself is not a danger to arteries. Many folks with high cholesterol live to be in their nineties with no ailments or medications. It is only after cholesterol has been attacked by ROS or free radicals that it becomes burned or oxidized (Editorial 1980, Steinberg 1989). Only then does it glue itself to the inside of arteries, plugging them up. But **unoxidized cholesterol** (if we have enough free radical quenchers on board, like vitamins A, C, E, and much more), **is harmless and cannot cause arteriosclerosis** (Esterbauer). Otherwise, **cholesterol is essential for life.**

ROS (reactive oxygen species or free radicals) create all disease: when they attract amyloid to the brain, we call that Alzheimer's. When they damage the function of genes we get the instructions to grow a cancer, or have autoimmune disease, etc. But we don't have to remain powerless until ROS cause damage. We know we are in trouble when the **cholesterol level warns us that ROS are on the warpath**. We know we had better shape up when laboratory tests confirm our SOD (super oxide dismutase, run by zinc, copper and manganese), LP (lipid peroxides, which need selenium for detoxification), 8-OhdG (a sign of gene damage that can lead to cancer) or GSH-Px (glutathione peroxidase, which needs selenium for detoxification) levels are rising, **signaling that we are working overtime fighting free radicals**.

For elevated levels of these parameters are sure signs that the body is paddling as fast as it can to get you out of trouble. It does not have enough antioxidants to combat the level of free radicals formed each day. Now you can see why the whole foods diet (that gets you off trans fats that cause high cholesterol that you already learned about in Chapter IV) reverses these signals of free radical overload and is so healing. That is also the beauty of these crystal ball tests in your **Cardio/ION**, but more about those in Chapter VII. Clearly once you know you are in the danger zone, it's time to change your diet, cleanse the gut, correct your nutrient deficiencies, detox your lifetime of accumulated chemicals (that also cause high cholesterol), improve environmental controls, and rev up antioxidant nutrients to even the score. There will be more on this subject to come later.

Government studies now show us that diet and environment contribute 95% to the cause of cancer and other diseases (Perrera, Lichtenstein). The mechanism is through the generation of reactive oxygen species or free radicals. The problem is all the **prescription cholesterol-lowering drugs also generate free radicals.** Clearly, instead of prescribing poisons for the body's cholesterol pathways, cardiologists should be prescribing anti-oxidants and measuring their effectiveness. They should be changing the diet (substituting trans fatty acids for cold pressed oils and more fresh fruits, vegetables, whole grains and beans that have their own high levels of built-in anti-oxidants) and lowering any chemical contamination that can also create free radical attack on blood vessel walls (starting with simple things like air purifiers and alkaline water filters). And they should show folks the non-prescription natural substances as well as the detoxification protocols that you'll learn about. Instead, **drugs turn off God's clever combined warning system and safety valve** that patches these arterial holes. Whole books have beautifully detailed and documented the idiocy of cholesterol-lowering drugs, some by MD-PhDs (Ravnskov), some written by previous editors of the *Journal of the American Medical Association* (Pinckney, Smith), and more.

So Why Do Folks Have a Heart Attack Who Don't Have High Cholesterol?

Vascular spasm and arrhythmia are common causes, and totally correctable nutrient deficiencies are most often the underlying causes of those. For example, the amino acid, arginine can fix vessel spasm (restore impaired endothelial dilatation of coronary circulation in folks with high cholesterol) (Drexler). Arginine makes spastic arteries relax and enlarge (allowing more nutrients and oxygen into the heart muscle) through producing more nitric oxide. And arginine dilates blood vessels even in folks with high cholesterol (Drexler, Kawano).

Excess cholesterol in the blood stream also activates one of the strongest blood-clotting substances, Thromboxane A2, which acts like a boa constrictor to heart blood vessels and turns on platelets to form clots (a potent vasoconstrictor and activator of platelet function). That's why after a high fat meal folks are more prone to a heart attack. But never fear, **Nature always has a cure.** The amino acid arginine also stopped all this with only 1000 mg twice a day (DeLorgeril, also much more in *The High Blood Pressure Hoax*). There are endless ways to keep vessels open and un-clogged. And I showed you earlier, how vitamins C and E protect against a heart attack after a fatty meal.

Reversing Cholesterol Plaque

What about folks who have coronary artery plaque with calcification, with or without high cholesterol? There are many ways to shrink that plaque or dramatically slow up its progression. Since it's not the focus of this book (but will be in future *TWs*), I'll just mention a few of them so that you have an idea of how crucial the total program is.

Arginine has even made existing cholesterol plaques shrink! In fact it led to comparable regression of arteriosclerotic lesions, as compared with lovastatin (Boger). In other words, arginine led to just as much dissolving of arterial plaque as did lovastatin (the prescription Lipitor). Do you know how much cheaper and safer and more health-promoting natural L-arginine is than the statin Lipitor?

Do You Need More Arginine Than Most?

It is important to know whether you are among the people who make a chemical (asymmetrical dimethyl arginine) in your blood that poisons the enzyme (nitric oxide synthase) that dilates our arteries and keeps plaque at bay. Fortunately there is a blood test to show if you are one of these folks. As just an example, in one study when people were **at the top of the *normal* level for**

ADMA, they had four times the average amount of heart attacks. If they were just a tad over the top of the normal level, they had a **27-fold increased risk of heart attack**. The beauty of **the ADMA test** is that it **identifies the people who need even more arginine** than regular folks. Make sure your doctor tests you with the blood test **ADMA** (metametrix.com). Arginine is crucial for keeping blood vessels healthy whether or not someone has high cholesterol (Boger, Drexler). This information has been in major cardiology journals for over a decade, yet very few cardiologists ever check it or recommend it.

In the meantime use **Arginine Powder** 500-7,000 mg twice a day (Carlson), depending on whether you are ADMA positive or not. Or for folks who want a lower dose sustained release form of arginine by a company that prides itself on avoiding toxic additives in their supplements, **Perfusia** (by Thorne, but use NEEDS, 1-800-634-1380, for Thorne does not sell to the public) one or two capsules twice a day is an excellent start. You can measure arginine levels in the **Cardio/ION Panel**. So why would anyone want to work blindly when this is so important? There are more details on this subject and these nutrients in *The High Blood Pressure Hoax* and as new data emerges, *Total Wellness*.

You have seen that many nutrients, like **vitamins D3 and K2 make plaque regress** or dramatically slow up. Start with **Vitamin D3 2000 mg** 1-2 a day and **Vitamin K2** 5 mg (Carlson) one daily. As well, **phosphatidyl choline** that you learned about in Chapter IV in the form of **PhosChol**, 1-3 tsp a day, **makes plaque regress** (Wojcicki, and see references in Chapter IV). It is the most potent form and with the most research behind it that I know of. For folks who may want to evaluate a liposomal form of PC, **Essential Phospholipids** (Allergy Research Group) uses this technology to deliver in one teaspoonful 900 mg of phospholipids; use 1-3 tsp. once or twice a day. There is more on this in Chapter VIII.

Taurine the Tower of Amino Acids

As new nutrients come along sometimes we forget about the old tried and true. Taurine is one of these, because it is not even considered an essential amino acid. I think you'll agree that it is extremely essential after you see what it does. First of all it is not only **the leading amino acid in the brain**, but **in the eye**, in **platelets that control clotting, and in the heart**. If that were not enough, it is extremely important for the developing fetus and young infant whose brains, eyes, and hearts are growing at enormous rates. But because it is also **crucial in making bile for digesting our fats, lowering cholesterol, helping magnesium get inside cells, and for detoxification** of our everyday onslaught of chemicals, it gets used up much too quickly.

That's why there are many papers and books about the ability of taurine to reverse many conditions which medicine never thinks of reversing. *Retinitis pigmentosa*, a cause of blindness, *congestive heart failure* which kills more people and more quickly than cancer each year, and *seizures resistant to all medications* are just a few of the things that can be turned around if taurine deficiency is investigated and corrected. In one study, 13 out of 15 people who were classified as severe heart disease so dramatically improved that they were upgraded to being only half as severe with four grams of taurine a day (Azuma). Meanwhile another study of patients using three grams of taurine a day plus three grams of l-carnitine and 150 mg of coenzyme Q10 also markedly improved their heart function (Jeejeebhoy). **It's almost criminal for a cardiologist to ignore assaying and correcting taurine, CoQ10, carnitine, arginine, etc., especially in someone dying** of heart failure. All these and much more are assayed in the **Cardio/ION**.

Taurine has been used to reverse, *heart failure, alcoholism, Alzheimer's, liver problems, cystic fibrosis, high blood pressure as well as other serious heart, eye and brain diseases, like macular degeneration, seizures, and depression.* And **taurine has re-**

versed high cholesterol. More important, never forget its role in *stabilizing the cell membrane*, which is like the computer keyboard for the entire cell, and in helping conserve magnesium. Taurine modulates calcium levels, mitigating the use of the brain-damaging calcium channel blockers, the number one prescribed drug by all cardiologists.

And remember in *DOD* (*Detoxify or Die*, 1-800-846-6687 or prestige publishing.com) how I showed you the evidence from leading cardiology journals that calcium channel blockers (Norvasc, Cardiezem, Procardia, etc.) are proven by MRI to shrink the brain causing loss of memory and thinking capacity within five years. But if the cell membranes that house the calcium channels are repaired with taurine, the right fatty acids, minerals like magnesium (which is nature's calcium channel blocker), etc., calcium channel blockers are not needed. And this is only one nutrient. Just imagine the power behind a balanced personalized program of nutrients.

There's more. Taurine is crucial for *fighting off infection* and neutralizing the effects of bacterial endotoxins, as well as protecting diabetics, protecting against blood clots, and much more. With the help of Vitamin B6 we make taurine in the body, but not nearly as much as we need in this century, and recall you cannot convert B6 to its useable form without enough zinc (which environmental toxins like plasticizers deplete). You begin to see how much healing power is in understanding, assaying and correcting the damaged molecular biochemistry of the human body. In the unprecedented toxic 21st century, we need taurine more than ever! Instead the focus is expensive drugs that work by poisoning a pathway to temporarily stifle the symptom.

And don't forget that hidden Candida (from antibiotics, sweets) lurking in the gut produces beta-alanine and acetaldehyde, as examples of several toxic organic acids in the bloodstream. Taurine neutralizes these. Yet when Candida is undiagnosed in the gut, the amount of beta-alanine that is sent out into the bloodstream can dramatically reduce the available taurine (Waterfield). This in turn makes the person more sensitive than everybody else to environmental chemicals. The most common symptoms are brain fog, exhaustion, plus muscle and joint aches. For without sufficient taurine folks cannot metabolize and detoxify everyday chemicals. This is just one more bit of evidence why many cannot heal anything from heart problems to chemical sensitivities until the gut is healthy first, as we described in Chapter V and further in *No More Heartburn*. It also explains why many people find a dramatic improvement in their chemical sensitivity once they get rid of their Candida. And through molecular mimicry, anti-Candida antibodies can destroy the thyroid, as can plasticizers (Vojdani). So what hope of healing does anyone have with yeasts lurking in the gut?

I've personally seen taurine be part of the prescribed nutritional program to successfully reverse congestive heart failure, drug-resistant arrhythmias, medication-resistant seizures (in adults as well as children), and macular degeneration, all of which were diagnosed as untreatable. Meanwhile, I can see no harm in a trial of 1000 mg of **Taurine** (from Metabolic Maintenance through Pain & Stress Center) 1-2 twice a day added to your cholesterol program. Certainly if you have any disease where the brain, eye, platelets, gall bladder, detox system or heart is failing, a trial of taurine and better yet, a measurement of taurine is essential.

Fine-Tuning Your Nutrient Needs

There are so many nutrients that help reverse damage done by cholesterol being deposited, like another methyl donor the body makes, **SAMe** (Rafique). And we will explore others in Chapter VIII. The plan is to impress upon you how many nutrients (some of which you may never have heard of or know very little about) all have a bearing on our overall health. Now the challenge is to pick from the most important ones to create a manageable program *for you*. And it can't be done without knowing your precise imbalances and deficiencies.

Obviously a deficiency is never solo. Using taurine as an example, in some studies researchers have found that taurine was low in the various conditions you just learned about. But many researchers miss the boat by trying to use a nutrient like a drug. Some were naive in thinking that taurine alone would cure the conditions. I guess they forgot their basic chemistry, for nutrients work in concert with each other in the body. It's a miraculous yet delicately balanced healing system built into our bodies. It would be very rare for taurine to be the only deficiency.

Everyone needs good biochemical guidance for identifying the complete carload of other deficiencies and to orchestrate a harmonious treatment program. That's why I would suggest the **Cardio/ION Panel.** It includes taurine, plus the indispensable red blood cell minerals like magnesium and zinc, copper, chromium, vanadium, and selenium, plus an assay of damaging trans fats and crucial fats like EPA and DHA, organic acids like d-arabinitol (produced only by yeasts like Candida, proving it's present even when stool studies are negative) and suberate, adipate and ethylmalonate that prove you need the vitamin-like substance carnitine (which is destroyed by plasticizers), amino acids like arginine and glycine, vitamins like D, A, E, plus risk indicators like fibrinogen, hsCRP, homocysteine (that are stronger risk determinants than cholesterol), other risk factors like testosterone, insulin, lipid peroxides (shows anti-oxidant need), 8-OHdG (shows gene damage), and much more.

It is so comprehensive that it takes me about an hour to review the over 10 pages with folks of their personal biochemistry on the phone to design and tailor a program to correct their individual deficiencies, dovetailing it with their personal medical history and symptoms (this service is not limited to our patients, but is available to our select readers and non-patients as well). It is a medical specialty, just as brain surgery is. Your physician has no hesitation to order an MRI even though he wouldn't do the brain surgery if it turned out to be a tumor. So don't get angry if he has not attended special courses, read and studied to learn this specialty. But do get concerned if he won't order it for you so you can get the assay interpreted elsewhere. How else are you going to benefit from the 21st century molecular biochemistry of human healing?

Clearly there are more beneficial nutrients than any one person could accommodate in their stomach. The point is to **(1) make sure you never fall for the old malarkey, "There is no known cause and no known cure for what you have," and (2) to give you a glimpse of the miraculous healing powers of nutrients** as opposed to drugs, which merely poison a natural pathway. And nutrients become even more powerful when combined with one another, as they were designed. The orchestration of synergistic nutrients can bring about unexpected healing in areas that you were not even focused on. I've given lots of spelled out basic protocols in the preceding chapters. Clearly, the best way to map out a plan for you personally is by first knowing all your deficiencies.

The Blind Cardiologist and the Cardio/ION

Clearly, as you saw in Chapter I, you have to be deficient in nutrients to get high cholesterol or to have a heart attack. And clearly statin drugs are known to create further deficiencies of folic acid, selenium, vitamin E, coenzyme Q10 and other nutrients crucial to a healthy heart. Therefore any physician prescribing statin drugs should be at least checking these nutrients. For once folic acid goes low, you raise homocysteine levels that then promote arteriosclerosis, thereby countering the very reason for which statins were prescribed. You have boarded **the medication merry-go-round**. Likewise with low selenium you set yourself up for cancers, hypothyroidism (which leads to high cholesterol), or chemical sensitivities, while low CoQ10 sets the patient up for congestive heart failure (with a median 5 year survival), cardiomyopathy, hair and teeth loss, depression, cancers, and more. Yet as you learned, sometimes very simple things like correcting a magnesium, niacin, omega-3, or an ascorbate deficiency can rectify the cholesterol problem (Lee, Chapters II, IV). But if the physician is not checking these, he is essentially working blindly. The patient is needlessly prescribed a lifelong course of statin drugs that guarantees a downhill course of more symptoms and more drugs.

When you find a physician who is up on 21st century molecular biochemistry of the human body, he will want to look at the pertinent biochemical information about your body's function and dysfunction. It is conveniently rolled into one test, the **Cardio/ION Panel**. In the meantime, a **3-part nutrient program** can be all the nutrients you need. For the odds are that just doing (1) the oil change that is spelled out in Chapter IV, (2) the mineral correction package in this chapter, plus (3) the select nutrients in Chapter II can bring about a huge change in not only your cholesterol, but also your general health, regardless of your medical label.

Executive Summary:
The Magic Package

I've only given you a brief example of a few vitamins, minerals, amino acids and fatty acids to demonstrate to you how important identifying and correcting your chemistry is for healing the human body, especially in cases where medicine has given up or decides you need a life-long sentencing to a drug. I would love to tell you in more detail about each of these plus the over 100 other nutrients that we have not even mentioned yet (some are in the next 2 chapters). But this is one book. I think you appreciate now how individual each of our biochemistries is. We all don't just look different we are different, chemically. That is why it is unthinkable that anyone would give up and merely drug someone for life, rather than get to the bottom of his or her symptoms and cure them. Start with the **Cardio/ION,** find your precise deficiencies and correct them first. Or you may be able to heal with the 3-part nutrient program above. That may be all you need to correct your cholesterol metabolism. And for folks with or without high cholesterol, correcting these is key to preventing cardiovascular disease, or slowing down and often reversing established disease.

Sources for this Chapter's Recommendations

- Methylcobalamin 5mg, Zinc Balance, BioSil, jarrow.com, or 1-877-VIT-AMEN
- Folixor 5mg, SilBoron, intensivenutrition.com, 1-800-333-7414
- NAC, DMG, davincilabs.com, or use NEEDS 1-800-634-1380
- Liposomal GSH, 1-877-VIT-AMEN
- LipoCeutical Glutathione, gshnow.com, 1-650-323-3238
- Recancostat, integrativeinc.com, 1-800-917-3690
- Cardio/ION Panel, Organic Acids, ADMA, metametrix.com, 1-800-221-4640
- Kyolic Liquid Cardiovascular, Kyo-Chrome, wakunaga.com, 1-800-421-2998
- Magnesium Chloride Solution 200mg/cc, windhampharmacy.com, 1-518-734-3033 (Rx required)
- Iodoral, Optimox, 1-800-223-1601, or 1-800-634-1380
- Vanadium 250 (from Vanadium Krebs), douglaslabs.com, 1-888-DOUG LAB
- IntraMin, druckerlabs.com, 1-888-881-2344
- Chelated Magnesium, Nutra Support Joint, Moly B, Chelated Zinc, E Gems Elite, Chelated Chromium, Biotin, Cod Liver Oil, Vitamin D3 2000 mg, ACES with Zinc, Chelated Selenium, Chelated Manganese, Chelated Copper, Vitamin B2, Glycine Powder, Vitamin K2, carlsonlabs.com, 1-800-323-4141
- Delta-Fraction Tocotrienols, allergyresearchgroup.com, 1-800-545-9960
- Essential Phospholipids, allergyresearchgroup.com, 1-800-545-9960
- Perfusia (Thorne, but they don't sell to the public), use NEEDS, 1-800-634-1380

References:

Lee KW, et al, The role of omega-3 fatty acids in the secondary prevention of cardiovascular disease, *Quart J Med*, 96:465-480, 2003

Richartz BM, et al, Reversibility of coronary endothelial vasomotor dysfunction in idiopathic dilated cardiomyopathy: acute effects of vitamin C, *Am J Cardio*, 88; 9:1001-05, Nov 2001

Chin JP, et al, HBPRCCA Astra Award. Therapeutic restoration of endothelial function in hypercholesterolaemic subjects: effect of fish oils, *Clin Exp Pharmacol Physiol*, 21; 10:749-55, Oct 1994

Goodfellow J, et al, Dietary supplementation with marine omega-3 fatty acids improve systemic large artery endothelial function in subjects with hypercholesterolemia, *J Am Coll Cardiol*, 35; 2:265-70, Feb 2000

Liu J, Atamna H, Kuratsune, Ames BN, Delaying brain mitochondrial aging with mitochondrial antioxidant and metabolites, *Ann NY Acad Sci*, 953:133-166, 2002

Fairfield KM, Fletcher R. H, Levinson W, Vitamins for chronic disease prevention in adults: Scientific review, *J Am Med Assoc*, 287; 23: 3116-3126, Jun 19, 2002

Fletcher RH, Fairfield KM, Levinson W, Vitamins for chronic disease prevention in adults: Clinical applications, *J Am Med Assoc*, 287; 23: 3127-29, Jun 19, 2002

Prasad KN, Cole WC, *Cancer and Nutrition*, IOS Press, Washington D.C., 1998

Moss RW, *Antioxidants Against Cancer*, Equinox Press, Brooklyn, 2000

Epstein SS, *The Politics Of Cancer Revisited*, East Ridge Press, Fremont Center, NY, 1998

Rogers SA, *Total Wellness 1999-2007*, prestigepubishing.com or 1-800-846-6687

Rogers SA, *Detoxify Or Die*, prestigepubishing.com or 1-800-846-6687

McCaddon A, Homocysteine and cognitive impairment; a case series in a general practice setting, *Nutr J*, 5: Feb 15, 2006

Sachdev PS, Homocysteine and brain atrophy, *Progr Neuropschopharmacol Biol Psychiatry*, 2005

McCaddon A, Davies G, Co-administration of N-acetylcysteine, vitamin B12 and folate in cognitively impaired hyper-homocystinemia patients, *Intern J Ger Psych*, 20:998-1000, 2005

Adair JC, et al, Controlled trial of N-acetylcysteine for patients with probable Alzheimer's disease, *Neurol*, 57: 1515-17, 2001

Naurath HJ, Joosten E, Riezler R, Lindenbaum J, et al, Effects of vitamin B12, folate, and vitamin B6 supplement in elderly people with normal serum vitamin concentrations, *Lancet*, 346: 85-89, July 8, 1995

Lietha R, Zimmerman M, Neuropsychiatric disorders associated with functional folate deficiency in the presence of elevated serum and erythrocyte folate: A preliminary report, *Journal Nutritional Medicine*, 4: 441-447, 1994

Narayanan BA, Narayanan NK, Reddy BS, Docosahexaenoic acid regulated genes and transcription factors inducing apoptosis in human colon cancer cells, *Internat J Oncol*, 19:1255-62, 2001

287

Peters JM, et al, Di-(2-ethylhexyl)-phthalate induces a functional zinc deficiency during pregnancy and teratogenesis that is independent of peroxisome proliferator-activated receptor-alpha, *Teratol,* 56:311-16, 1997

Pelton R, et al, *Drug-Induced Nutrient Depletion Handbook,* (1-877-837-5394)

Brownstein D, *Drugs That Don't Work and Natural Therapies That Do!,* Medical Alternatives Press, West Bloomfield, MI 48323, 1-888-647-5616

Rogers SA, Zinc repairs 33 genes and shrinks cancers, *Total Wellness,* July 2005, prestigepublishing.com or 1-800-846-6687

Chinetti G, et al, PPAR: nuclear receptors at the crossroads between lipid metabolism and inflammation, *Inflamm Res,* 49; 10:497-505, 2000

Fong LYY, Zhang L, Jiang Y, Farber JL, Dietary zinc modulation of COX-2 expression and lingual and esophageal carcinogenesis in rats, *J Natl Ca Inst,* 97; 1:40-50, Jan 5, 2005

Fong LY, Nguyen VT, Farber JL, Esophageal cancer prevention in zinc to-deficient rats: rapid induction of apoptosis by replenishing zinc. *J Natl Ca Inst,* 93: 1525-33, 2001

Khalfoun B, Thibault R, Watier H, et al, Docosapentaenoic and eicosapentaenoic acids inhibit in vitro human endothelial cell production of interleukin-6, *Adv Exp Med Biol,* 400B: 589-97, 1997

Raederstorff D, Pantze M, Bachmann H, Moser U, Anti-inflammatory properties of docosapentaenoic and eicosapentaenoic acids in phorbol-ester-induced mouse ear inflammation, *Int Arch Allergy Immunol,* 111; 3:284-90, Nov 1996

Fibrinogen References:
Palmieri V, Celentano A, Roman MJ, et al, Relation of fibrinogen to cardiovascular events is independent of preclinical cardiovascular disease: the Strong Heart Study, *Am Heart J,* 145; 3:467-74, Mar 2003

Green D, Hull RD, Brant R, Pineo GF, Lower mortality in cancer patients treated with low molecular weight versus standard heparin, *Lancet,* 339; 8807: 1476, June 13, 1992

Leveau B, Chastang C, Brechot JM, et al, Subcutaneous heparin treatment increases survival in small cell lung cancer. "Petites Cellules" Group, *Cancer,* 74; 1:38-45, Jul 1 1994

Coppola G, Rizzo M, Abrignani MG, et al, Fibrinogen as a predictor of mortality after acute myocardial infarction: a forty-two-month follow-up study, *Ital Heart J,* 6; 4:315-22, Apr 2005

Danesh J, Lewington S, Thompson SG, et al, Plasma fibrinogen level and the risk of major cardiovascular diseases and nonvascular mortality: an individual participant meta-analysis, *J Am Med Assoc,* 294; 14:1799-809, Oct 12, 2005

Packard CJ, O'Reilly DS, Caslake MJ, et al, Lipoprotein-associated phospholipase A2 as an independent predictor of coronary heart disease. West of Scotland Coronary Prevention Study Group, *New Engl J Med,* 343; 16:1148-55, Oct 19, 2000

Bordia AK, The effect of vitamin C on blood lipids and fibrinolytic activity and platelet adhesiveness in patients with coronary artery disease, *Atherosclerosis,* 35; 2:180 1-87, Feb 1980

Vanschoonbeek K, Feijge MA, Paquay M, et al, Variable hypocoagulant effect of fish oil intake in humans: modulation of fibrinogen level and thrombin generation, *Arterioscler Thromb Vasc Biol,* 24; 9:1734-40, Sep 2004

Philipp CS, Cisar LA, Saidi P, Kostis JB, Effect of niacin supplementation on fibrinogen levels in patients with peripheral vascular disease, *Am J Cardiol,* 82; 5:697-99, A9, Sep 1998

Johansson JO, Egberg N, Splund-Carlson A, Carlson LA, Nicotinic acid treatment shifts the fibrinolytic balance favorably and decreases plasma fibrinogen in hypertriglyceridemic men, *J Cardiovasc Risk,* 4; 3:165-71, Jun 1997

Calder PC, N-3 polyunsaturated fatty acids and inflammation: from molecular biology to the clinic, *Lipids,* 38; 4:340 3-52, Apr 2003

Chromium References:
Abraham AS, Brooks BA, Eylath V, The effects of chromium supplementation of serum glucose and lipids in patients with and without non-insulin dependent diabetes, *Metabolism,* 41:768-71, 1992

Gaby A, Chromium, *Integrative Medicine,* 5; 4:22-26, Aug/Sep 2006

Preuss HG, et al, Effects of different chromium compounds on blood pressure and lipid peroxidation in spontaneously hypertensive rats, *Clin Nephrol,* 47; 5:325-30, 1997

Riales R, Albrink MJ, Effect of chromium chloride supplementation on glucose tolerance and serum lipids including high density lipoproteins of adult men, *Am J Clin Nutr,* 34; 12: 2670-78, 1981

Press RI, et al, Effect of chromium picolinate on serum cholesterol and apolipoprotein fractions in human subjects, *West J Med,* 152; 3: 41-45, 1990

Magnesium References:
There is much more in many of the books. Start with *Depression Cured At Last!,* as magnesium deficiency is common to every disease.

Ma J, Folsom AR, Metcalf PA, et al., Association of serum and dietary magnesium with cardiovascular disease, hypertension, diabetes, insulin, and carotid artery wall thickness: the ARIC study. Atherosclerosis Risk in Communities Study, *J Clin Epidemiol,* 48: 927-40, 1995

Gartside PS, Glueck CJ, The important role of modifiable dietary and behavioral characteristics in the causation and prevention of coronary heart disease hospitalization and mortality: the prospective NHANES I follow-up study, *J Am Coll Nutr,* 14: 71-79, 1995

Rayssiguier Y, Gueux E, Magnesium and lipids in cardiovascular disease, *J Am Coll Nutr,* 5: 507-19, 1986

Ravn HB, Vissinger H, Husted SE, et al, **Magnesium inhibits platelet activity**--an infusion study in healthy volunteers, *Thromb Haemost,* 75: 939-44, 1996

Altura BM, Altura BT, Cardiovascular risk factors and magnesium: relationships to atherosclerosis, ischemic heart disease and hypertension, *Magnes Trace Elem,* 10: 1 82-92, 1991

Marier JR, Magnesium content of the food supply in the modern-day world, *Magnesium,* 5: 1-8, 1986

Almoznino-Sarafian D, et al, Magnesium and C-reactive protein in heart failure: it's an anti-inflammatory effect of magnesium administration? *Europ J Nutr*, 46:230-37, 2007

Cleveland LT, Goldmann JD, Borrud LG, *Data tables: Results from USDA's 1994 Continuing Survey of Food Intakes by Individuals* and *1994 Diet and Health Knowledge Survey*, Riverdale MD, Agricultural Research Service, USDA, 1996

Nielsen F H, et al, Dietary magnesium deficiency induces heart rhythm changes, impairs glucose tolerance, and increases serum cholesterol in postmenopausal women, *J Am Coll Nutr* 26:121-132, 2007

Arginine/taurine References:
Boger RH, et al, Asymmetric dimethylarginine (ADMA): a novel risk factor for endothelial dysfunction: its role in hypercholesterolemia, *Circulation*, 98: 1842-47, 1998

Drexler H, et al, Correction of endothelial dysfunction in coronary microcirculation of hypercholesterolemia patients by L-arginine, *Lancet*, 338:1546-50, 1991

De Lorgeril M, Dietary arginine and the prevention of cardiovascular diseases, *Cardiovasc Res*, 37:560-3, 1998

Boger RH, Bode-Boger SM, Brandes RP, Phivthong-Ngam L, Bohme M, Nafe R, Mugge A, Frolich JC, Dietary L-arginine reduces the progression of atherosclerosis in cholesterol-fed rabbits: comparison with lovastatin, *Circulation*, 96:1282-90, 1997

Drexler H, Zeiher AM, Meinzer K, Just H, Correction of endothelial dysfunction in coronary microcirculation of hyperchoesterolaemic patients by l-arginine, *Lancet*, 338:1546-50, 1991

Kawano H, et al, Endothelial dysfunction in hypercholesterolaemia is improved by L-arginine administration: possible role of oxidative stress, *Atherosclerosis*, 161; 2:375-80, Apr 2002

Mochizuki H, Oda H, Yokkogoshi H, Amplified effect of taurine on PCB-induced hypercholesterolemia in rats, *Adv Exp Med Biol*, 442: 285-290, 1998

Satoh H, Cardio-protective actions of taurine against intracellular and extracellular Ca 2+-induced effects, *Adv Exper Med Biol*, 359: 181-196, 1994

Satoh H, et al, Review of some actions of taurine on ion channels of cardiac muscle cells and others, *Gen Pharmacol*, 30: 451-63, 1998

Waterfield CJ, Turton JA, Scales MD, Timbrell JA, Reduction of liver taurine in rats by beta-alanine treatment increases carbon tetrachloride toxicity, *Toxicology*, 77: 7-20, 1993

Jeejeebhoy F, et al, Nutritional supplementation with MyoVive repletes essential cardiac myocyte nutrients and reduces left ventricular size in patients with left ventricular dysfunction, *Am Heart J*, 143:1092-1100, 2002

Azuma J, et al, Therapy of congestive heart failure with orally administered taurine, *Clin Ther*, 5: 398-408,1983

Other References:
Tamura T, Turnland JR, Effect of long-term, high-copper intakes on the concentrations of plasma homocysteine and B vitamins in young men, *Nutr*, 20: 757-59, 2004

McNulty H, et al, Riboflavin lowers homocysteine in individuals homozygous for the MTHFR 677C-T polymorphism, *Circulation,* 113:74-80, 2006

Plotnick GD, Corretti MC, Vogel RA, Effect of antioxidant vitamins on the transient impairment of endothelium-dependent brachial artery vasoactivity following a single high-fat meal, *J Amer Med Assoc*, 278; 20:1682-6, 1997

Nathens AB, Neff MJ, Jurkovich GJ, et al, Randomized, prospective trial of antioxidant supplementation in critically ill surgical patients, *Ann Surgery*, 236: 8 14-8 22, 2002

Porter JM, Ivatury RR, Azimuddin K, et al, Antioxidant therapy in the prevention of organ dysfunction syndrome and infectious complications after trauma: early results of a prospective randomized study, *Am Surg*, 65: 4 78-4 83, 1999

Cowley HC, Bacon OJ, Goode HF, et al, Plasma antioxidant potential in severe sepsis: a comparison of survivors and nonsurvivors, *Crit Care Med*, 24: 1179-83, 1996

Gokce N, Keaney JF Jr, Frei B, et al, Long-term ascorbic acid administration reverses endothelial vasomotor dysfunction in patients with coronary artery disease, *Circulation*, 99: 3234-40, 1999

Taddei S, Virdis A, Ghiadoni L, et al, Vitamin C improves endothelial-dependent vasodilatation by restoring nitric oxide activity in essential hypertension, *Circulation*, 97: 2222-29, 1998

Hackman DG, et al, What level of plasma homocysteine should be treated? Effects of vitamin therapy on progression of carotid atherosclerosis, *Am J Hypertens*, 2000 Jan, 13; 1 Pt 1:105-10

Rasouli ML, et al, Plasma homocysteine predicts progression of atherosclerosis, *Atherosclerosis*, 2005 Jul, 181; 1:159-65

Tsimikas S, et al, Oxidized phospholipids, Lp(a)lipoprotein, and coronary artery disease, *N Engl J Med,* 2005 Jul 7, 353;1:46-57

Ginter E, Ascorbic acid in cholesterol and bile acid metabolism, *Ann NY Acad Sci*, 1975 Sept 30, 258:410-21

Glueck CJ, et al, Evidence that homocysteine is an independent risk factor for atheroscleriosis in hyperlipidemic patients, *Am J Cardiol,* 1995 Jan 15, 75; 2:132-6

Turley SD, et al, The role of ascorbic acid in the regulation of cholesterol metabolism and the pathogenesis of atherosclerosis, *Atherosclerosis,* 1976 Jul; 24; 1-2:1-18

Kaul D, Baba MI, Genomic effect of vitamin 'C' and statins with human mononuclear cells involved in atherogenic process, *Eur J Clin Nutr,* 2005 Aug; 59; 8:978-91

Rubins HB, et al, Distribution of lipids in 85,000 men with coronary artery disease, *Am J Cardiol,* 1995 Jun15, 75; 17:1196-1201

Rafique S, et al, Reversal of extrahepatic membrane cholesterol deposition in patients with chronic liver diseases by S-adenosylmethionine, *Clin Sci,* 83:353-6, Sep 1992

291

Stein J, Antioxidants slow progression of transplant atherosclerosis, *Internal Med World Rep*, pg 7, Feb. 2001

Delpre G, Stark P, Niv Y, Sublingual therapy for cobalamin deficiency as an alternative to oral and parenteral cobalamin supplementation, *Lancet,* 354; 9180:740-1, Aug 28, 1999

Craig G, Elliot C, Hughes K, Masked vitamin B12 and folate deficiency in the elderly, *Br J Nutr,* 1985; 54:613-619

van der Mei IAF, et al, The high prevalence of vitamin D insufficiency across Australian populations is only partly explained by season and latitude, *Environ Health Persp*, 115: 1132-39, 2007

Vieth R, et al, Efficacy and safety of vitamin D3 intake exceeding the lowest observed adverse effect level, *Am J Clin Nutr*, 73; 2: 288-94, 2001

Holick MF, Sunlight and vitamin D for bone health and prevention of autoimmune diseases, cancers, and cardiovascular disease, *Am J Clin Nutr,* 80 (suppl 6): 1678s-88s, 2004

Holick MF, Vitamin D: importance in the prevention of cancers, type 1 diabetes, heart disease, and osteoporosis, *Am J Clin Nutr,* 79; 3:362-71, 2005

Holick MF, High prevalence of Vitamin D inadequacy and implications for health, *Mayo Clin Proc*, 81; 3:353-73, Mar 2006

Hollis BW, Circulating 25-hydroxy vitamin D levels indicative of vitamin D insufficiency: implications for establishing a new effective dietary intake recommendation for vitamin D, *J Nutr,* 135; 2:317-22

Zitterman A, Vitamin D in preventive medicine: are we ignoring the evidence? *Brit J Nutr,* 89; 5:552-70 2, 2003

Watson KE, et al, Active serum vitamin D levels are inversely correlated with coronary calcifications, *Circulation,* 96; 6:1755-60, Sept 16, 1997

Zittermann A, et al, Vitamin D and vascular calcification, *Curr Opin Lipidol,* 18; 1:40 1-6, Feb 2007

Martins B, et al, Prevalence of cardiovascular risk factors and the sum levels of 25-hydroxyvitamin D in the United States, *Arch Intern Med,* 167:1159-65, 2007

Goreleijnse JM, et al, Dietary intake of menaquinone is associated with a reduced risk of coronary heart disease: the Rotterdam Study, *J Nutr,* 134; 3:3100-3105, Nov 2004

Goreleijnse JM, et al, Inverse association of dietary vitamin K-2 intake with cardiac events and aortic atherosclerosis: The Rotterdam Study, *Thrombosis Haemost,* (suppl July): 473, 2001

Kawashima H, et al, Effects of vitamin K2 (menatetrenone) on atherosclerosis and blood, coagulation in hypercholesterolemia, rabbits, *Jpn J Pharmacol,* 75; 2:135-43, Oct 1997

Spronk HM, et al, Tissue-specific utilization of inadequate menaquinone-4 results in the prevention of arterial calcification in warfarin-treated rats, *J Vasc Res* 40; 6:531-37, Nov-Dec 2003

Vermeer C, et al. Role of K vitamins in the regulation of tissue calcification, *J Bone Min Metab*, 19; 4:201-06, 2001

Shearer MJ, Vitamin K, *Lancet,* 345; 8944: 229-34, Jan 28, 1995

Shurgers LJ, et al, Novel conformation-specific antibodies against matrix gamma-carboxy-glutamic acid (Gla) protein: undercarboxylated matrix Gla protein as marker for vascular calcification, *Arterioscler Thromb Vasc Biol,* 25; 8:1620 9-33, Aug 2005

Oral anticoagulant treatment: friend or foe in cardiovascular disease? *Blood,* 104; 10:3231-32, Nov 15, 2004

Berkner KI, et al, The physiology of vitamin K nutriture and vitamin K-dependent protein function in atherosclerosis, *J Thromb Haemo,* 2; 12: 2118-32, Dec 2004

Naito Y, et al, Tocotrienols reduce 25-hydroxycholesterol-induced monocyte-endothelial cell interaction by inhibiting the surface expression of adhesion molecules, *Atherosclerosis,* 180:19-25.2005

Parker RA, et al, Tocotrienols regulate cholesterol reduction in mammalian cells by post-transcription suppression of 3-hydroxy-3 methylglutaryl coenzyme A reductase, *J Biol Chem,* 268, 11230-8, 1993

Song BL, et al, Insig-dependent ubiquitination and degradation of 3-hydroxy-3-methylglutaryl coenzyme A reductase stimulated by delta- and gamma-tocotrienols, *J Biol Chem,* 281:25054-61, 2006

Chao JT, et al, Inhibitory effect of delta-tocotrienol, a HMG COA reductase inhibitor, on monocyte-endothelial cell adhesion, *J Nutr Sci Vitaminol* (Tokyo), 40:332-7, 2002

Cook NR, et al, A randomized factorial trial of vitamin C and E and beta-carotene in the secondary prevention of cardiovascular benefits in women, *Arch Intern Med,* 167:1610-18, 2007

Ford ES, et al, *Obesity,* 15:1139-46, 2007

Richards BJ, *Fight For Your Health, Exposing the FDA's betrayal of America,* wellnessresourcesbooks.com, Minn MN, 2006

DeRijke YB, et al, The redox status of coenzyme Q10 in total LDL as an indicator of in vivo oxidative modification: studies on subjects with familial combined hyperlipidemia, *Atherosclerosis, Thrombosis and Vascular Biology,* 17:127-33, 1997

Vanadium References:
Verma S, et al, Nutritional factors that can favorably influence the glucose/insulin system: vanadium, *J Am Coll Nutr,* 17; 1:11-18, 1998

Natesampillai S, et al, Vanadate elevates lipogenicity of starved rat adipose tissue: mechanism of action, *Endocrinol,* 139; 5: 2514-18, 1998

Cohen N, et al, Oral vanadyl sulfate improves, hepatic and peripheral insulin sensitivity in patients with non-insulin-dependent diabetes mellitus, *J Clin Investig,* 95: 2501-09, June 1995

Noda C, et al, Vanadate improves cardiac function and myocardial energy metabolism in diabetic rat hearts, *Jpn Heart J,* 44:745-57, 2003

Green A, The insulin-like effect of sodium vanadate on adipocyte glucose transport is mediated at a post-insulin-receptor level, *Biochem J,* 238:663-69, 1986

Chapter VII

The Toxic Connection

There is one more cause of high cholesterol that is greater than food, greater than nutrient deficiencies, and often greater than even hidden bugs. This is the category of everyday toxins that we slowly tank up on throughout our lives. The scientific evidence for what I'm about to tell you is in the last two books and the last few years of *Total Wellness* newsletters, so I won't make this chapter any larger by adding those hundreds of scientific references, although my obsessive-compulsive nature will lead me to include quite a few key references in this chapter.

First, for the naysayers who insist that (1) toxicity is overblown, and (2) we get such minute doses that they are inconsequential, and (3) if it were important their doctors would check it, let me give you folks who are not up on it a crash course in reality.

1. We are the **first generation of people ever exposed to such an unprecedented number of toxins**. Right now government studies show that every human in the United States has measurable levels of a symphony of toxins, which are now called **ubiquitously unavoidable xenobiotics.** And how they interact with one another in the body is insidiously catastrophic. Let's take a look.

The number one pollutant in the human body, plasticizers, are over 10,000 times higher in humans than all other pollutants put together. Phthalates or plasticizers get into our air and water supplies from incinerators and industrial exhaust. But the number one route of pollution is foods. Plastic wrap around fruits, vegetables and meats actually permeates into the foods and then gets stuck in our body chemistry. Likewise plastic bottles used for sodas, fruit juices, spring water, infant formula, milk and other beverages also leach plastics into the liquid and then it gets stuck in our body chemistry. And many canned foods' linings, prescription medications (slow-release coatings), plus our textiles, detergents, toiletries, cosmetics, car interiors, furnishings and construction materials outgas to contribute further phthalates to the human body.

2. We are so polluted that **the average U.S. baby now is born with measurable levels of Teflon, plasticizers, fire retardants, pesticides, and heavy metals** like mercury, lead, arsenic and cadmium.

3. We have so polluted the world via our smokestacks that the **Arctic polar bears**, which have the cleanest air, food, and water, **have osteoporosis and hypothyroidism from our chemicals**. These are new diseases for them.

4. When EPA scientists measured the exhaled breath of Americans, they found perchloroethylene was in 93% of them, while benzene (a known cause of leukemia, common in vehicle and industrial exhaust) was in 89% of common folks.

5. Scientists have repeatedly shown that **low doses** of many of the most common environmental chemicals **are actually more dangerous than high doses.**

6. Furthermore, no one has ever studied the total effect of the combination of all of the unwanted chemicals in the human body.

7. Most physicians are as unknowledgeable regarding pollutant chemistry and environmental medicine as the layperson.

8. Worst of all, these toxins overload our innate ability to detoxify, so they bioaccumulate. The bottom line is we slowly tank up on enough until we get a disease. It is as simple as that.

9. In the body heavy metals kick minerals out of enzymes, chemicals poison proteins, and act like a broken key in membrane receptors, and both damage our chemistry in a multitude of other ways.

10. The good news is you can get rid of them, thus turning back the hands of time. You can watch disease melt away, and for many, experience a body healthier than it ever was before.

One big problem is that these unavoidable pollutants (that are everywhere) damage our chemistry in a staggering number of ways, one of which is to create high cholesterol. Let's take a look at some of the evidence.

Teflon Creates Hypercholesterolemia

Many only think of Teflon in regard to a frying pan that's easy to clean because food doesn't stick. But Teflon is part of the family of fluorinated chemicals that are used everywhere in our home carpets and furnishings and even clothes to make them stain resistant. Nearly every restaurant and factory food has traces as well as many machines for heating water for coffee, etc.. We are exposed to so much Teflon in our air, food, and water that we all have it in us. Even the newborn baby has measurable levels of Teflon in his umbilical cord blood at the moment of birth. And when scientists drop helicopters into pristine areas and shoot wild animals with a tranquilizer gun to draw their blood, they find Teflon in every species, from fish and frogs to four-footed furbearers.

It turns out that as **Teflon levels slowly accumulate** in the human body throughout a lifetime, **they damage many genes including those that govern the metabolism of lipids, like cholesterol** (Guruge). This eventually leads to high cholesterol that resists any type of treatment other than getting the damaging Teflon out of the body. How **Teflon** affects one person may be totally different from another. In rat studies it **turns on 106 genes and turns off 38 genes**. And whether you look at the genes of animals in the wild or humans in captivity, the metabolism of lipids (fats like cholesterol) appears to be the major target (Guruge, Heuvel). Unfortunately, scientists have found that **humans are often more sensitive to hidden chemicals than rats used in experiments** (they eat a better diet, for one!) (Stahlhut).

Sadly, one of the most important facts about Teflon is it is what's called an unavoidably **persistent environmental pollutant.** In other words, we cannot escape from it and the body has no way of metabolizing it thoroughly to get rid of it. It is designed to never degrade or break down; consequently **it stays in us forever.** The damage it wreaks is not fully discovered, but for starters it **damages the receptors for vitamin A** and the **chemistry to make**

more DHA, the most important fatty acid in our arterial cell membranes. We need both to protect against heart disease, in our brains to protect against Alzheimer's, and in other cells to protect against cancer. And remember, we cannot escape Teflon. The newborn baby to the very old have measurable levels, and we progressively tank up on more as we go through life. Fortunately there is one way to get it out of the body, which I'll show you shortly.

If your cholesterol is very resistant, remember **fluoride is in Teflon** molecules. **Cogimax** is a special form of silicon that can help displace fluoride and can reduce the amount the body absorbs. Take 1-3 a day. Next, reducing the heavy metal load is key for many folks, since they are closely tied in with Teflon molecules. We'll talk about how to get Teflon and heavy metals out later.
.

In the meantime, heavy-duty German **Silit** fry pans, pots, and a Silit pressure cooker (from natural-lifestyle.com) are great substitutes for your cheapo Teflon pans. It always amazes me that people will spend $100 or more for a dinner of processed, non-organic foods, but not buy a superior cooking pan that they'll use three times daily for a lifetime and that assures better health.

The Teflon Tragedy

I remember when Teflon was introduced. It was the hottest new thing in cooking because you never had to scrub a pan again, just merely rinse it out. No matter how bad a cook you were you could hardly burn anything and nothing stuck to the bottom. Since then it has been added to all sorts of textiles, fabrics and more to make them stain resistant. We even wear the stuff. Because of this technology we all now have Teflon in us, including newborn babies and the polar bears and fish in the remote Canadian Arctic.

Studies show that this category of PFOA (perfluorooctanoic acid) that is part of a larger category called PFCs (perfluorochemicals, which include Scotchguard, etc.), causes cancer, damages the immune system **bringing on allergies, recurrent infections, and destroys hormones**, plus **Teflon triggers autoimmune problems where the body attacks its own cells as in rheumatoid arthritis, lupus, arteriosclerosis, diabetes, colitis, thyroiditis, and much more.** In other words, it does all the stuff that the plasticizers, PCBs, pesticides and many of the other unavoidable environmental pollutants do as well. And Teflon damages the liver and blood vessel linings encouraging the body to make more cholesterol. Yet no one has ever looked at the combined effect of all these toxins.

If that were not enough, PFOA are loaded with fluoride that damages the brain and promotes bone loss as well as tooth discoloration and premature aging. Like many of the other persistent environmental pollutants, there is absolutely no evidence that they ever fully degrade or get out of us. All we do is progressively keep tanking up on more. A sad fact is the highest levels are in kids. And considering that it never goes away, you can understand why more children and young adults now are getting diseases of old age like diabetes, cancer, hypertension, depression, joint replacements, defective brains and even high cholesterol.

Like so many other pollutants, Teflon-type chemicals add to the total load accelerating disease and aging. All cures can be stalled indefinitely until there is sufficient unloading of the total body burden of damaging pollutants. How do you get rid of them? The protocols in *Detoxify or Die* followed by *The High Blood Pressure Hoax* guide you more explicitly through detoxification, depending upon how much you need. And subsequent *TW's* will keep you abreast of newer finds, cheaper sources of therapeutic agents, and ways to make the program easier and more efficient. But buck up, I'll give you a simplified version here.

Start by using one **Iodoral** daily, the best form of iodine/iodide that I know of, a mineral to keep the fluoride part of Teflon moving out of your body (if it can break free of this nasty molecule). Next, I suggest you throw out the Teflon cookware. Unfortunately, most food manufacturers and restaurants still use it and I don't foresee them getting rid of it. I'll show you the rest of the program shortly.

Plastics Cause High Cholesterol

Plastics also damage cholesterol metabolism, and like Teflon, PCBs, trans fats and other hidden yet potent causes of high cholesterol, they too are ubiquitous and unavoidable. There is just plain too much in our air, food, and water in this era. We are the first generation and the experimental generation. There are numerous ways the plastics damage our cholesterol metabolism, but I know you don't want to become a molecular biochemist (Xu). So suffice to say, as with all the other environmental pollutants we actually have an average daily intake of plastics of around 19 µg/kilogram body weight per day (Kavlock). But if you have an IV in the hospital or outpatient chelation with plastic tubing, for example, it can increase your plastic level to way over 160 mcg per day. This is especially scary when you think about a newborn on IVs who has a more immature detoxification system than the adult (Latini). If that weren't bad enough, the plastics tend to preferentially go right from the mother into the placenta and fetus. The high level of plastics from IVs explains why many people with prolonged exposure to IVs such as with chelation, or prolonged hospitalizations with lots of IVs never get completely well or go on to have more serious problems. They never got the plastics out!

What else do plastics do in the human body? They are called **environmental endocrine disruptors because they damage hormones and make hormones act unpredictably.** For example, they can damage the thyroid hormone without damaging the tests that doctors normally use to diagnose thyroid problems. And don't forget **that a low thyroid can create high cholesterol. Likewise plasticizers lower testosterone, which also creates arteriosclerosis. This also creates diabetes, metabolic syndrome also called Syndrome X (which accelerates aging), increases weight**

that just will not budge, promotes prostate and breast cancers, and much more.

You see plastics are not only hidden in our foods from containers and plastic wraps, but they're also in cosmetics, shampoos, soaps, lubricants, pesticides, paints as well as polyvinyl chloride. So they outgas from the electrical wiring in our appliances, computers, homes, offices and cars. They're unavoidable. That's why they are the #1 pollutant in the human body. Yet they are still considered inert even though **they clearly create diabetes, low testosterone, low thyroid function, insulin resistance, and high cholesterol, all of which promote cardiovascular disease** (Stahlhut). And much research published in the government's leading environmental journal now proves that **low doses are even more damaging than high doses** (vom Saal, Rogers).

If that still weren't enough, plastics do a lot more once they are in the human body. As I began to show you in the last chapter, a major problem is that **phthalates cause a zinc deficiency** (Peters). This is especially dangerous in the fetus of a mother drinking from plastic water bottles, or feeding her newborn from plastic formula bottles. This deficiency in the adult goes on to cause numerous diseases and symptoms because zinc is in over 200 enzymes (Rogers). Most important is probably the DNA polymerase, which is the main gene repair enzyme in the body and is highly zinc dependent. Without enough zinc, we get cancer. As well, the **phthalates decrease catalase, one of many specialized detoxifying enzymes** we make in our bodies to protect us from our daily onslaught of environmental chemicals, so that they do not go on to cause more serious diseases like cancers (Magliozzi). The bottom line is **we are lucky if all we get is high cholesterol. Because if high cholesterol is used as a warning, as it should be, smart folks will go on to get rid of the underlying causes and not just try to beat it to death with a statin drug that ushers in faster aging and more diseases.**

Plastics basically damage peroxisomes (organelles inside our cells), which control the genes that control the metabolism of all of your cholesterol. But worse, they also damage control for all fatty acids and phospholipids for the cell membrane, hormones, immune system, and much more (Beier, Ram, Bell, Kliewer). And they create inflammation, the basis of not only arteriosclerosis but also chronic fatigue, other chronic diseases and aging (Chinetti, Melnick).

Why are they so unavoidable? Over 97% of human urines studied contained detectable levels of plastic metabolites in one government study of over 2500 samples (Silva). Remember, phthalates (dialkyl or alkyl/aryl esters of 1,2-benzenedicarboxylic acid) are used as plastic softeners, and are hidden in detergents, soaps, cosmetics, shampoos, solvents and perfumes, additives and hairsprays, lubricants, insecticides, residential and commercial construction materials, automobiles, floorings, paints, carpet backings, adhesives, wood finishers, vinyl seat covers, clothing, purses, notebooks, toys, pens, and wallpaper, PVC products, medical tubing, and more. Now you see why they are unavoidable. The levels inside new cars are the highest levels measured in any indoor environments, up to 34 mcg per cubic meter.

And they are even higher in folks who have had IVs, especially infants. It can bring on a life of medical misery, creating nutrient deficiencies, hormone problems and mysterious symptoms that defy diagnosis or cure (Shea, Barry, Roth, Loff, Cullum). **Yet the average physician knows nothing about them and their ability to bring on every type of abnormality on the body, much less how to diagnose it and get rid of them.**

Luckily the same route that we use to remove Teflon, PCBs, pesticides and more from the body that you will learn about also removes the plastics. But we also have to make a concerted effort to reduce our consumption of them starting with avoiding all plastic containers as much as possible. For starters, buy some spring water in glass bottles with a screw on cap so that now you have a glass bottle that you can carry wherever you go (or for more fun, make it a screw-cap empty glass wine bottle for carrying your good water, and see what kind of looks you get on the tennis court). Keep one at your desk, one in the boudoir for a nighttime drink, one in your car, and take it to your courts and courses. Fill it with good water from your **alkaline water machine** or other water filter that you have at home. You can get cute little containers at the local wine shop, for example, that protect against glass spatter should you drop and break the bottles. Call the **American Environmental Health Center** (aehf.com) to get glass baby bottles with safe nipples for the newborn.

Plastics Cause High Insulin

Bisphenol A (BPA) is one component of the plastics that we get from our plastic water bottles and plastic wrap on foods. It causes a rapid drop in glucose that then **causes a dramatic rise in plasma insulin.** After as little as four days of treatment with plastic (BPA), mice have developed chronic hyperinsulinemia. As you recall, having **elevated insulin not only makes it impossible to lose weight, but can bring out all sorts of other common maladies like high blood pressure, diabetes, hypoglycemia, chronic fatigue, unwarranted mood swings, high triglycerides, abnormal thyroid function, prostate and breast cancers, ovarian malfunction as in endometriosis, polycystic ovary disease, and early coronary artery disease**.

Clearly **plastics cause high cholesterol by multiple mechanisms**. For example, the addition of high insulin is like adding oil to a fire, accelerating arteriosclerosis, diabetes, obesity and more. It doesn't end. Plastics provide a perfect example of how one unavoidable environmental exposure creates common diseases that medicine treats as a deficiency of the latest drug. **Phthalates create diseases that folks are told are chronic and have no known cause and no known cure.** Obviously you are now too smart to fall for that malarkey ever again. The cure is to get the poisons out of the body.

BPA is one of the most common forms of phthalates and we are all exposed, humans and animals alike from our air, food and water. They leach out of food containers of all sorts (coatings inside food cans, plastic food containers, even cellophane windows of cookie boxes), IV tubing, dental sealants, construction materials, computers, cars, couches and carpets. When their residues are spewed over the earth via incinerators, scientists find wild animals in remote pristine areas of all species have plasticizers in them. They not only damage hormones but the very chemistry of every cell membrane. This one type of plastic, BPA, is one of the highest volume chemicals produced in the world and is found in government studies in over 95% of urine and blood samples of people in the United States.

The European Commission's Scientific Committee on Food reports a tolerable daily intake of 10 µg/kg/day, but the US EPA considers a level 5 times more potent to be safe, using 50 micrograms per kilogram per day as their reference. Unfortunately this antiquated "standard" is based on studies performed in 1980s before technology revealed the true dangers of plastics and how they can create nearly very chronic disease known to medicine and even "mysterious" new ones.

BPA at doses about a thousand-fold less than the LOAEL (lowest observable adverse effect level) level established by the US EPA damages blood sugar control and wildly raises insulin, both contributing to arteriosclerosis that cholesterol is blamed for. Meanwhile, longer **exposure to phthalates increases pancreatic beta-cell insulin content and creates hyperinsulinemia and peripheral insulin resistance or Syndrome X, complete with inability to lose weight or inability to control diabetes, hypertension and/or dyslipidemia (high cholesterol, triglycerides).**

As **plastics poison the thyroid** (without damaging common tests of thyroid function, see *Detoxify or Die*), **hypothyroidism also creates high cholesterol.** Other symptoms of subclinical hypothyroidism include dry skin, poor memory, fatigue, constipation, muscle cramps, constipation, hoarseness, cold intolerance, muscle weakness, slow thinking, inability to lose weight, impotence, infertility, erectile dysfunction, heart failure, cramps, shortness of breath, and unwarranted depression (see *DOD*), inviting even more drugs.

As further evidence of how inadequate the "safe" cut-off for plasticizer is, **a dose lower than the level found in the blood of human babies at birth produces a 2.5-fold increase in insulin and a 20% decrease in blood glucose.** Translation: this is enough to deprive the innocent newborn's brain of sugar and lead to irritability, seizures, poor brain function, abnormal development, and more. A low dose of plasticizer of 10 µg/kilogram/day (a five times weaker dose than the EPA considers safe) can also change insulin content. A higher dose of 100 µg (twice the US reference) dramatically increased pancreatic insulin content after only four days of exposure creating marked insulin resistance (Metabolic Syndrome X). I repeat some of these facts to make learning easier for you, for this is crucial information for a generation at risk.

The bottom line is that the health of our children and grandchildren is in a much more dangerous situation than we could have ever imagined. We're already seeing unprecedented epidemics of obesity and diabetes and cancers among children, as well as more congenital defects and impaired behavior and intellect. In fact, now we even know that mothers passing on their phthalates to their male fetuses and then further feeding them from plastic bottles are setting them up for enlarged prostates and increased cancer risk when they reach adulthood (Richter) (there is much more information for concerned grandparents who want to make a difference in *Total Wellness* 2000 to present).

PCBs Create High Cholesterol

Most people were not born with high cholesterol, but they developed it as adults. So for starters let's look at how we get 500 rats in the lab with high cholesterol so that we can do experiments with cholesterol-lowering drugs. One easy way is to give them **PCBs** (Mochizuki). Polychlorinated biphenyls are man-made chemicals created as a by-product from manufacturing myriads of things that we consider indispensable. PCBs are a family of many types of chemicals that are eventually spewed into the air from industrial exhausts, thus permeating our air, food, and water. EPA studies show that **100% of U.S. humans have PCBs stored in our their bodies**. So anyone of us can develop high cholesterol or any of the other staggering symptoms that PCBs cause, including cancers, at any time. PCBs silently stockpile in our bodies over the years until they finally damage enough of our chemistry to create a disease, but more on this later, and more importantly how to remove them to reverse disease.

The lead story on the front page of *USA Today* a couple of years ago told about one of the cousins of PCBs, PBDE. *USA Today* showed the world that the stockpiling of chemicals in the human body is a seriously cascading yet "invisible" problem (Weise, Petreas, Herrick, Rogers). The unsuspected environmental chemical they were talking about this time was the **flame retardant (PBDE**), which has been found to be **20 times higher in U.S. breast milk** than in the breast milk of European nursing mothers. And this applies to all people, since breast milk is just an example of an easy way to assay fat without a biopsy. Flame retardants stockpile in breast milk and damage children's brains.

Why is PBDE dangerously 20 times higher in US citizens? Because we're one of the few countries foolish enough to be convinced that they need to legislate a known carcinogenic chemical for use in everyone's mattresses so some drunk having a cigarette doesn't burn himself up. As a result, this nasty carcinogenic chemical called a flame retardant outgases from our sofas and chairs, couches, pillows, car seats, plane seats, mattresses, and most stuffed furnishings as well as foam products, and the casings and wires in electrical products like computers.

The interesting thing is only 3000 people die in fires each year and the Chemical Manufacturers Association estimates the number would be 960 people higher without the flame retardant. Big deal. For this we poison everyone with a known carcinogen? **PBDE is a cousin to PCBs, which are the most cancer-causing man-made chemicals on the face of the earth.**

The scariest part is that **the levels of PBDE in US humans is doubling every two years,** promising a nation of more maladies requiring all sorts of prescription drugs. These chemicals that have permeated the environment have *caused brain damage with low levels of exposure.* Fire retardants damage literally every part of the body, including cholesterol metabolism. Disease doesn't just appear for no reason. Ubiquitous flame-retardants are in the air of every home, office, institution and vehicle. The national solution for chemicals that permeate the environment, produce disease in even very low levels, and unavoidably stockpile the body? Government-sponsored agencies are going to study it. Do they ever tell you anything about how to get the chemicals out of your body? Not a whiff. Lucky for you however, there's one proven way of getting these chemicals out of the body, as described here and in more thorough detail in *Detoxify or Die* (prestigepublishing.com or 1-800-846-6687). Even after disease has occurred, it's not necessarily too late to get the causative element out, in fact it's even more important than ever.

If you want to really be concerned about future generations, remember the average baby spends the majority of his time swaddled in this chemical, a known carcinogen that has been legislated into our everyday environments. For PBDE outgases from the innocent infant's crib mattress, crib bumpers, car seat, and playpen. He never gets a breath of fresh air. And this is looking at only one chemical in his toxic environment (see *DOD*).

Furthermore this government study (U.S. EPA 1984) showed **100% of human fat samples contained stored <u>xylene</u>,** another unavoidably common hydrocarbon that can interfere with cholesterol chemistry (from gasoline, auto exhaust, paints, glues, plastics, mattresses, furnishings, cleansers, degreasers, laboratory fixatives, office and home construction materials, new carpeting, etc.). And most of us also possess another carcinogen <u>**1,4-dichlorobenzene**</u> (from home and commercial deodorizers ("plug-ins"), moth balls, sanitizers in textiles for furnishings, bedding, clothes and many other products) (U.S.D.H.H.S. 1998). It doesn't end.

Heavy Metals Damage Cholesterol Enzymes

Since the **liver makes 80% of the cholesterol regardless of what your diet is,** it shouldn't come as a surprise that if you go on a torturous low cholesterol diet, the liver just compensates and puts out more cholesterol (Kuntz). But God's miraculous body design has a mechanism for controlling and neutralizing excess cholesterol. The enzyme **lecithin: cholesterol acyltransferase, abbreviated LCAT, pulls access cholesterol out of arterial tissues and binds it to the good or happy cholesterol, HDL.** The HDL carries the excess cholesterol to the liver where it is turned into the bile. As bile acid, it is now used to:

- Enhance absorption of crucial essential fatty acids, as well as fat-soluble vitamins, like vitamins A, D, E, K, and beta-carotene, CoQ10, and more.
- Plus bile is used for food digestion.
- And it is a major detoxifier in the gut (Madani, Bruce, Park).

But don't forget that by taking a statin cholesterol-lowering drug, you turn off the production cholesterol, which turns off the production of bile, which then decreases your absorption of fat-soluble vitamins and ability to detoxify (Kuntz). In short, you dig a hole for yourself.

So if **LCAT is the hero and gets rid of excess cholesterol**, why isn't it doing its job? The answer is easy. In the laboratory if we want to turn off that enzyme so that we can create high cholesterol in animals for experiments, a quick way to do it is to **poison the LCAT enzyme with mercury or other heavy metals like cadmium and lead,** all three of which are in all of us.

Now since these heavy metals also poison a number of other enzymes and can lead to literally many other diseases as well as accelerate aging, the smart thing would be to get rid of the mercury and other heavy metals. And luckily there are several ways that I'll show you to do this, because we need all of them. For heavy metals are not the only culprits. When researchers want to create animals with high cholesterol, they can dose them with pesticides that are also in all of us. We will never run out of toxins again.

Fortunately, once you put the body level of unwanted chemicals and heavy metals back to where it was before you had high cholesterol, it's **like turning back the hands of time**. Not only have you cured your cholesterol problem but many other symptoms. I believe it is literally the closest thing to the **"fountain of youth"** that we currently have.

Epidemics Out of Control

We are engulfed by epidemics out of control. As one small example, the US government's CDC tells us that diabetes has doubled in the last quarter-century in Americans. Some schools even report that as much as one in eight children have some form of diabetes. Yet the "authorities" totally ignore teaching folks about all the data proving that the phthalates or plasticizers, which permeate our foods, are one of the most potent causes of diabetes.

Another silent cause of diabetes is arsenic that we also cannot escape, since it's a common pesticide for poultry, as an example, and a common contaminant of rice, drinking water and more (Lasky). It is a blatant carcinogen triggering cancers of the skin, lung (in non-smokers), bladder, and in non-lethal concentrations disrupts the endocrine system (Kaltreider) and can trigger breast and prostate cancers. As we showed in past issues of *TW*, it's one of the heavy metals that can cause prostate cancer to become resistant to all forms of chemotherapy. And for our purposes in this book, you should know that arsenic is another cause of heart disease (Mumford). Furthermore, arsenic clearly interferes with the ability of human fat cells to regulate their blood sugar (Paul). Via several pathways, **arsenic leads to diabetes, which then in turn is fertilizer for arteriosclerosis and puts patients on a fast track for early heart death, regardless of their cholesterol level.**

This is just one more tiny example of why we all need to do a home detox program to get rid of the plasticizers, followed by oral and rectal home chelations to get rid of arsenic, lead, mercury and other heavy metals that create our diseases that resist medicines. There's no medicine that can unblock pathways poisoned by pollutants. You just plain have to get them out of the body

Let's Create High Cholesterol

Where do you think researchers get all those rats and other laboratory animals with high cholesterol to do their drug experiments on? If we knew how to create high cholesterol, it sure would give us a handle on healing it. As with cancer, Parkinson's, thyroiditis, depression, and any other disease, we can create them all with sometimes as little as one dose of some common unavoidable chemical that we are all exposed to every day (Betarbet, Rogers).

Creating high cholesterol or high triglycerides is easy. For starters, we can dose the little buggers with **mercury**, which is in all of us

(Sood). In fact mercury contamination is so prevalent in the human body that zero is no longer the "normal" level for a laboratory test. Instead, we use the "population average". In other words, do you have more or less than the "average" person has. Of course this is meaningless in terms of whether or not it produces symptoms, because (1) we are all biochemically unique, so the level that causes high cholesterol in you may not be the same one that does it in me. (2) How many symptoms and which ones a particular chemical produces in each person is dependent on their individual total load of all the other hidden chemicals that they have accumulated in their lifetime. (3) This in turn is largely dependent on their nutritional levels, especially those that run the detoxification pathways of the body. We may both be equally exposed, but one of us may get rid of most of the chemical, while the other may silently store most of it until the day it finally rears its ugly head and creates a recognizable disease.

We get mercury from our dental "silver" fillings which daily add to our load throughout the years as long as it is in our teeth (*DOD*). We get it from fish and other seafood, because industrial and incinerator exhaust and coal-fired electricity plants pollute the water and soil where it is then taken up by the plants (and animals) we eat. The front page of *The Wall Street Journal* showed us we don't even have to have mercury amalgam fillings or eat seafood to get mercury toxicity. We have sent so much manufacturing to China that they have had to dramatically increase the number of coal-burning power plants to supply electricity for these factories. **Mercury is released as a result of coal burning** and US meteorological agencies have traced the mercury rain out to the US. Fifty percent of US mercury comes via the clouds from China.

Mercury Creates Heart Disease by Multiple Routes

In one study, hair mercury content was assessed in 1,014 men ages 42-60 years. **One of the strongest predictors of who would get arteriosclerosis over the next four years was who had the high-**

est hair mercury levels (Salonen). Yet how many internists, neurologists, or cardiologists assess mercury burden in someone with high cholesterol, much less someone complaining of dwindling brain function, dizziness, Parkinson's, ALS, Alzheimer's, neuropathy, or headache? Instead, we wait until worse heart or brain symptoms emerge like a heart attack or stroke, and then begin a life sentence on expensive drugs that do not cure, but are guaranteed to bring new problems. Mercury has long been known as a potent trigger to cardiovascular disease (Virtanen).

Mercury, in our food and air is also intentionally put in the body as the preservative in immunizations (thiomerosal) as well as outgassing from our silver amalgam dental fillings with every bite. It can create autoimmune diseases like MS, ALS (Havarinasab), damage the calcium channels (Goth), or cause autoimmune thyroid problems that in turn cause high cholesterol. Doing the heavy-metal provocation test in *The High Blood Pressure Hoax* will show you if you should have your Mercury removed. And the urine test **Porphyrin Profile** will show if your load of heavy metals or plastics is actually silently damaging you. More on this later.

Mercury in the mouth isn't the only oral cardio-toxin. We have acrylic glues and dental adhesives that have caused heart attacks (see *DOD*), plus porcelain crowns contain cadmium, while heavy metals are hidden beneath root canals, and white composite fillings leach plasticizers. Don't forget that these **toxic teeth are connected to acupuncture meridians, which in turn provide access to every other organ in the body.** And these are just some of the toxins in the teeth. See *Pain Free In 6 Weeks* for the map of acupuncture meridians and body parts that are affected by each tooth. For example, getting rid of a mercury filling or hidden infection in a root canal tooth or cavitation that was in the heart meridian has cleared angina, a painful shoulder, or other heart problems.

Mercury is a major culprit that can create heart disease by many mechanisms. First, it promotes free radicals that drill holes in cell membranes, which can be measured by raised lipid peroxides (Gualler). Through lipid peroxidation mercury accelerates aging and **mercury oxidizes LDL cholesterol, making it act like sticky glue, adhering plaque to the arteries. It also makes platelets stick together and clot, leading to strokes and heart attacks.** And mercury damages the lining of blood vessels, making it easier for them to go into spasm. In fact, higher mercury levels in hair predict progression of arteriosclerosis in the carotids (neck arteries), which then leads to strokes (Haystack). But medicine merely sees all these conditions as deficiencies of statins, Plavix, nitroglycerine, other medications, or surgery.

As for the dentists who strongly argue against mercury being a problem, we described in *TW* studies done at national dental meetings where the dentists who still use mercury were found to be more prone to having depression and hand tremor, just the kind of guy you want working in your mouth! For it is well known that **brain mercury levels can increase threefold with only five amalgam (silver) fillings** (Eggleston). Memory loss, depression, insomnia, emotional instability, headache, fatigue, impotence, hearing loss, unsteady walking and loss of coordination, tunnel vision, tremors, muscle weakness, joint pains and stiffness, tingling and numbness, chemical sensitivities, and depression are the tip of the iceberg for some of the almost **endless symptoms that mercury toxicity can cause**, as well as paralyzing enzymes and promoting free radicals that lead to arteriosclerosis.

It's interesting that one tiny mercury spill can cause a school to be evacuated, and hospitals and dental clinics have to pay professional licensed toxic waste haulers to remove it. When you go to have a mercury filling either put in or taken out the dental assistant is gowned, gloved and masked as though ready for bioterrorism or a hazmat operation. Yet you're supposed to have it in your mouth forever. Another "disconnect" in medicine.

Mercury makes platelets stick together thereby increasing the chance of heart attack (Kostka, Wierzbicki) and it **accelerates the progression of arteriosclerosis** (Salonen). **Mercury also binds selenium and depletes glutathione peroxidase.** It not only inactivates the major detoxifier glutathione, but catalase and superoxide dismutase (the last two are actually improved with alkaline water and your detox cocktail takes care of the glutathione). **Mercury levels have been directly associated with a risk of having a heart attack, yet good healthy levels of DHA (in your cod liver oil) can protect against that** (Bolger). Even trace amounts of mercury can trigger **autoimmune** diseases as well as damage the **calcium channels** in heart cells, leading to all sorts of cardiovascular symptoms which are then inappropriately treated with calcium channel blockers to purposely poison those already poisoned channels (Goth), and rot the brain.

Aluminum is another common heavy-metal, hidden in city water supplies, processed foods, aluminum cookware (common in restaurants and factory food processing), coffee pots, hot water heaters, baking powder, it's added to salt and sugar so they pour easily, etc. and accumulates in the brain. Aluminum triggers Alzheimer's, arteriosclerosis, aging and much more.

Any of the other myriad of everyday pollutants that EPA studies show we all have in us, like plasticizers, PCBs, heavy metals or organic hydrocarbons can cause high cholesterol, arteriosclerosis, and any form of heart disease, with just one dose alone! (Mochizuki, Bond, Levine) **Taking a cholesterol-lowering drug does not guarantee you won't go on to get arteriosclerosis,** since you have done nothing to correct the underlying chemical glitch caused by abnormal amounts of chemicals gumming up the proper metabolism of cholesterol. And the chemicals don't even have to cause high cholesterol. They can just generate enough free radicals in the arterial wall to cause lesions that plug up the coronaries (with soft plaque that doesn't calcify or show on Ultrafast Heart Scan) without ever having produced cholesterol elevation.

Get the Lead Out

O.K., I can hear you saying, "Alright, I get the picture, already!" but please let me just tell you a smidge about one more important heavy metal. Lead can also mimic any heart disease, blood vessel disease, autoimmune problem, infertility, high blood pressure, kidney disease, or cancer. **Lead raises homocysteine, creates arrhythmia, angina, cardiomyopathy, heart failure, and high cholesterol.** Some people have a lead line, which is a dark line at the junction of the teeth and gums (Marsden), also seen with mercury that migrates from a mercury amalgam filling. As well, lead can mimic Alzheimer's in adults or learning and behavior problems in children (Lustberg).

Physicians from Johns Hopkins University have found that the old cutoff for a " safe lead level" is grossly inadequate. For example, if a person has **"normal" blood lead levels** (< 30 mcg per dl) they have a walloping **68 % increase in deaths due to cancer** and a **46% increase in deaths due to heart disease.** With even lower "normal" levels of 10 to 20 mcg/dl they have a 46% increase in death from cancer compared with folks whose levels are less than 10. Studies show that there is no evidence for the currently accepted "safe" standard or threshold, because **early deaths occur even at concentrations well below the current "safe" EPA standard** (Schwartz, Hong, Shafer, U.S. GAO). Scientists agree that **there is really no safe level of lead.** Clearly **anyone with any heart disease, metabolic syndrome, arrhythmia, and of course high cholesterol deserves appropriate study of their lead levels** (Park).

"How can my child be high in lead when we do all that is recommended in this country to protect them?" many patients ask. We must remember that chemical pollution is a global problem. We are no longer capable of protecting ourselves since we rely on so many things outside of U.S. jurisdiction. *The Wall Street Journal* had been inundated last year alone with articles showing heavy metal contamination of children's toys, foods (chocolate), pet foods, and even garden hoses. These products, contaminated with lead and other toxins, were from foreign countries where we have no control and they have no interest in environmental medicine.

For example, Matel recalled over a million Sesame Street toys because they were contaminated with lead paint. That means the children mouthing these toys or even playing with them and then touching their hands to their mouths secretly got increased lead from a seemingly harmless toy. And Matel had been doing business with this company for over 15 years (*WSJ*, 8-2-07). Kids suffer permanent loss of intellect from much lower levels. And these were only the folks who got caught. **Our only real protection comes down to each individual, and his knowledge and dedication to a detoxification program** like you will learn here.

As Harvard studies show, having lead on board is a major risk factor for coronary heart disease (Jain). Furthermore blood levels are only useful for acute poisoning over the last few days or weeks. **So don't be fooled when your Cardio/ION lead levels look normal.** To find our lifetime accumulations you need to do the heavy-metal provocation test, which is fully explained in *The High Blood Pressure Hoax*. And if you're in doubt that lead is damaging your cells, the **Porphyrin Profile** that you will learn about exposes lead's damage beautifully. The sad fact is that **lead has been known as a cause of every phase of cardiovascular disease including high cholesterol plus heart disease and premature death with or without high cholesterol for over two decades,** yet still it is not routinely checked by the conventional cardiologist.

And the mechanisms of lead toxicity, like those of plastics, extend far beyond damaging cholesterol metabolism. Let me give you just a sampling of the other mechanisms that overlap to contribute to cardiovascular death. **Lead's deadly mechanisms include:**

- Poisoning the detox system (cytochrome p450, CYP)
- Which in turn raises LDL oxidation (the process that allows cholesterol to glue itself to the arterial wall)
- Lead raises homocysteine (and is 4x more a potent predictor of death than cholesterol)
- Lead lowers zinc, copper, and detox SOD
- Lead promotes high blood pressure, osteoporosis, dementia (rotting the brain at any age)
- Lead poisons other enzymes for proper blood vessel chemistry: All roads can lead to vascular disease and a heart attack (Jain, Kuntz, Rogers, Hu, Shih, Navas-Acien, Moller).

Superoxide dismutase or SOD is one of the major antioxidants that we make in the human body to protect the blood vessel wall. One of lead's many damaging mechanisms is that **lead lowers superoxide dismutase (SOD) levels**. Studies right out of the cardiology journals show that folks with coronary artery disease have substantially reduced SOD and that that deficiency in antioxidant control contributes to creating coronary artery disease (Landmesser, Wang).

It makes sense to be sure you have healthy levels of manganese, copper and zinc since they are needed to make SOD. But remember that not only lead but also the unavoidably ubiquitous plasticizers lower zinc and copper. Luckily, you can supplement SOD with a sublingually absorbed **SOD**. Use five drops under the tongue twice a day (but keep it in the refrigerator). It contains 5380 units of SOD derived from bovine liver.

Unfortunately, lead is in everyone and blood levels are meaningless (unless extremely elevated) without a provocation test (to prove the body is trying to get rid of it) or a **Porphyrin Profile** (to get a snapshot view of the current damage it is doing in your body). In essence, **scientists can create any disease they want by merely using the chemicals that we're all exposed to** in our everyday air, food, and water. Although we can reduce our intake, we cannot avoid them. And once environmental toxins become locked in the body, all bets are off as to what diseases they will trigger in each person. For we all have our own special blend of toxic soup intricately intertwined with our own special blend of depleted nutrients. Don't forget that not only are we the first generation of man exposed to such a high level of toxins, but **only you have the power to reverse the irreversible**. Even Mayo Clinic studies have shown that end-stage congestive heart failure, for which there are no further drugs or surgeries, can be reversed. Likewise a multitude of other end-stage medical labels are meaningless once you realize you have the power to reverse the actual underlying toxic causes.

Lead Toxicity Can Stop Pain Treatments From Working

Having lead on board has far-reaching effects above and beyond cholesterol metabolism or even cardiovascular disease. As one example, for years patients and readers have had great success with a far infrared/electromagnetic field pad that accelerates healing and pain relief in recalcitrant conditions. It was first tested in experimental animals given methanol (wood alcohol), a known cause of blindness. It actually prevented the blindness in animals whose eyes were treated with the pad. Since then it has been proven to work by more than one mechanism, one of which is to increase a detox enzyme cytochrome C oxidase.

I have personally seen it make second-degree burns disappear within four hours, tennis elbow can clear in six hours versus six weeks, various joint pains in knees, hips, elbows, backs, necks, shoulders heal as does plantar fasciitis and lots of other musculoskeletal conditions. And I've even seen it rescue teeth from root canals or extraction. It accelerates the healing of surgical sites as well as orthopedic injuries. No home should be without the **Lumen** (much more information, all the references, and how to obtain it are in *TW* 2005-2007). The point is if the person has enough lead on board to secondarily create a silent copper deficiency, there is not sufficient copper to make cytochrome C oxidase, hence annihilating the effectiveness of this indispensable device. This is just one small example of how undiagnosed and untreated heavy metal toxicity extends to everything.

Having High Cholesterol is One of the Luckiest Things That Ever Happened to You

Think about it. If you did not have high cholesterol, you probably wouldn't be reading this book. But because you are, you can from this point on own your health. No HMO, no insurance company, no doctor, no pharmacist, no hospital owns your health, but you do and you are the only person who can make or break it. Let's face it. We are all like a time bomb waiting to go off. No one knows the exact number and amounts of these chemicals that each one of us has accumulated that will finally turn on some horrible life-ending disease. **The mean daily cadmium intake for each of us is 0.3 mcg /l.** This doesn't sound like much but is enough over time to create high cholesterol, kidney damage, prostate cancer, arthritis, osteoarthritis, and much more. **The mean daily OP pesticide intake is 2.55 mcg /l.** Again, this doesn't sound like much, but can create Parkinson's or autoimmune diseases as an example. **But the mean daily phthalate intake (and this is only *one* of several esters) is 176 mcg /l., while the average total daily phthalate intake is 3 mg which is <u>3000 mcg</u>.** Yes, the levels of plastics in the body are our highest pollutant.

We do know that many diseases are becoming epidemic and can all be traced to an environmental overload in the human body. As an example, when I was in my 3rd year of medical school 40 years ago, cancer was rare. You hardly ever heard about it in a child. Now it is the number one disease to kill children ages 1-15 and young adults 25-45. And it is the number two cause of death for all other adult age ranges. In fact a significant percentage of lawsuits stem from the fact that physicians are so unaccustomed to thinking of young women in their early 20s as possibly having breast cancer that they have missed the opportunity to properly diagnose it early.

Now you can begin to see why it is so ludicrous to see children brought up on plasticizers hidden in their infant formula bottles from day of birth. This one pollutant alone seriously damages the normal chemistry of fatty acids. As a result, right now the obesity epidemic has hit even toddlers, whereby kids as young as four years old have high insulin levels, a precursor to diabetes as well as abnormal liver functions (*Investor's Business Daily*, A2, 5/6/03). All this abnormal chemistry can lead to high cholesterol as well.

Diagnosing Toxic Overload

According to government studies now, it is a given that we're all loaded with these environmental toxins. And the biochemical evidence clearly shows that these are a major cause of every disease and ailment as well as accelerated aging. Wouldn't it be great if we could actually determine if chemical toxicity is currently causing measurable damage in our bodies? Well we can. A test called **Porphyrins Profile** shows if your chemistry is currently being damaged by heavy metals especially arsenic, mercury and lead (which are unavoidable in this era) and/or organotoxins like hexachlorobenzene (in room air fresheners), methyl chloride, dioxins, polyvinyl chloride (plastics) and PCBs. Once you find abnormalities on the **Porphyrins Profile**, then you definitely want to do the **Cardio/ION Panel** to identify your nutrient deficiencies to avoid their hampering proper detoxification. **You need to make a dedicated effort to have an expert interpretation and correction of your imbalances and deficiencies, for then you are ready to start a three-pronged detoxification program.** And keep in mind, to the uneducated eye, your Cardio/ION may look quite normal. You must factor in government-controlled new standards, your environmental history, and the priceless clues supplied by organic acids and combined biochemical parameters.

319

I know I've given you a huge amount of information about many of our environmental pollutants, and especially the heavy metals. The reason is simple. Getting rid of them can actually cure lots of conditions that we are still telling folks have no known cause and no known cure. One particular drawback is the plethora of physicians who know little about these toxins and even deny their importance. So let's take a peak at some of the important information you will get from your **Porphyrin Profile** that proves your damage.

We all know that we make hemoglobin in our red blood cells that carries life-giving oxygen to our other cells. It turns out that this system is very sensitive to being poisoned by mercury and other toxins. The beauty is we can tell which toxins have poisoned us by where the damage is in the heme pathways. Knowing which metabolic by-products (porphyrins) are produced luckily tells us which actual toxins have been the culprits. For example, elevation of penta- and copro-porphyrins is a specific mercury damage marker (Pingree). And as folks are detoxified with chelators as you will learn about here, they actually remove mercury from the kidneys and lower their porphyrin markers of damage. Or let's look at another equally unavoidable heavy metal, arsenic (leading to diabetes, prostate cancer resistant to chemo, etc.). Arsenic raises proto-, uro- and copro- porphyrins, while polyvinyl chloride plastics raise coproporphyrins (Wang, Lord). We can identify them all, lead, dioxin, PCBs, etc., plus it won't surprise you that many prescription drugs do their damage here also (Doss, Creighton, Lord, Moore).

But the use of pohphyrins extends far beyond heavy metals and damaged oxygen-carrying capacity of red blood cells. Besides hemoglobin, other heme proteins include cytochrome p450 proteins. Why are these important? These are what detoxify our bodies against all types of toxins. They determine whether we get disease or premature aging or not. If that were not crucial enough to our disease-free survival, another heme protein includes our mitochondrial cytochromes. Translation: these are the very structures in our cells that make energy. But poor energy is blamed on everything from chronic fatigue to old age. We don't have to fall for that any more.

You don't have to be a molecular biologist to see that disturbance in **porphyrin metabolism is a revolutionary biomarker** of:

- Damaged oxygen delivery (translated into common symptoms like fatigue, shortness of breath, heart failure, etc.)
- Damaged detoxification (any symptom from Parkinson's, autism or ALS to heart disease, cancer, etc.)
- Damaged energy (ATP) synthesis
- Aging and all disease in general, including deadly heart disease (Fowler).

So regardless of a person's complaint, whether some bizarre neurological disease, undiagnosable muscle and joint aches, confusing sweating, weakness, lost concentration or memory, or whatever, the **Porphyrin Profile** can target the cause (Lord).

In addition, this test measures where environmental toxins (PCBs, plastics, heavy metals, etc.) dramatically change our chemistry, and **can also prove cellular damage even before the person has a symptom, yes, in "healthy" people** (Woods). And isn't that a much better place to start from than with a list of symptoms?

Detoxification is the Key

Don't you wish there was a way to reverse this chemical overload in our bodies? Don't you wish there was a way to turn back the hands of time and put our bodies back where they were when we were more youthful? Well there happens to be not just one way, but several ways of detoxifying the body. And it's a good thing we have so many ways, because it's not a question of which ones will we choose, but more accurately how often do we have to do all of them. For **we are so polluted that we need multiple ways, and it is an ongoing process**.

The Colors of Toxicity

For the naysayer who still can't believe that the human body stockpiles chemicals that it is unable to detoxify every day, let me give you a few simple examples from my patients. One gal had been on the macrobiotic diet for four months. It cleared all seven of her symptoms but for two weeks her hands were oozing purple, as was the skin over her neck and over her liver. Then she took her bed sheets and pillowcases out of a shopping bag and spread them out on the examination table in my office. They were stained purple. Purple was the color of the permanent wave solution that she used with her bare hands on patrons for 18 years as a hairdresser. Because the macrobiotic diet is so cleansing, its last duty is to get rid of chemicals that have created disease.

For folks who want to use the macrobiotic diet to improve their health, start with *You Are What You Ate*, and then proceed directly to the sequel *The Cure Is In the Kitchen*. Also read *Macro Mellow*. These constitute the "Macro Trilogy" with which people have successfully turned their cancers around after everything in medicine had failed. Now you can begin to see why something as simple as a diet is able to reverse cancer. It merely detoxifies the body and corrects the nutrient deficiencies. For more details call or use the web site to get the free sample issue of *Total Wellness* (December 2006) that describes one of the best documented cases of a **complete cure of wildly metastatic cancer**, given just days to live, bed-ridden and on oxygen. This cancer conqueror is extremely well over 12 years later.

As another example, one gal had a black tongue for three days every time she used the far infrared sauna detoxification protocol that is detailed in *Detoxify or Die*. This was the color of the hair dye that she used for over 15 years on her prematurely gray hair.

And a nurse, poisoned with cold sterilization solution in the operating room, put out odorous yellow-brown stain on her clothes for months during her detox. A construction worker discharged barely visible fibers from the skin (? insulation). Another person used a different detox protocol for ankle arthritis of over a year's duration. Not only did the arthritis totally disappear never to return again, but also the color of the toenail polish that she formerly used suddenly appeared on three toenails just distal to the ankle arthritis and could not be removed with polish remover or even scraped off with a scalpel. The discolored toenails had to grow out over six months (details in *TW* 2003).

After 38 years of seeing people discharge all sorts of colors, substances, and odors, I'm convinced that **our toxic overload is at the root of all "incurable" symptoms.** So let's take a look at some of the protocols that you can do, starting with simple and working up toward the more sophisticated for those who have heavily entrenched disease.

Step One: The Far Infrared Sauna

Clearly, we must get the chemicals out. God fortunately has provided one mechanism: sweat. For example, Mayo Clinic studies have shown that end-stage congestive heart failure patients, for whom there are no further drugs or surgeries, can be reversed. Normally heart patients are the first people to die from a heat wave, so a sauna would be unthinkable. But the special low-temperature far infrared sauna has enabled folks on death's doorstep to sweat out their chemicals, thereby actually reversing "irreversible, end-stage" heart disease, even after everything medicine has to offer had failed. These folks did the impossible: they reversed heart failure and dropped medicines while their heart function improved and returned to more youthful levels. There's much more and all of the details (plus scientific backup and medical references) are described in *Detoxify or Die*. **Medical labels become**

meaningless once you realize you have the power to reverse the actual underlying toxic causes of most diseases.

Detoxify or Die spells out the protocol for safely getting rid of all your toxins, all with non-prescription items, at your convenience, in the privacy of your home. And you can even accomplish work so that there's no time lost while you are getting healthier. As well, the entire family can benefit from it, from infants to the elderly. So think twice before you ever believe anything is incurable. The **far infrared sauna** is available from High Tech Health, hightech-health.com or 1-800-794-5355. You must follow the protocols in *Detoxify or Die* to avoid sweating out precious minerals that could lead to arrhythmia, seizure, severe muscle cramps or seizures. Don't jump in without adequate preparation and knowledge.

Step Two: Rectal Chelation

Chelation caution: Chelation has been a life-saver for folks with emergent cardiovascular or neurologic problems caused by heavy metals, like serious congestive heart failure, angina, depression, paralysis, etc. If the person has dangerously high levels of cadmium, mercury, lead, arsenic, or other heavy metals causing severe symptoms, then it makes sense to have them sit for four hours of intravenous chelation several times a week for months on end to reduce the load as quickly as possible. Or consider the rapid IV technique of Dr. Gary Gordon (*TW*).

However, if the problem is not emergent, it makes a lot more sense to do the far infrared sauna protocol instead. Why? Because no one has just heavy metal problems, so you might as well do the only proven therapy that is not only safe for the heart and also removes not only heavy metals, but other nasty chemicals that are not removed by chelation. For **chelation does not remove pesticides, volatile organic hydrocarbons, the phthalates or plasticizers, Teflon, VOHs, cancer-causing PCBs and dioxins and other xenobiotics**. But the far infrared sauna removes all of these things, including heavy metals. Plus it is safer and in the long run is infinitely cheaper.

And there is the more deleteriously counter-productive problem with **intravenous or IV chelation. It actually tanks up the body with more plasticizers from the IV tubing and the plastic intravenous fluid bags**. Once inside humans, plasticizers damage the peroxisomes, little organelles inside the cells that are responsible for cholesterol metabolism among other things. When our peroxisomes become loaded with plastics, it makes it impossible to lower cholesterol, lose weight, or regain normal hormone functions, because plastics in the body can present as anything from testicular cancer in young males or breast development and menstrual periods in 6-month-old girls, to infertility, loss of libido, diabetes, and numerous other divergent symptoms and diseases. The problem is anyone diagnosing any of theses problems will not think of removing plastics as the underlying cause.

But now back to chelation. It is the best way of removing heavy metals. Sure, the far infrared removes some heavy metals, but it may take us too long. We may not live long enough. We are all so loaded with such a chemical soup of pollutants that it makes sense to **lower the total body burden of plasticizers, pesticides, etc. with sauna and add targeted chelation for the heavy metals**. This can be accomplished with rectal suppositories of the same chemical used in the IV (intravenous, meaning injected into the vein) chelation, EDTA. It is far safer to not force EDTA by IV (which also loads us up on plastics), but to gently use whatever dose you need by rectal suppository, as with, for example, one-quarter the dose, 750 mg. For in IV chelation usually 3000 mg are forced through every organ of the body over 1-3 hours. This can damage kidneys. But by using the suppository, you tailor the dose to your tolerance and schedule. More importantly, when you avoid the IV, you don't load the body with enormously more damaging plasticizer. The chelation suppositories are non-prescription, inserted before bed, and gently chelate while you sleep. There is also a 1500 mg dose, but requires your doctor's prescription.

A.M.-P.M. Nutrients

The protocol for using **Detoxamin** rectal suppositories (detox-amin.com or 1-877-656-4553) is fully described in *The High Blood Pressure Hoax*. But for starters, remember how in Chapter VI you made up all your nutrients once a week? Now you want to put them in the 2 rows of ice cube trays or in two bottles for each day, marking them A.M. and P.M. **In the A.M., you put any nutrient with a mineral.** Then carry it in your pocket or have it on your desk so you can whittle away at it throughout the morning (spread them out to maximize absorption). In the P.M. bottle, you put vitamins and other non-mineral supplements, taking them after 3 P.M. For the A.M. group, try to finish the last ones before 3 P.M. By taking your supplements that contain minerals in the morning, by nighttime, your chelation suppository is removing your heavy metals, not your mineral supplements.

The Detoxamin folks are beginning research to discover more about the mechanisms and benefits of this rectal EDTA. Their first experiment was done using radioactive Detoxamin on rats showing that the rectal dose provides 36% of the IV dose, but the rectal route actually delivered three times the levels to the prostate as compared with the IV route (Ellithorpe). Further studies for which I have seen the medical journal drafts used patients who were antibiotic treatment failures for their chronic pelvic pain syndrome from chronic prostatitis with calcifications. **Detoxamin** treatment along with tetracycline to break through the biofilms of resistant organisms significantly reduced the pain and in some cases improved libido and erectile function. In *Total Wellness* I'll be reporting on the latest developments regarding their research, showing it does more than we ever dreamed of.

Another source, available in 450 and 900mg (or 1200 mg with your doctor's prescription) of calcium disodium EDTA (ethyl-enediaminetetraacetic acid) suppositories (in the same cocoa-butter base with the same methocel E4M premium USP for a time-release effect) is called **Kelatox.**

Step Three: Oral Chelation

With our bodies tanked up with mercury, cadmium, lead, arsenic, bismuth, aluminum, and other heavy metals, we need more than one way to remove heavy metals. DMSA (dimercaptosuccinic acid) was discovered to be among the most potent oral chelators for mercury and other heavy metals. It is non-prescription as Cap-tomer, and the exact same chemical is also prescription (and 10 times more expensive) as Chemet®. You must be extremely care-ful and knowledgeable before using **Captomer** (thorne.com or 1-800-228-1966 or for non-physicians NEEDS, 1-800-634-1380). Also **DMSA** capsules are available from Vitamin Research (vrp.com). Be sure not to take any nutrients containing minerals for the few days each month you are on it. Many folks can tolerate 500 mg twice a day, days 1-3 and 15-17 of each month. The pro-tocol is fully described in *The High Blood Pressure Hoax.*

Some might rightly ask why they have to do so many types of che-lation. It's because there's much evidence to show that different agents have different access to our heavy metal storage sites in the body (Lee). Furthermore, we have too many yet unknown toxins from the over 1000 chemicals that the average person is exposed to daily. If nothing else, we should at least be concerned about our heavy metal levels because they rot the brain at any age (Hu, Shih, Kosnett). Unfortunately, in infancy we chalk it up to genetics or birth defects, or a Ritalin deficiency as they get older, while on the other end of the spectrum we chalk it up to Alzheimer's or old age, while never getting to the reversible root of the cause. And that is just one example of a toxin that is in all of us. We are the first experimental generation. But I think you'll agree with me that the evidence is clear that we had better **detoxify or deteriorate.**

Step Four: The Ongoing Program

Basically, we need an ongoing detoxification program for life. There are many ways to do it. One example protocol would be:

- Far infrared sauna 3-6 days a week,
- EDTA rectal suppositories 1-2 before bed 1-3 weeks a month, remembering to take no minerals after about 2 p.m.
- Oral DMSA 1-4 days every 2-6 weeks, remembering to take no minerals when on it.
- Detox Cocktail should be done every day, regardless of which protocol you are doing.

<u>Warning</u>: I have seen folks, including several physicians, who thought they knew enough to jump in and use these tools without proper knowledge. It has produced seriously disastrous results with incapacitating pain, severe arthritis, and more as heavy metals were chelated out of storage and released into other organs where they got "stuck". It took 1-2 years to straighten them out, depending on the a mount of damage. So please read both *Detoxify or Die* and *The High blood Pressure Hoax* before you plunge into detoxification. As important as it is you must remember, we are the first generation experiencing this and we don't have a lot of physicians trained in it to help you. This is a major reason why you have to become extremely knowledgeable.

Step Five: Assessment

Long before you embark on a detoxification program, it would be best to assay all your minerals, vitamins, fatty acids, amino acids, organic acids and cardiovascular risk factors like homocysteine, fibrinogen, hsCRP, testosterone, insulin, and more. You will find all this neatly rolled into one blood test, the **Cardio/ION Panel** (metametrix.com or 1-800-221-4640). After 38 years in medicine, I can safely say it is the best single tool to show why folks are not healing. An even more important reason for getting it **before you embark on a detoxification program** is that **you need to be sure your deficiencies are corrected and that your detox system is maximally prepared to handle the onslaught of chemicals** that will be presented to it. As I said earlier, I have seen folks, including physicians, get into serious medical trouble who jumped into detox programs without first being sure their detox nutrients were ready for peak performance.

Furthermore, after you have been doing any detox program for 3-9 months, it is wise to re-assess your levels, because **we lose good minerals as we get rid of heavy metals and other pollutants**. You may not have to do the whole Cardio/ION, but at least check the **RBC (erythrocyte) Minerals**.

You may have noticed I omitted showing the dangers of smoking, for example, or the benefits of exercise. These are self-evident. I want to focus on things that are stronger risk factors and that you may not be exposed to elsewhere.

Getting Your Blood Tests Done, And Avoiding the Perils of an Inferior Interpretation

The Cardio/ION Panel is in my opinion the most important crystal ball test in all of medicine at this point in time, because it finds the causes of symptoms and points you toward the cures for every disease. If your physician is unknowledgeable about the test, (1) ask the lab to send your physician information about the test and ask the lab to send him a copy of one of my latest publications in a peer-reviewed medical journal for physicians, entitled, Using organic acids to diagnose and manage recalcitrant patients (*Alternative Therapies*, 12; 4:44-53, July/August 2006, or 1-760-633-3910 or 1-866-828-2962 or alternative.therapies @innerdoorway.com). With 132 references it spells out why it borders on malpractice not to order the organic acids, as they are the only way available to diagnose many "incurable problems". As well, he can get continuing medical education credits for reading this article and taking the test at the end of the article. (2) Call the lab, MetaMetrix 1-800-221-4640, to see who in your area does order the test. Also, (3) chiropractors and naturopaths can order it.

For interpretation, there are various levels, from the abbreviated guide that comes with the report to two books available through the lab, the *ION Handbook* (Roberts MM, Lord RS) and the much more detailed, **Laboratory Evaluations in Molecular Medicine** (Bralley JA, Lord RS). And a new version of that great and indispensable text is in press, so check with them, plus they present courses for physicians on interpretation. I also have scheduled non-patient phone consults for select readers who want to brainstorm with me personally and/or want me to interpret their Cardio/ION and collate with their medical records and history.

Whatever interpretation modes you use for this 10 page report of highly technical state-of-the-art molecular biochemistry of your body, bare in mind several facts: (1) You must remember that "normal" is a relative designation. For some values you want to be in the highest percentile, for others, the lowest. For example, the average American diet provides only 40% of the magnesium you need in a day, so you want to be in the top percentile since most folks are deficient, and you are being compared with them. You are not normal if your magnesium is in the fourth quintile or lower, and it is O.K. to be above the $95^{th}\%$. And remember that the government periodically makes labs re-establish the norm for tests. With nutrients, they take hundreds of samples of a nutrient, for example magnesium, and see where 95% of folks fall. Unfortunately this is not a great idea, because the norm for magnesium in 2006 was 40-80 and in 2007 it dropped to 15-35 ppm packed cells. There are many reasons why this method was chosen, but remember it is chosen by the very folks who have not even determined if there is an RDA for half the minerals so crucial to health. In addition, these regulators are the same folks who don't change the RDAs in a timely manor to reflect the last ten years of research. So interpretation must be done by someone knowledgeable to factor all of this into results that may look quite normal, but in truth hide the secrets to getting well.

(2) You must compensate for the items that are not yet measured, for example, if fatty acids are deficient, then phosphatidyl choline that the fatty acids embrace in the cell membrane are deficient, for there is nothing to hold them in place. PhosChol must be added if EPA or DHA are in the 3rd quintile or normal. Plus even though vitamin E may look normal, it's measuring predominantly a tocopherol. You still want all 8 forms as Chapter II showed.

(3) The balance between complementary nutrients must be interpreted. For example, even if the zinc level is in the normal range, if beta-carotene is high normal and vitamin A is low normal, even though all three are in the normal range, this person is functionally zinc deficient. How do we know? Because the enzyme that converts a molecule of beta-carotene into two molecules of vitamin A is zinc-dependent, and can't work without it. Furthermore, when we correct zinc, the ratios improve, as does health.

(4) You often must heal the gut first in order to absorb the other nutrients. If the organic acid D-arabinitol is high, the gut is full of yeast. This can delay healing indefinitely. Likewise, an elevated indican shows bad bugs in the upper intestine that may interfere with the production of digestive pancreatic enzymes. Look for other clues for why corrections may be resistant. For example, an elevated tricarballyate is an organic acid from too much of another bad bug in the gut. It acts as a claw and chelates magnesium right out of the gut before it gets absorbed. So magnesium may never correct until the gut is healed first (see *No More Heartburn*) and tricarballyate is normalized.

(5) The interpreter must be tested. How else are you going to know if he/she is any good? Before you two even open your report, innocently ask your doctor, "What nutrient is low if a beta-hydroxy-iso-valerate is elevated?" If he doesn't immediately know that it reflects a deficiency of biotin, he may be deficient in more important parameters. If he is honest and says he doesn't know but will look it up right now, keep him. He is trying to learn and is honest.

(6) Watch out for those resorting to the "drug mentality". For example, some docs when they see low sulfation, merely tell folks to take sulfur products. But that won't cure the detox deficiency until you get rid of the plasticizers that cause low sulfation (*TW* 2008).

(7) And by all means, **just because all your heavy metals are in the normal range does not mean they are OK.** See details in *The High Blood Pressure Hoax.*

(8) Patterns or groupings of abnormalities that provide clues, for example, elevated behenic, lignoceric, and arachidic acids suggest heavy damage from plasticizers, and it is even a stronger association when DHA is lower in proportion to EPA. I say all this not to confuse you, but to warn you that many folks have shown the 10-page report to physicians who took one glance and said it looked "O.K." while the report, which takes about an hour to go over, was loaded with abnormalities that screamed for correction and clearly explained why the person was at a healing impasse.

After the First Heart Attack, You Must Detox

Anyone who has followed the reading to this point realizes that **we must all take a year or two out of our lives for a serious, concentrated detox program to reverse the hands of time. It's our only recourse** against the epidemic degenerative diseases that escalate with age. For once someone has had a heart attack and then either surgery or stents, they become almost a prisoner of the medical system. Aspirin and Plavix plus the calcium channel blockers, beta-blockers and other medications are foisted on them, along with the inevitable statin drug, even if they don't have high cholesterol. So let's look at how these folks, who are worse off than those of us who have not yet had a heart attack, can immensely improve their chances of a healthful life.

First let's make sure that you understand some of the basic facts. After six months of a drug-coated stent there were more heart attack deaths or need for new surgery in those who had drug coated stents that in those who had plain metal stents (Lagerqvist). Second of all, many people who have medicated stents are part of an experiment since the United States Food and Drug Administration only approved them for a single vessel blockage and no more than two stents per patient. As a result, 60% of stents that are coated with a drug consist of off-label use, which includes putting them in people with multiple other medical problems that also added to their increased death rates (Chappell).

But the data gets worse. In another study **patients treated with medications alone did better than those treated with stents**, whether or not it had a drug in it (Hochman). In fact that entire issue of *The New England Journal of Medicine* (March 8, 2007) was practically devoted to the higher cardiovascular risk and death rates of coated stents.

But it continues to get even worse. Clopidogrel is the generic name for Plavix, the around $4/capsule that most all cardiologists prescribe after anyone who has had a stent. Unfortunately, you do not get your money's worth because **Plavix has been proven to be no better than aspirin** and this was even published in the 1996 *Lancet.* I don't understand how these facts can be published in the leading journals to guide cardiologists in their work, but they seem to be selectively ignored. Furthermore, when researchers compared Plavix plus aspirin to aspirin alone in another study, the difference in death rate was extremely small (Yusuf). For the expense and the questionable benefit as well as the risk of dying from brain hemorrhage, this drug looks even worse than the Nexium scam (remember page 215?).

Now, let's look at the other benefits of EDTA (the chemical that is in chelation therapy) in its much safer, cheaper, more physiologic form, the suppositories that you just learned about. **EDTA** not only chelates heavy metals, but **EDTA inhibits unwanted clotting**. Add this to the benefit of getting rid of the underlying causes of all sorts of heart disease, like hidden mercury, lead, cadmium, and arsenic and it makes even more sense to use the detox program you just learned about (Chappell, Kindness, Menke, Cranton).

And last but not least, a beautiful study was done on 220 patients with known cardiovascular disease and who were followed for three years. One group had EDTA chelation while the other group did not. For the **folks who do not have EDTA, 22% had to have repeat angioplasties versus only 4% who had EDTA** treatments needed repeat angioplasties. And nearly **12% of them without EDTA required bypass surgery versus none required bypass surgery that had EDTA**. And don't forget, most of those doing EDTA do not give their patients the benefit of a Cardio/ION Panel nor a more complete detox program as well as safer suppositories. The bottom line is twofold: (1) **34% of patients treated with angioplasties required another surgical procedure within three years.** (2) **Chelation cut the need for repeat angioplasties fivefold** and more than double that for bypass surgery. And these EDTA chelations were not done under the most optimum conditions that you are learning about here, namely preceded by a comprehensive Cardio/ION Panel with expert interpretation and correction, followed by a **tri-partite detoxification program** that includes far infrared sauna, safer EDTA suppositories and DMSA to optimize detoxification of the varied types of toxins through multiple pathways.

Clearly a heart attack is a warning. You had better get serious about the detox program and learning about all the nutrition and more that is in this book if you want to cut your chances of recurrence.

Protect Yourself

Government studies now confirm that the multitude of environmental toxins that we all have in us create everything from high cholesterol to diabetes, cancer and much more. They've explored the mechanisms and seen how environmental toxins poison the LDL receptor activity and create not only high cholesterol and triglycerides, but damage the chemistry of other phospholipids. This creates arteriosclerosis, early heart attacks and much more even without producing high cholesterol (Ha, 2007). The air surrounding us now contains far too many chemicals continually damaging our DNA and overloading its ability to repair itself (Brauner). It's clear from just these last two references that auto and industrial exhausts trigger heart attacks, lung cancers and more. It's surprising that it has been in *The New England Journal of Medicine* because so few doctors deal with it (Peters). Environmental toxins work by many mechanisms, but fortunately the effects can be measured such as elevation of lipid peroxides, 8-OhdDG, hsCRP, and fibrinogen and more, all of which are in the **Cardio/ION Panel**. In addition, the **Porphyrin Panel** confirms that you have current damage and had better take measures to reverse it, which is what this book is all about.

We know that **diesel exhaust can elevate the fibrinogen and make the blood more eager to clot** and it's right out of major cardiology journals (Mills). Likewise Harvard studies of the **trucking industry show that truckers have a 41% increased heart attack rate** (and increased lung cancer) primarily from vehicle exhausts (Laden). Furthermore another Harvard study and others confirmed increased odds of a heart attack while driving in heavy traffic; sometimes triple (Peters, Tonne). And bear in mind that **one out**

335

of four people who have a heart attack have no symptoms. It's what we call a silent myocardial infarction (Kannel).

Therefore, I highly recommend using a car air filter that plugs simply into your car cigarette lighter. And be sure to recirculate the air in the car versus pulling in vehicle exhaust fumes from the highway. The E.L. Foust Co. has made such a car filter for decades that has withstood the test of time (1-800-EL-FOUST or www.foustco.com). The **Foust Auto Air Cleaner** absorbs toxins from the vehicle's interior air, allowing you to breathe far less toxic air than everyone else around you on the highways. I highly recommend one, and if not for yourself, what about the kids and grandkids?

Overwhelmed? Don't Be

Sure you're overwhelmed. So is the average physician. Sadly you now know more about healing than the vast majority of them. But you now have control. Sure, you'll have to go back and reread several times. Do you think we read something just once in medical school? No, we read until it was memorized, hopefully forever.

So whenever you feel there's a big knowledge gap, terms you're not familiar with, or you feel overwhelmed, just keep plowing through. Later on you may want to go to the other books and past years of *Total Wellness* newsletter to fill in the blanks. I don't want to bore the faithful readers by repeating things that they have learned in the previous books and newsletters. Knowledge, like health, is built up over time and it would be extremely rare to get everything you need from just one book, with just one reading of it. Learning about health is a process that rewards you as nothing else can. Don't forget most folks know infinitely more about some team's scores than they do about creating their own health. **You now have the evidence and direction to empower yourself more than you ever have in your life. You can own and control your health, if you choose.** Remember the journey of a thousand miles begins with just one step. Take as many or few baby steps as you need. Perhaps you may not even get to a detox program until next year. So be it. Whatever you start with is a positive.

But just think of one simple example of why we are such a sick nation. The number one pollutant in the human body, plasticizers in our homes, offices and travel air, foods, and water, can create anything from diabetes to cancer and even high cholesterol (Chinetti). And the phthalates or plasticizers do much more, like create a hidden zinc deficiency which then turns on inflammation, another mechanism for arteriosclerosis (Fong). And this is right out of the *Journal of the National Cancer Institute*. But medicine wants us to think that high cholesterol is a Lipitor deficiency and inflammation is a Celebrex deficiency. And even though many folks who died of a heart attack didn't even have high cholesterol, physicians rarely recommend something as simple as cod liver oil to raise the HDL, even though this was published in the *New England Journal of Medicine* over 18 years ago (Pekkanen). Truly medicine has a different agenda for our health.

Busy Executive Summary

We are all progressively tanking up on more environmental chemicals, beginning with the moment we are conceived in the uterus. They are the major cause of abnormal body chemistry that we label as various diseases that are then seen as a deficiency of the latest drug or have no known cause, and no know cure! The truth is there are proven ways to get hidden toxins out of the body and thereby reverse disease. For starters, the worst end-stage heart failure patients were used who had nothing else that could be done for them, medically or surgically. By all medical standards, these Mayo Clinic patients were "done". But with the far infrared sauna protocol, they reversed this "irreversible" condition, dropping medications and symptoms. And heavy metal detoxification protocols added to this in the combined forms of rectal suppositories and oral chelation have restored health in the most recalcitrant cases. This is the closest we will come to the **fountain of youth** in this era, for it is the only proven way to actually reverse the major underlying causes of disease. First use the 3-part nutrient correction program in the preceding chapter. When your detox system is healthier (1-6 months usually), then do the 3-part detox program in this chapter.

Sources for this Chapter's Recommendations

- Porphyrin Profile, Cardio/ION Panel, metametrix.com, 1-800-221-4640
- Far Infrared Sauna, hightechhealth.com, 1-800-794-5355
- Detoxamin, detoxamin.com, 1-877-656-4553
- Kelatox, kelatox.com, 1-866-707-4482
- Captomer (Thorne), call NEEDS, 1-800-634-1380
- DMSA, vrp.com, 1-800-877-2447
- Silit pans and pressure cooker, natural-lifestyle.com, 1-800-752-2775
- Cogimax, optimox.com, 1-800-223-1601 or 1-877-VIT-AMEN
- Lumen, lumenphoton.com, 1-828-863-4834
- SOD sublingual, intensivenutrition.com, 1-800-333-7414
- Foust Auto Air Cleaner, foustco.com, 1-800-EL FOUST

References:

Over 1300 references for this chapter are in: Rogers SA, *Detoxify or Die*, 2002, and *The High Blood Pressure Hoax*, both from Prestige Publishing, Syracuse NY, prestigepublishing.com or 1-800-846-6687

Rogers SA, *Total Wellness* 2000-2007, prestigepublishing.com or 1-800-846-6687

Sood PP, et al, Cholesterol and triglyceride fluctuations in mice tissues during methylmercury intoxication and monothiols and vitamin therapy, *J Nutri Environ Med*, 7; 3:155-162, 1997

Tonne C, et al, A case-control analysis of exposure to traffic and acute myocardial infarction, *Environ Health Perspect*, 115:53-57, 2007

Kannel WB, et al, Incidence and prognosis of unrecognized myocardial infarction, *New Engl J Med*, 311; 18:1144-47, 1984

Peters A, et al, Exposure to traffic and the onset of myocardial infarction, *New Engl J Med*, 251; 17: 1721-30, 2004

Bell FP, Effects of phthalate esters on lipid metabolism in various tissues, cells and organelles in mammals, *Environ Health Persp*, 45: 41-50, 1982

U.S. EPA, *National Human Adipose Tissue Survey, Vols. I-V*, EPA-560/5-84-003 through 87-035, 1984-1987

Kaloyanova F, El Batawi MA, *Human Toxicology of Pesticides*, CRC press, Boca Raton FL, 1991

U.S. Environmental Protection Agency, *Broad scan analysis of the FY82 National Human Adipose Tissue Survey Specimens*, EPA-560/5-86-035, Dec 1986; *Characterization of HRGC/MS unidentified peaks from the analysis of human adipose tissue*, EPA-560/5-87-002A, May 1987

Eggleston D, et al, Correlation of dental amalgam with the mercury in brain tissues, *J Prosthetic Dentistry*, 58; 6:704-07, 1987

Guallar E, Sanz-Gallardo MI, Kok FJ, et al, Mercury, fish oils, and the risk of myocardial infarction, *New Engl J Med*, 347; 22:1747-54, Nov. 28, 2002

Solonen JT, et al, Intake of mercury from fish, lipid peroxidation, and the risk of myocardial infarction and coronary, cardiovascular, and early death in eastern Finnish men, *Circul*, 91:645-55, 1995

Vimy M, et al, Mercury released from the dental "silver" fillings provokes an increase in mercury and antibiotic-resistant bacteria in oral and intestinal flora of primates, *Antimicrob Agents Chemother*, 37:825-34, 1993

Crinnion WJ, Long term effects of chronic low-dose mercury exposure, *Alt Med Rev*, 5; 3: 209-223, June 2000

Sood PP, et al, Cholesterol and triglyceride fluctuations in mice tissues during methylmercury intoxication and monothiols and vitamin therapy, *J Nutri Environ Med*, 7; 3:155-162, 1997

Kolata G, New suspect in bacterial resistance: amalgam, *New York Times*, Apr. 24, 1993

Salonen JT, et al, Mercury accumulation and accelerated progression of carotid atherosclerosis: a population-based prospective 4-year follow-up study in man in eastern Finland, *Atheroscler*, 148:265-273, 2000

DeSouza Queiroz ML, Pena SC, Saller TSI, et al, Abnormal antioxidant system in erythrocytes of mercury exposed workers, *Human & Exp Toxicol*, 17: 225-30, 1998

Shenker BJ, Guo TL, Shapiro IM, Low-level methylmercury exposure causes human T-cells to undergo apoptosis: evidence of mitochondrial dysfunction, *Environ Res*, 77: 149-59, 1998

Bond JA, Gown AM, Juchau MR, et al, Further investigations of the capacity of polynuclear aromatic hydrocarbons to elicit atherosclerotic lesions, *J Toxicol Environ Health*, 7: 327-35, 1981

Levine RJ , Andjelkovich DA, Kersteter SL, et al, Heart disease in workers exposed to dinitrotoluene, *J Occup Med*, 28: 8 11-16, 1986

Mochizuki H, Oda H, Yokogoshi H, Amplified effect of taurine on PCB-induced hypercholesterolemia in rats. *Adv Exper Med Biol*, 442: 285-290, 1998

Danielson H, et al, Effect of biliary drainage on individual reactions in the conversion of cholesterol to taurocholic acid, *Europ J Biochem*, 2: 44,1967

Levy TE, *Stop America's #1 Killer*, 2006, LivOnBooks.com, 1-800-334-9294

Bruce B, Spiller GA, Klevay LM, Gallagher SK, A diet high in whole and unrefined foods favorably alters lipids, antioxidant defenses, and colon function, J *Amer Coll Nutr*, 19; 1:61-67, 2000

Betarbet R, Sherer TB, Greenamyre JT, Chronic systemic pesticide exposure reproduces features of Parkinson's disease, *Nature Neurosci*, 3; 12:301-1315, Dec 2000

Kihara T, Biro S, Imamura M, Yoshifuku S, Takasaki K, Ikeda Y, Tei C, et al, Repeated sauna treatment improves the vascular endothelial and cardiac function in patients with chronic heart failure, *J Am Coll Cardiol*, 39; 5:754-9, Mar 2002

Rundle A, Tang D, Perera FP, et al, The relationship between genetic damage and polycyclic aromatic hydrocarbons in breast tissue and breast cancer, *Carcinogenesis*, 21; 7: 1281-89, 2000

Bahn AK, Mills JL, Snyder PJ, et al, Hypothyroidism in workers exposed to polybrominated biphenyls, *New Engl J Med*, 302; 1: 31-33, 1980

Kilburn KH, Warsaw RH, Shields MG, Neurobehavioral dysfunction in firemen exposed to polychlorinated biphenyls (PCBs): Possible improvement after detoxification, *Arch Environ Health*, 44; 6:345-350, 1989

Meining GE, *Root Canal Cover-UP*, Bion Publishing, Ojai AS, 1994, or PPNF 1-800-366-3748

Lustberg M, Silbergeld E, Blood lead levels and mortality, *Arch Intern Med*, 162; 2443-49, 2002

Guallar E, Sanz-Gallardo I, Van't Veer P, et al, Mercury, fish oils, and the risk of myocardial infarction, *New Engl J Med*, 347; 22: 1747-54, 2002

Bolger PM, Schwetz BA, Mercury and health, *New Engl J Med*, 347:22:1735-36, 2002

Wiseman H, Halliwell B, Damage to DNA by reactive oxygen and nitrogen species: role in inflammatory disease and progression to cancer, *Biochem J*, 313:17-29, 1996

Salonen JT, Seppanen K, Kaplan GA, et al, Mercury accumulation and accelerated progression of carotid atherosclerosis: a population-based perspective 4-year follow-up study in man in eastern Finland, *Atherosclerosis*, 148: 265-73, 2000

Kostka B, Kinetic evaluation of ADP-induced platelet aggregation potentiation by methylmercuric chloride, *J Tr Elem Exper Med*, 4:1-9, 1991

Weirzbicki R, Prazanowski M, Mielicki WP, et al, Disorders of blood in humans occupationally exposed to mercuric vapors, *J Tr Elem Exper Med*, 15: 21-9, 2002

Schwartz J, et al, The concentration-response relation between PM 2.5 and daily deaths, *Environ Health Persp*, 110: 1025-1029, 2002

Hong YC, Lee JT, Kim H, Kwon HJ, Air pollution, a new risk factor in ischemic stroke mortality, *Stroke*, 33: 2165-21 69, 2002

Shafer KS, Kegley SE, Persistent toxic chemicals in the U.S. food supply. *J Epidemiol Commun Health*, 56: 813-817,2002

U.S. GAO, Report to the chairman, Subcommittee on Oversight and Investigations, Committee on Energy and Commerce, House of Representatives. *Pesticides. Adulterated Imported Foods Our Reaching U.S. Grocery Shelves*, GAO/RCED-92-205

Waldman P, EPA bans staff from discussing issue of perchlorate pollution, *Wall St J,* A3, April 28, 2003

Weise E, Flame retardant found in breast milk, U.S. levels highest in the world study says, A1, A 10, *USA Today*, Sept. 23, 2003

Petreas M, et al, High body burdens of 2,2', 4, 4'-tetrabromodiphenyl ether (BDE-47) in California women, *Environ Health Perspect*, 111; 9:1175-59, 2003

Buckeley WB, Small town is furious at IBM, once local hero, *Wall Street Journal,* B1-2, July 31, 2003

Herrick T, As flame retardant builds up in humans, debate over a ban, *Wall St J,* A1, A10, Oct 8, 2003

Bell FP, Effects of phthalate esters on lipid metabolism in various tissues, cells and organelles in mammals, *Environ Health Persp* 45: 41-50, 1982

Kliewer SA, Fatty acids and eicosanoids regulate gene expression through direct interactions with PPAR, *Proc Nat Acad Sci* 94:4318-23, 1997

Chinetti G, et al, PPAR: nuclear receptors at the crossroads between lipid metabolism and inflammation, *Inflamm Res*, 49; 10:497-505, 2000

Kihara T, Biro S, Imamura M, Yoshifuku S, Takasaki K, Ikeda Y, Tei C, et al, Repeated sauna treatment improves the vascular endothelial and cardiac function in patients with chronic heart failure, *J Am Coll Cardiol,* 39; 5:754-9, Mar 2002

Ellithorpe R, et al, Comparison of the absorption, brain and prostate distribution, and elimination of CaNa2 EDTA of rectal chelation suppositories to intravenous administration, *J Am Nutraceut Assoc,* 10; 2: 1-8, 2007

Goth SR, et al, Uncoupling of ATP-mediated calcium signaling and dysregulated IL-6 secretion in dendritic cells by nanomolar Thiomerosal, *Environ Health Persp,* (available at http://dx.doi.org/ online 21 March 2006

Virtanen JK, et al, Mercury, fish oils, and risk of acute coronary events and cardiovascular disease, coronary heart disease, and all-cause mortality in men in eastern Finland, *Arterioscl Thromb Vascul Biol*, 25:220 8-33, 2005

Lord RS, Bralley JA, Urinary porphyrin profiling, *Laboratory Evaluations in Functional and Integrative Medicine*, chap 8, 2007, metametrix.com

Stahlhut RW, et al, Concentrations of urinary phthalate metabolites are associated with increased waist circumference and insulin resistance an adult US males, *Environ Health Persp,* 115:876-82, 2007,

Guruge KS, Yeung LWY, Yamashita N, et al, Gene expression profiles in rat liver treated with perfluorooctanoic acid (PFOA), *Toxicolog Sci*, 89; 1:93-107, 2006

341

Heuvel JPV, et al, Differential activation of nuclear receptors for perfluorinated fatty acid analogues and natural fatty acids: a comparison of human, mouse, and rat peroxisome proliferators-activated receptor -(alpha), -(beta), and -(gamma), liver X receptor -(beta), and retinoid X receptor-(alpha), *Toxicol Sci*, 92; 2: 476-89, Aug 1, 2006

US EPA, Preliminary Risk Assessment of the Developmental Toxicity Associated with Exposure to Perfluorooctanoic Acid and its Salts, US Environmental Protection Agency, Office of Pollution Prevention and Toxics, Risk Assessment Division, Apr. 10, 2003

Brucker DF, Effects of environmental synthetic chemicals on thyroid function, *Thyroid*, 8:827-56, 1998

O'Reilly DS, Thyroid function tests--a time for reassessment, *Brit Med J*, 320:1332-4, 2000

Robbins J, Factors altering thyroid hormone metabolism, *Environ Health Perspect*, 38:65-70, 1981

Skinner G, et al, Thyroxine should be tried in clinically hypothyroid but biochemically euthroid patients, *Brit Med J*, 314:1764, 1997

Mya MM, et al, Subclinical hypothyroidism is associated with coronary artery disease in older persons, *J Gerontol Biol Sci Med Sci*, 57; 10:658-9, 2002

Shea KM, Pediatric exposure and potential toxicity of phthalates plasticizers, *Pediat*, 111; 6:1467-74, June 2003

Barry YA, et al, Perioperative exposure to plasticizers in patients undergoing cardio- pulmonary bypass, *J Thorac Cardiovasc Surg*, 97:900-905, 1989

Roth B, et al, Di-(2-ethylhexyl)-phthalates as a plasticizer in PVC respiratory tubing systems: indications of hazardous effect on pulmonary function in mechanically ventilated preterm infants, *Europ J Pediat*, 147:41-46, 1988

Loff S, et al, Polyvinyl chloride infusion lines exposed infants to large amount of toxic plasticizers, *J Pediat Surg*, 35:1775-1781, 2000

Cullum ME, Zile MH, Acute polybrominate biphenyl toxicosis alters vitamin A homeostasis and enhances degradation of vitamin A, *Toxicol Appl Pharmacol*, 81: 177-181, 1985

Silva MJ, Barr DB, Calafat AM, et al, Urinary levels of seven phthalate metabolites in the U.S. population from the National Health and Nutrition Examination Survey (NHANES) 1999-2000, *Env Health Perspect*, 112: 3 31-38, 2004

Xu Y, et al, Effects of di-(2-ethylhexyl)-phthalate (DEHP) and its metabolism on fatty acid homeostasis regulating proteins in rat placental HRP-1 trophoblast cells, *Toxicol Sci*, 84: 287-300, 2005

Kavlock R, et al, NTP Center for the Evaluation of Risks to Human Reproduction: Phthalates expert panel report on the reproductive and developmental toxicity of of di-(2-ethylhexyl)-phthalate, *Reprod Toxicol*, 16:529-50 3, 2002

Latini G, Potential hazards of exposure to of di-(2-ethylhexyl)-phthalate in babies. A review, *Bio Neonate*, 76:269-76, 2000

Magliozzi R, et al, Effects of the plasticizer DEHP on lung of newborn rats: Catalase immunocytochemistry and morphometric analysis, *Histochem Cell Biol*, 120: 41-49, 2003

Peters JM, et al, Di-(2-ethylhexyl)-phthalate induces a functional zinc deficiency during pregnancy and teratogenesis that is independent of peroxisome proliferator-activated receptor-alpha, *Teratol*, 56:311-16, 1997

Melnick RL, Schiller CM, Mitochondrial toxicity of phthalate esters, *Environ Health Perspect*, 45:51-56, 1982

Beier K, et al, Suppression of peroxisomal lipid B-oxidation enzymes by TNF-a, *FEBS Lett*, 310:273-8, 1992

Ram PA, et al, DHEA 3 B-sulfate is an endogenous activator of the peroxisome-proliferator pathway: Induction of cytochrome P450 4A and Acyl-Co oxidase mRNAs in primary rat hepatocyte culture and inhibitory effects of Ca++ channel blockers, *Biochem J*, 301:753-8, 1994

Bell FP, Effects of phthalate esters on lipid metabolism in various tissues, cells and organelles in mammals, *Environ Health Persp*, 45: 41-50, 1982

Kliewer SA, Fatty acids and eicosanoids regulate gene expression through direct interactions with PPAR, *Proc Nat Acad Sci*, 94:4318-23, 1997

Chinetti G, et al, PPAR: nuclear receptors at the crossroads between lipid metabolism and inflammation, *Inflamm Res*, 49; 10:497-505, 2000

Kato K, Silva MJ, Calafat AM, et al, Mono (2-ethyl-5-hydroxyhexyl) phthalate and nono-(2-ethyl-5-oxohexyl) phthalate as biomarkers for human exposure assessment to di-(2-ethylhexyl) phthalate, *Env Health Perspect*, 112:327-30, 2004

Kuntz E, Kuntz HD, *Hepatology, Principles and Practice*, Springer Medizin Verlag, Wetzlar Germany, 2006

Alonso-Magdalena P, Morimoto S, Ripoll C, Fuentes E, Nadal A, The estrogenic effect of bisphenol A disrupts pancreatic beta-cell function *in vivo* and induces insulin resistance, *Environ Health Persps* 114; 1: 106-112, 2006

Richter CA, et al, Estradiol and bisphenol A stimulate androgen receptor and estrogen receptor gene expression in fetal mouse prostate mesenchyme cells, *Environ Health Persp*, 115:902-08, 2007

Park MSC, Kudchodkar BJ, Liepa GU, Effects of dietary animal and plant proteins on the cholesterol metabolism in immature and mature rates, *J Nutr* 117:30, 1987

Madani S, Frenoux JM, Prost J, Belleville J, Changes in serum lipoprotein lipids and their fatty acid compositions and lipid peroxidation in growing rats fed soybean protein versus casein with or without cholesterol, *Nutr*, 20:554-563, 2004

Bruce EC, Chouinard RA, Tall AR, Plasma lipid transfer proteins, high-density lipoproteins, and reverse cholesterol transport, *Ann Rev Nutr*, 18: 297-330, 1998

Havarinasab S et al, Immunosuppressive and autoimmune effects of Thiomerosal in mice, *Toxicol Appl Pharmacol*, 204:10 9-21, 2005

Havarinasab S, et al, Alteration of the spontaneous systemic autoimmune disease in(NZBxNZW)F1 mice by treatment with Thiomerosal ethyl mercury, *Toxicol Appl Pharmacol*, in press

Goth SR, et al, Uncoupling of ATP-mediated calcium signaling and dysregulated IL-6 secretion in dendritic cells by nanomolar thiomerosal, *Environ Health Persp*, March 2006

Abramson JJ, et al, Thiomerosal interacts with the Ca2+ release channel ryandine receptor from skeletal muscle sarcoplasmic reticulum, *J Biol Chem*, 270: 29644-47, 1995

Carnaris GJ, et al, The Colorado Thyroid Disease Prevalence Study, *Arch Intern Med*, 160: 526-34, 2000

McDermott MT, Ridgway EC, **Subclinical hypothyroidism is mild thyroid failure and should be treated,** *J Clin Endocrinol Metab,* 86; 10: 4585-90, 2001).

Mya MM, Aronow WS, **Subclinical hypothyroidism is associated with coronary artery disease in older persons,** *J Gerontol Biology Sci Med Sci*, 57; 10: 658-9, 2002

Mya MM, Aronow WS, Increase prevalence of peripheral arterial disease in older men in women with subclinical hypothyroidism, *J Gerontol Biology Sci Med Sci*, 58; 1: 68-9, 2003

Jain NB, et al, Lead levels and ischemic heart disease in a prospective study of middle-aged and elderly men: the VA normative aging study, *Environ Health Persp*, 115:871-75, 2007

Navas-Acien A, et al, Lead exposure and cardiovascular disease a systematic review, *Environ Health Persp*, 115; 3: 472-82, 2007

Hu H, et al, The epidemiology of lead toxicity in adults: measuring dose and consideration of other methodologic issues, *Environ Health Persp*, 115:455-62, 2007

Shih RA, et al, Cumulative lead dose and cognitive function in adults: a review of studies that measured both blood lead and bone lead, *Environ Health Persp*, 115; 3: 483-92, 2007

Lee BK, et al, Provocative chelation with DMSA and EDTA: evidence for differential access to lead storage sites, *Occup Environ Med*, 52; 1:13-19, 1995

Kosnett MJ, at al, Recommendations for medical management of adult lead exposure, *Environ Health Persp*, 115; 3: 463-71, 2007

Hu H, et al, Fetal lead exposure at each stage of pregnancy as a predictor of infant mental development, *Environ Health Perspect*, 114: 1730-35, 2006

Shih RA, et al, Environmental lead exposure and cognitive function in community-dwelling older adults, *Neurology*, 67; 9:1556-62, 2006

Menke A, et al, Blood lead below 0.48 micromol/L (10 µg/dL) and mortality among US adults, *Circulation*, 114: 1388-94, 2006

Cranston EM, *A Textbook I EDTA Chelation Therapy*, 2nd ed, Charlottesville, VA, Hampton Roads Publishing Company 2001

Chappell LT, Should EDTA chelation be used instead of long-term clopidogrel plus aspirin to treat patients at risk from drug-eluting stents?, *Alt Med Rev*, 12; 2: 152-58, 2007

Chappell LT, et al, Subsequent cardiac and stroke events in patients with known vascular disease treated with EDTA chelation therapy, *Evid Based Integr Med*, 2:27-35, 2005

Mills ML, et al, Diesel exhaust inhalation causes vascular dysfunction and impaired endogenous fibrinolysis, *Circulation,* 112: 3930-36, 2005

Laden F, et al, Cause-specific mortality in the unionized US trucking industry, *Environ Health Persp,* 115: 1192-96, 2007

Brauner EV, et al, Exposure to ultraviolet particles from ambient air and oxidative stress-induced DNA damage, *Environ Health Persp,* 115: 1177-82, 2004

Peters A, et al, Exposure to traffic and the onset of myocardial infarction, *New Engl J Med,* 351: 1721-30, 2004

Pekkanen J, Linn S, Heiss G, et al, *N Engl J Med,* 322: 1700-0 7, 1990

Chinetti G, et al, PPAR: nuclear receptors at the crossroads between lipid metabolism and inflammation, *Inflamm Res,* 49; 10:497-505, 2000

Fong LYY, Zhang L, Jiang Y, Farber JL, Dietary zinc modulation of COX-2 expression and lingual and esophageal carcinogenesis in rats, *J Nat Ca Inst,* 97; 1:40-50, Jan 5, 2005

Paul DS, et al, Molecular mechanisms of the diabetogenic effects of arsenic: inhibition of insulin signaling by arsenite and methylarsonous acid, *Environ Health Persp,* published online January 29, 2007

Mumford J, et al, Chronic arsenic exposure and cardiac repolarization abnormalities with QT interval prolongation in a population-based study, *Environ Health Perspect,* published online Feb 14, 2007

Lasky T, et al, Mean total arsenic concentrations in chickens 1989-2000 and estimated exposures for consumers of chicken, *Environ Health Perspect,* 112:18-21, 2004

Kaltreider RC, et al, Arsenic alters the function of the glucocorticoid receptor as a transcription factor, *Environ Health Perspect,* 109:24, 5-51, 2001

Moller L, et al, Blood lead as a cardiovascular risk factor, *Am J Epidemiol,* 136;9: 1091-1100, 1992

Wang XL, et al, Plasma extracellular superoxide dismutase levels in an Australian population with coronary artery disease, *Arterioscler Thromb Vasc Biol,* 18:1915-21, 1998

Landermesser U, et al, Vascular extracellular superoxide dismutase activity in patients with coronary artery disease, relation to endothelium-dependent vasodilatation, *Circulation,* 101: 2264-70, 2000

Park SK, et al, Low-level lead exposure, metabolic syndrome, and heart rate variability, *Environ Health Perspect,* 114: 1718-24, 2006

Pingree SD, et al, Quantitative evaluation of urinary porphyrins as a measure of kidney mercury content and mercury body burden during prolonged methylmercury exposure in rats, *Toxicolog Sci,* 61:234-40, 2001

Wang JP, et al, Porphyrins as early biomarkers for arsenic exposure in animals and humans, *Cell Mol Biol,* 48; 8:835-43, 2002

Woods JS, Altered porphyrin metabolism as a biomarker of mercury exposure and toxicity, *Can J Physiol Pharmacol,* 74:210-15, 1996

345

Fowler BA, Porphyrinurias induced by mercury and other metals, *Toxicol Sci,* 61:197-98, 2001

Lord RS, Bralley JA, Urinary Porphyrin Profiling, in *Laboratory Evaluations in Functional and Integrative Medicine,* chap 8, Toxicants and Detoxification, metametrix.com, 2008

Creighton JM, et al, Drug-induced porphyrin biosynthesis, VII. Species, sex, and developmental differences in the generation of experimental porphyria, *Can J Physiol Pharmacol,* 50; 6:485-89, Jun 1972

Doss MO, Porphyrinurias and occupational disease, In: Silbergeld E FB, ed. *Mechanisms of Chemical-Induced Porphyrinopathies,* 204-18, 1987

Moore MR, et al, Drug-induction of the acute porphyries, *Adv Drug Reac Ac Pois Rev,* 2:149-89, 1983

Chapter VIII

Creating Your Cholesterol Reversal Plan and More

Are you overwhelmed? Don't be. Just rejoice in the fact that you have so many empowering evidence-based options for a healthier life, more than most of your doctors and cohorts. For with or without high cholesterol, we all need these tools. Sure, no one needs everything in this book. But no one knows (yet) the exact balance you need, so we need to make you as smart as possible in as few pages. So let's break it down into some workable options for you.

- For **fast results**, lower your cholesterol with **Kyolic Formula 107 Red Yeast Rice** 600 mg. If not improved in a month, add Niacin-Time, then proceed to add Policosanol, Tocotrienols and Tocopherols, Magnesium, Vitamin C, etc. (all detailed in Chapter II)
- In the meantime start to correct the underlying causes by beginning with a **diet** of whole foods, alkaline water, and an oil change with "no trans fats", remembering never to trust those words "no trans fats" on a label (Chapter IV).
- **Infection** control starting with improved oral hygiene and a month trial of Kyolic Liquid, probiotics, detox cocktail, detox enema, immune boosters.
- **Nutrient** corrections preferably beginning with the **Cardio/ ION Panel**. If your physician resists, remind him of an article in the *Journal of the American Medical Association* over a decade ago showing anti-oxidants were necessary to slow down coronary artery disease, the number one cause of death. How does he propose to prescribe nutrients when he has not yet determined which ones and how much you need? (Hodis HN, Mack WJ, LaBree L, et al, Serial coronary angiographic evidence that antioxidant vitamins intake reduces progression of coronary artery atherosclerosis, *J Am Med Assoc*, 273: 1849-54, 1995).

- **Toxin** identification with the **Porphyrin Profile** followed by reduction of toxins with the far infrared sauna plus oral and rectal heavy metal home chelations (Chapter VII).

- **Evaluation**. The two most important initial tests are (1) the Ultrafast Heart Scan to determine your coronary calcium score, and (2) the Cardio/ION Panel to show all your nutrient deficiencies and imbalances that need correction before the body can heal. After 3-9 months of home chelation you will need to at least check your **RBC Minerals** (separately or as part of the Cardio/ION), since the good minerals get lost with heavy metal chelation. When you are ready, you can start to explore the many other options in here and ongoing in your monthly referenced newsletter, *Total Wellness*. For this can bring you to even higher levels of wellness for only $1 a week! How can you afford to be without this empowering?

Emergency Medicines to Have on Hand

Since **half the people who have a heart attack die before they ever make it to the hospital**, there are some prescription items that you should carry with you that just may save your life. Let's look at the rationale for them.

First, it is screamingly ludicrous now that all sorts of public facilities have to have a defibrillator on hand. As well, folks who can afford one either purchase them for personal use or have them implanted in their bodies. The rationale is that when a person goes into serious cardiac arrhythmia like ventricular fibrillation, you can shock the heart back into a normal sinus rhythm and save their life. However, the reason that it's not universally effective is that you can electrocute a heart all day long, but if it's magnesium deficient, as one example, it won't respond until you give enough magnesium to allow the heart muscle fibers to contract in sequence once more. Studies show that one of the major differences between those who survive a heart attack and walk out of the hospital versus those who are carried out in a body bag to the morgue is the amount of magnesium they came in with. In other studies, **those who were given an injection of magnesium when they entered the emergency room were less likely to die from the heart attack** and had fewer arrhythmias as complications when they did survive.

Second, when someone does have a heart attack one of the first medications given in the emergency room is one of the many "clot busters". You have learned how many nutrients do a superior job at clot preventing, so you want to keep them up. But for an emergency, heparin is the cheapest, easiest, and safest clot dissolver you can give.

Third, when coronary arteries are plugged up with clot, you want them to expand. You want to dilate them so that hopefully some blood can get through to the heart muscle.

Therefore it makes sense to ask your doctor for small prescription of the following:

1. Six nitroglycerin sublingual tablets 0.3 mg so that you could slip one or two under the tongue in attempt to provide vasodilatation.
2. A small vial of heparin (clot-dissolver) so you could inject 5000-10,000 units subcutaneously (in your skin).
3. A vial of magnesium sulfate 2 g to inject 1 cc in each thigh (the reason we don't inject the whole 2 cc in one spot is that it stings for about 20 minutes, so it's better to separate the magnesium sulfate into two smaller amounts).

When you weigh the pros and cons of teaching folks to give these simple treatments, especially if they are 10 minutes or more away from emergency medical treatment, the benefits far outweigh the risks. The package of a tiny 1 cc syringe, a tiny vial of heparin and magnesium and the teeny nitroglycerin tablets can fit into any standard pocket and could even be cleverly added to a slightly oversized cell phone case.

Emergency Heart Attack Medicines

There are all sorts of drugs to thin the blood and stop clotting on the market now. The reason is simple. We have too many processes going on in the body that promote abnormal clotting. From trans fatty acids, Teflon and plastics in our foods to unhealthy guts which don't make enough of vitamin K (yes it's needed for proper clotting and to inhibit abnormal clotting), to a host of other nutrient deficiencies as well as toxicities. They all result in way too many free radicals that promote clotting and abnormal chemistry. If that weren't enough, we're putting so many foreign objects right inside the body, like the epidemic insertion of coronary artery stents, that the body has to protect itself and wall them off with clotting. Plus **many other things promote abnormal clotting, such as the NSAIDs** (stands for "non-steroidal anti-inflammatory drugs", like Motrin, Aleve, ibuprofen, Celebrex, and more). You might think NSAIDs only cause increased intestinal bleeding. But remember the old Vioxx was removed from the market for quadrupling the rate of heart attack? Because many NSAIDs are non-prescription, folks often have a false sense of safety concerning them. But becoming OTC (available over-the-counter) is not a safety issue, but marketing. Why else would many prescription medications from Prilosec to Motrin suddenly no longer need a prescription as soon as their patents expired?

It started out innocently enough with aspirin decades ago. And I've shown you how vitamin E in the form of **E-Gems Elite**, 2 a day, **Kyolic Liquid**, and other nutrients are far superior to put the brakes on unwanted clotting. Because Heparin is so inexpensive and not patentable, all sorts of heparin replacements have come on the market. But these stripped down synthetic agents are associated with abnormal reactions where they can actually trigger antibodies that cause clotting, so you actually get the exact opposite effect that you want.

Then there are other types of drugs to stop clots like the direct thrombin inhibitors, one of which is argatroban. But do not let that big name fool you. It's a small molecule actually derived from L-arginine, the inexpensive amino acid you learned about in *The High Blood Pressure Hoax,* which God uses to create healthful vasodilatation, relaxation and healing inside of our blood vessels. As usual when medicine gets stuck, they look at how God heals things and then try to genetically engineer it, changing it into something that is similar but can be patented and sold at obscene profits. The problem is that by altering the molecule you then bring on abnormal side effects that you don't get with more natural products.

In past *TW* issues I showed you some of the evidence for the dangers of some of the more commonly used "blood thinners" **like warfarin (Coumadin), guaranteed to create osteoporosis and accelerate arteriosclerosis, aspirin which doubles the risk of stroke, and Plavix which was found at the American College of Cardiology meeting to be no better than aspirin, and in fact in folks who had not yet had a heart attack, it gave them a 50% increased risk of having one.**

Various enzymes like **Wobenzyme, Ananese, Lumbrokinase**, or **Nattokinase** as well as a special proprietary form of aged garlic extract, **Kyolic,** have properties that make blood less likely to abnormally clot. And I've shown you how, for example, **Gamma Tocopherol** is also important in decreasing hypercoagulability, but needs to be balanced daily with all of the other seven parts of vitamin E (see Chapter II).

So why are we prescribing so many blood thinners? They are prescribed whenever anything foreign is put in the body, like a joint replacement, heart valve replacement or a stent. They are also prescribed when there's an abnormal heart rhythm that could throw clots such as atrial fibrillation. And if you have a heart attack and end up in the emergency room, clot-busters to dissolve the clots are rapidly prescribed. But since **half the people who have a heart attack die before they get to the emergency room,** I'd like to make a plea for you to have your own little emergency box of things that just might save your life.

Making Your Own Cardiac Emergency Drug Box

What should we include in this box? A tiny vial of heparin pre-scribed by your doctor and a couple of 1 cc syringes would be very important to have on hand. If you had a heart attack and especially if you were far away from treatment, I would suggest you slip 2 prescription 0.3mg **Nitrostat** (nitroglycerine tablets) under the tongue. Next inject 10,000 units of **Heparin** under the skin imme-diately. Then into the muscle of an arm or leg (or just the skin) I would give 2 cc of **Magnesium Sulfate** (divided into two 1 cc in-jections since it stings for 20 minutes if given in one spot). If your doctor won't give you a prescription for the magnesium injections, at least have him give you a prescription for the best absorbed oral form, **Magnesium Chloride Solution 200 mg per cc** (windham-pharmacy.com, directions in Chapter II). This works almost as well as an IV and you can dump half a teaspoonful under the tongue and let it get absorbed like sublingual nitroglycerin. Re-member, one of the deciding factors of who walks out of a hospital a week after a heart attack versus who is carried out in a body bag is how much magnesium they had on board when they entered. The high magnesium guys get to walk out.

Two other harmless non-prescription nutrients can rescue the heart in trouble. I would use a huge scoop of **Arginine Powder** (Carl-son), since it can **cut the chance of further thrombosis or clot by two-thirds.** Seven grams (7000 mg) twice day is usually tops, and of course balanced with other nutrients you will need less. I have described that at length along with the entire scientific backup in *The High Blood Pressure Hoax.*

So let's go to the next item: two huge scoops of **Corvalen** (D-ribose). The reason? It too has an enormous volume of scientific medical data behind it, proving that it supplies the needed energy that the damaged heart requires to heal (Pliml, Seifert). In the prestigious *Lancet* over 15 years ago they showed how D-ribose thwarts angina (Pliml). But most cardiologists are not even aware of it, and you never hear of it being prescribed. The exceptions are cardiologists like Dr. Stephen Sinatra and Dr. James Roberts who are trying to educate the others on the benefits of metabolic cardiology versus drugs only (Sinatra and Roberts). If all cardiologists would merely read the volumes of studies on D-ribose it looks like it should border on malpractice to fail to recommend or include it in just about any heart program (Omran, Pauly, Sinatra).

For starters, **Corvalen makes the damaged heart recover six times faster regardless of cause or diagnosis.** Clearly this is the difference between life and death (Pauly, Ingwall). If that were not enough, **for folks having revascularization procedures, the hearts were 49% stronger than those who did not have D-ribose** (Perkowski). And even after someone has had a heart attack or has had a silent one (no pain, does not know they've damaged their heart), Corvalen (D-ribose) rescues heart functions so well that it even helps to identify what is called **hibernating myocardium. In other words, it literally brings damaged heart muscle that no physician could rescue** (with cardioversion or drugs) **back to useful life** (Wilson). The best form I know of for D-ribose is from the company that has dedicated itself to the research (not just being a copy-cat), **Corvalen.** Use 2-7 gm twice a day for maintenance, but 10 gm for emergency twice a day.

Because none of these will be given in the emergency room and they have a long track record of (1) **improving coronary artery blood flow,** (2) **reducing the size of the area of heart damage**

from the heart attack, (3) **and speeding healing,** you must take the initiative. Upon questioning, you may be surprised to find that most cardiologists never intended to give you many of these, and in fact do not even know about them. I'll give you more on other things that are needed after the acute emergency in future *TW* issues. I cannot conceive of any problem stemming from the use of these that would negate their benefits. If your doc refuses to prescribe the three Rx items, heparin, magnesium sulfate and nitroglycerin, plus a few 1cc syringes for administering the heparin and magnesium sulfate, he should start to bring himself into the 21st century with *The High Blood Pressure Hoax.*

So if someone drops over dead from a heart attack, first thing you want to do is the Heimlich maneuver to make sure they weren't choking if it happened during a meal (directions in *TW* 2007), and start CPR to keep the blood flowing to the brain and the heart. Next slip a couple of Nitroglycerin under the tongue and give the heparin and magnesium injections. If the victim is awake, also give a big scoop each in a glass of water of **Arginine Powder** and **Corvalen Powder** as you head to the emergency room as fast as you can. If you can fit it in, about six enzymes, in the form of **Nattokinase** or **Wobenzyme-N,** would be great as well.

There are other items that could be added that we'll review in *TW*. For example, adding carnitine can also dramatically reduce the size of the infarct at the time of the heart attack. Translation: the size of the area of the heart that was damaged was smaller because carnitine provided enough energy for the cells to protect themselves from death. Also **during the next 28 days the amount of angina was half**, and as well there was a marked reduction in heart failure, arrhythmias and other sequelae **when carnitine was added** (Singh). I would use 1 twice a day of **GPLC** since it is closest to the form used in most research. And of course the adequacy of this dose can also be checked through your **Cardio/ION**. And carnitine has many other benefits, such as lowering triglycerides (Clark), an independent cardiovascular risk factor (Cullen). And carnitine is needed for vitamin E absorption, a nutrient you recall that is lowered by statins. Unfortunately, carnitine synthesis is another of the pathways damaged by phthalates (plasticizers you learned about in the last chapter) once they get stuck in our chemistry. So whether healing from a heart attack or trying to prevent one, and especially if you have any evidence of fatty acid disturbance on your Cardio/ION, think of including a form of carnitine like **GPLC**.

For now this plan is a lot healthier start than just showing up in the ER! This combination, even if you cannot get all the components, makes a lot more sense than a mere defibrillator, as well. Defibrillators promote a false sense of security. You can sit there and electrocute somebody's heart all day long, but if they don't have enough magnesium or D-ribose, for example, on board you may not get the heart started again. Likewise if the heart has a huge clot, where are you going? I would suggest you and your spouse rehearse this combo so that when the event occurs, you are well-rehearsed. **Rehearse or end up in a hearse**. Remember, one out of every two who has a heart attack does not survive. Only 50% make it to the ER. Let's make sure you are a survivor.

Crucial Steps After Heart Surgery

(1) Diet, of course, is major. Because it is so healing, Dr. Dean Ornish modified the macrobiotic diet. With food he accomplished what no medication is capable of, for he was able to bring about regression (melting away) of coronary atherosclerosis after one year on the diet, along with a **91% reduction in angina** (Ornish 1998). **In contrast, the folks who were not on the diet had no decrease in angina, but instead had an enormous 186% increase in angina.** No medication has this power to dissolve away plaque, and no time is more important than after surgery, since studies show **within six months folks already have evidence of re-clotting their new vessels.** In contrast, this diet keeps shrinking away arteriosclerosis. After five years, those who were not on the diet had an increase of 11.8% of compromised blood flow in-

side the vessel due to build up of plaque, while **those on the diet reduced their initial plaque by 3.1%.**

Dr. Ornish added nightshades (tomatoes, peppers, chilies, cayenne, etc.) to the macrobiotic diet to give it more pizzazz. However if you have arthritis, you had best read *Pain Free in 6 Weeks* first before you do this diet. You may need to do the more strict macrobiotic diet, like the one folks used to successfully reverse cancers when everything else has failed. Start with *You Are What You Ate* and progress to *The Cure is in the Kitchen* (1-800-846-6687 or prestigepublishing.com). And if you ever get into serious trouble, remember, it's the same diet that folks have reversed end-stage cancers with. When they were told there was nothing more that medicine could offer, and they were given only days to live, some bed-ridden on oxygen, these folks kicked death in the teeth and healed their cancers with a mere diet (*Tired or Toxic?* explains many of the mechanisms of how it works). Many went on to live decades more, medication-free, and very healthfully.

(2) Check your **Cardio/ION Panel**. In fact it would be fun for you to ask your cardiologist what blood tests he plans on using to check your progress. If they merely include a chemical profile, CBC and the lipids (which is standard), I would fire him. You want someone who's going to check all of these bare minimum, but also the more serious risk factors, like the hsCRP, RBC magnesium, fibrinogen, insulin, Lp(a), vitamin E, homocysteine and lipid peroxides, testosterone, etc.. And you must know the status of the fatty acids and their balance, your zinc, whether the hospital antibiotics and sugar IVs have created a yeast overgrowth in the gut, and so much more. It is all in the Cardio/ION Panel and more.

Don't forget, we're talking about the rest of your life. You just had a $55,000 operation that only put four new vessels in. What about the miles of other vessels that are most likely similarly damaged in your body, or in your brain, or in your pelvis? How many times do you think your body can heal from this type of surgery? Now is the time to make or break your future and **all the control lies within your grasp**. No one else is going to grab you by the arm and make you do these state-of-the-art tests. Most cardiologists are totally unaware of them, but if you find one who recommends this program, don't ever let him/her go. You have hit the jackpot.

(3) Last but not least, read *Detoxify or Die* followed by *The High Blood Pressure Hoax* to learn how to get the underlying heavy metals and lifetime accumulation of heart-damaging, clot-forming chemicals out of your body. Learn how to turn the hands of time back. You need a heart as clean as it was in your twenties. This is the only proven method. You have to start by getting rid of the causes. Only you control your future.

I recall the shock about Darryl Kile, the Cardinals' 33-year-old pitcher who died of a heart attack. Autopsy showed 60-90% occlusion of two coronary arteries. Too bad he wasn't a reader of *Total Wellness*, at least for the July 2001 (or April 2007) issues. For this may have spurred him on to get the Ultrafast Heart Scan that could have shown these plugs. You would think that baseball clubs insuring these players for millions of dollars would at least want to keep up with the latest and greatest advances in medicine. I'm sure they'll think twice from now on when it comes to taking more responsibility for their knowledge of medicine, and not relying on "medical experts". Certainly even if you didn't have enough regard for your own body, when your business depends heavily on the health of folks whose diets you have no control over, it behooves you to know as much as possible and take control.

Unfortunately the conventional management in cardiology is still a "wait and see if you get symptoms" game, and once you do, any symptom suddenly becomes a deficiency of drugs and surgery. But we know that within six months those who have had either new vessels or roto-rooting (angioplasty) of the old ones are already reclotting their new vessels, because they have not done **what is necessary to reverse the chemistry of coronary artery**

357

disease: change the diet, get the chemicals out, measure and restore the nutritional deficiencies, and turn off the molecular cascade that creates disease.

After half a century we still haven't learned. In 1954, the *Journal of the American Medical Association* reported a high percentage of autopsies on 18-year-old U.S. soldiers killed in the Korea battle showed they already had arteriosclerosis. Heart disease isn't something that comes on suddenly in our 40s and '50s, it begins in youth. It just usually takes that long for it to develop into noticeable symptoms. But with our "modern" diets higher in trans fatty acids, sugars including high fructose corn syrup, bleached white flour products, nutrients processed out of the foods and a slew of additives, dyes, preservatives, pesticides, plasticizers and other chemicals added to the foods, this speeds things up. We are seeing degenerative diseases in folks in their 20s and 30s that we never used to see until old age.

Reversing Heart Disease

I've referenced Dr. Dean Ornish who has reversed heart disease with a modified macrobiotic diet (*Journal of the American Medical Association*). In *The High Blood Pressure Hoax* we explained arginine, vitamins K2, C, E and other nutrients that contribute to reversing coronary plague, as well as chelation done at home. Cardiologists Dr. Sinatra and Dr. Roberts told of other nutrients that you learned about here like D-ribose, carnitine, CoQ10, etc. (Sinatra S, Roberts JC, *Reverse Heart Disease Now*, J Wiley & Sons, 2007). The bottom line is the very things that you have learned about here are a composite, because there is no one formula for everyone. But once you understand the process and the rational for various supplements and the crucial role of detoxification, you will also realize that the starting point is to know your individual deficiencies and toxicities. I know of no better start than with the **Cardio/ION** followed by the **Porphyrin Profile**.

The Hospital: Not a Place to Heal

Those of us who have had (and cured) chemical sensitivities know that one of the unhealthiest places you can go is to the hospital. And now 30 years later scientists and clinicians are "discovering" this fact for the first time (Lazarou, Weinhold, Ebbesen). I recall many a night in the 70s and 80s walking down hospital corridors, which reeked of industrial strength floor cleaners and polishes, to make rounds on my patients. I vividly see in my mind's eye the surprised looks on the faces of asthmatics who couldn't believe that other medical specialists (even pulmonologists!), nurses, orderlies, and venipuncture technicians would wear smelly perfumes, deodorants, hairsprays, aftershaves and clothes that smelled grossly of cigarette smoke, fabric softener, or formaldehyde wrinkle-proof finish into their rooms when they were struggling to breath.

I remember one gal whose allergic target organ was her uterus. Instead of having spasm of vessels in the coronaries to cause angina, or spasms of arteries in the brain to cause migraine or stroke, or spasms of bronchioles in the lung to cause asthma, her spasms were in the uterine muscle. This led to abnormal bleeding and cramps whenever she was exposed to high enough doses of common chemicals. When she got pregnant, she had to be particularly careful of abnormal exposures. In those days we didn't know nearly as much about getting well as we know now, so environmental controls were particularly important.

When she was on the verge of a spontaneous abortion with serious bleeding and uterine cramps during her first pregnancy, her gynecologist asked me to consult on the case. With the help of her husband we put air cleaners in her hospital room plus non-toxic bed linens and she had a healthful diet as opposed to the dead, processed, overcooked foods from the cafeteria. Among the many orders I wrote that night in her chart was one that simply asked the hospital to get her large room window unlocked so that she could have fresh air. You wouldn't believe the excuses the hospital came up with. After three days they still could not handle such a sophisticated order and she aborted. The window never was unlocked.

On the flip side, another gal was smart enough to get all of her nutrients assayed after she had failed miserably at the medical school fertility clinic. Within less than six months of correcting her nutrients and doing environmental controls, she was pregnant for the first time in her life. And when she delivered a beautifully healthy baby boy nine months later, her husband sent me the flowers instead of his wife. Again I can't impress upon you that:

> **No healing should be labeled impossible until you have looked at all the chemistry of the human body, including undiagnosed nutrient deficiencies, allergies and toxicities.**

A recent article in the government's National Institutes of Health journal states that "according to the EPA, *indoor air pollution in buildings* of all types ranks among *the top five environmental health risks to public health.*). And **hospitals have even more contaminants than most buildings** with the laboratory chemicals, latex gloves and catheters, PVC intravenous tubes, potent disinfectants and many other contaminants. Of the 500 criteria for hospitals to get for their certification, only a handful deal with indoor air quality. No one looks at vinyl flooring or thinks twice about not painting indoors with sick patients present who are trying to heal.

Phthalates, toluene, mold retardants and other pesticides are among the many chemicals that outgas into hospital air. **In 1995, a report from the New York Attorney General found 33 active pesticides were applied in health-care facilities and most hospitals** throughout the state, yet less than half of them provided any type of notice to the patients or employees. Pesticides can cause any neurologic symptom and damage you can think of (Parkinson's, ALS, MS, neuropathy), and the heart's nervous system is no exception. The autonomic nervous system of the heart can be the target organ. For example, pesticides can mimic the flu with total body

360

pain, cause serious headaches, cause any gastrointestinal symptoms, or mimic a heart attack with chest pain. Pesticides are notorious for impairing the immune system or ability to fight off infection, a major cause of death in the hospital.

Only now 30 years later are a few hospital systems even thinking about trying to reduce their chemical overload, however the time will come like all good things. But progress is slow. I vividly recall when I had asthma in 1972 and would walk out of hospital staff meetings when 300 doctors would light up their cigarettes after our staff dinner. They thought I was strange. It was over 20 years later before smoking was banned in my hospital, supposedly a haven for the healing.

The well-known statistics of over 100,000 in hospital deaths from drugs makes drugs the fourth cause of death. But when you remember that heart attacks are number 1, cancers are number 2 and strokes are number 3, you realize that heart attacks and strokes are the same pathology, arteriosclerotic vascular damage. That moves drug reactions up to the number 3 cause of death. And you have learned how it's really #1. Pretty scary, isn't it?

And if you get stuck, you can always go to the **American Environmental Health Foundation and Unit** (1-800-428-2343, 8345 Walnut Hill Lane, Dallas, TX 75231, aehf.com) created and directed for decades by cardiovascular surgeon, Dr. William J Rea, M.D. This unit is where folks who have been therapeutic failures from all over the world have gone to be rescued and learned how to reverse their diseases. Dr. Rea has not only trained many physicians, but many physicians owe him a huge part of our restored health. He also is the author of the 3 volumes, *Chemical Sensitivity*, has an annual scientific conference for physicians from all over the world for over a quarter of a century, a catalog of products for healthful living from air cleaners, saunas and safe everyday products to books, nutrients and much more.

361

Can You Believe the News?

What about all the things you read about that are contrary? Progressively more books are coming out showing how professional journalists no longer report the facts and events objectively, but slant their reporting according to agendas. Lifelong CBS news reporter Bernard Goldberg has written *Bias. A CBS insider exposes how the media distort the news.* And he is not alone, as William McGowan, former reporter for *Newsweek*, the BBC, and a regular contributor to the *Wall Street Journal* wrote *Coloring the news. How crusading for diversity has corrupted American journalism.* Meanwhile, Tammy Bruce wrote *The New Facts Police. Inside the left's assault on free speech and free minds.* And William Proctor wrote, *The Gospel According to The New York Times. How the world's most powerful news organization changes your mind and values.*

But even more important than the imbalance in journalists' personal views are the views of those who pay their salaries and actually dictate the thrust and tone of articles. The pharmaceutical companies' control of the media has been thoroughly exposed in numerous books whose authors include editors for *The New England Journal of Medicine*, professors of medical schools, congressmen, etc. (Angell, Haley, Cohen, Epstein, Moss, Breggin, Glenmullen, Moore, Richards). And one of many reasons why drug profits are so enormous is they have cleverly managed to get us, yes you and I, to pay for much of their research. For if you read the fine print of scientific papers you find the money comes from US government research grants.

Is Your Doctor Working Blind?

It is an understatement to say that to put anyone on statin drugs without first at least measuring, bare minimum, their red blood cell minerals and fatty acids is not good medicine. In fact, it is the poorest medicine I can think of. First of all, Harvard researchers from the School of Public Health have been teaching for decades that trans fatty acids are a major cause of high cholesterol, high LDL triglycerides and low HDL (the good) cholesterol. So where are you going without measuring your trans fatty acids? And while you are at it, you might as well measure all of the fatty acids since hypercholesterolemia reflects a damaged fat chemistry.

Furthermore most people cannot heal until at least their mineral deficiencies are found and corrected. **RBC (red blood cell) Minerals with Heavy Metals** measures magnesium, zinc, chromium, copper, manganese, selenium, plus heavy metals like cadmium, aluminum, mercury, arsenic and lead which are notorious for damaging proper cholesterol metabolism. (And again, I warn you not to let your doc fall for the commonest mistake in interpreting the heavy metals. That is to call them normal just because they all fall in the "normal range". He must read *The High Blood Pressure Hoax*.) Furthermore, you learned how medications and just the body's work of detoxifying this world could cause vitamin deficiencies. Yet you saw how just pennies of vitamins (some articles right out of the *Journal of the American Medical Association*) not only reverse Alzheimer's but slow the progression of coronary artery disease, while with more sophisticated applications of this knowledge even reverse it.

You know by now also that whomever you choose to interpret your **Cardio/ION** should be sure to incorporate crucial nutrients that are not yet assayed but that complement the missing ones. For example, the **enzyme LCAT that drags plaque off the arterial wall is extremely dependent on phosphatidylcholine** (Parks). Certainly if there are any abnormalities in the cell wall fatty acid constituents or vitamin E, **PhosChol** should be a part of your prescription.

And last but not least, you've learned that **cholesterol is one of the most minor bit players when it comes to cardiovascular disease. Much more important are parameters controlled by nu-**

trients such as homocysteine, hsCRP, fibrinogen, insulin, testosterone, lipoprotein(a), and more. The beauty is that all of this has been rolled into one comprehensive 10-page report called the **Cardio/ION**.

You can, if you choose, go the route bought and paid for by the extremely powerful chemical/pharmaceutical industry that controls medicine, medical education, medical research, and media advertising and even medical boards. You can spend thousands of dollars a year on prescription medicines that will inevitably lead to other diseases and require careful monitoring of your liver and other organs functions. Granted it's very enticing to take the easy way out with paid doctor visits and paid prescriptions and the seduction of leaving all the thinking to your doctor.

Or you can choose to find the cause and the cure of your high cholesterol and get rid of it once and for all in a healthful way that promotes your longevity in a multitude of areas. If you are really lucky, you will even find a doctor who is aware of all of this or at least is eager to start to learn and become a partner with you in your quest for drugless health.

Drugs are indispensably great for emergencies, but for chronic conditions, you have learned that **high cholesterol is not a deficiency of cholesterol-lowering drugs.** But you get what you pay for, for drugs inevitably lead to an avalanche of symptoms starting with nutrient deficiencies then rolling into cardiac disease, suicidal depression or any illness you can imagine. Your body was designed to be healthy and to be able to heal against all odds. It was not designed for drugs that literally poison and turn off natural God-designed pathways. Remember **health cannot be bought, but it can be taught**. You are now smart enough to take on the challenge, for you have all the tools at your fingertips.

Practicing Medicine By the Book

Does your doctor practice medicine by the book? The *PDR (Physician's Desk Reference)* is the main book describing all prescription drugs. If you want to know how a drug works, you are generally out of luck, because for most drugs it says, "the mechanism of action is unknown". But it tells how to dose it and then gives page after page of side effects. Can you imagine we use these when no one knows how they work and when they have an arm's length of serious consequences? But that's the way we are all brainwashed from the moment we enter medical school to the last day we practice, to treat every disease as though it is a deficiency of some drug.

How can folks get off the medicine merry-go-round, which always depletes further nutrients, adds more toxins, and eventually triggers more symptoms, calling for more drugs? Luckily there is a much more scientific way to help folks get rid of symptoms. And at the same time they learn how to avoid drugs while they actually learn how to find the causes and cures. Even Columbia College of Physicians and Surgeons medical researchers have shown that over **95% of all disease has only two fundamental causes: diet and environment.** Translation: nutrient deficiencies and unwanted stockpiled toxicities.

Most all drugs work by poisoning an enzyme or metabolic pathway in the body. But smart medicine focuses on (1) finding why the pathway is malfunctioning and (2) repairing that malfunction once and for all. With drug medicine, because you didn't fix what was broken, symptoms pile on. For example, magnesium deficiency is extremely epidemic since government studies confirm the average person doesn't even get half the magnesium he needs in a day. So magnesium deficiency may go on to cause your elevated cholesterol, angina, hypertension, fatigue, PMS, or depression. But by resorting to Prozac, the magnesium deficiency is not corrected and may then cause insomnia, back spasms in an old injury, hypertension, migraines or atrial fibrillation or other arrhythmia. **The ultimate magnesium deficiency is sudden cardiac death.** And that doesn't even begin to look at the damage from the 3 molecules of fluoride that each molecule of Prozac put in the body.

On the flip side, when you use **smart medicine versus drug medicine**, you find the cause of every symptom. The side effects in this simplified example are that in correcting the magnesium deficiency you may also find you have improvement in insomnia, memory, chronic pain, constipation, mood, or loss of bowel spasms, angina or hypertension. Harmful side effects tank up in the body as nutrients get depleted and toxic drug metabolites accumulate in drug medicine. **But beneficial side effects stockpile in smart medicine, as many unexpected things heal.**

The difference between the two ways to practice medicine refers back to the books. If a doctor is drug-oriented, the *PDR* is his guiding light, and it makes it quick and easy to get on to the next patient. Remember **the average office visit is seven minutes**. The doctor relying purely on drugs doesn't have to delve into a complicated history; consequently he can get on to the next patient more quickly.

But in **smart medicine**, extensive time is needed to learn about the patient and his symptoms, including diet, environment, even his pesticide and dental histories. The point is to find out how the body got so damaged in order to repair God's miraculous chemistry. For we have been cleverly designed to heal, even cancers and diagnoses that to this day still proclaim there is no known cause and no known cure. As evidenced in previous *TW*s, most diseases are reversible, but the earlier the better. Rheumatoid arthritis, juvenile or adult, multiple sclerosis, autism, macular degeneration, depression, schizophrenia, GERD, ADD, atrial fibrillation, angina, hypertension, irritable bowel, chronic fatigue, fibromyalgia, cancer... **the diagnostic label is inconsequential**. It is just a name. **What matters is how far you have to go to find the repairable cause.**

Some are incredibly easy and others very complex. No two people have identical causes, even if they have the same symptoms or disease label.

But even for cancer, as a dreaded example, once you dissolve the suit of armor off the cancer cells (*TW* 2006), heal the gut that houses half the immune and detox systems (*No More Heartburn*), identify and correct nutrient deficiencies, get rid of hidden toxins (*The High Blood Pressure Hoax*), infections, biofilms, etc., you can unload the body enough so that it heals itself. That's the beauty of the miraculous design as well as harmonization with food components, like the carrot juicing in *Wellness Against All Odds* that makes the cancer p53 gene revert back to normal. There is no drug in the world that does that, but God designed food to be healing. Likewise, zinc is one example that I've referenced in 2005 *TW* that makes 33 cancer genes go back to normal, while it makes cancers shrink.

The "Disconnect" in Medicine

Yet even though the beta-carotene research was done at Harvard and the zinc study was published in the *Journal of the National Cancer Institute* (with our money!), they are conveniently ignored. Instead, drugs that can cost $500-$12,000 a shot and only give 2-4 weeks of extra life to the cancer victim are pushed on folks. Follow the buck and you'll understand why pennies of zinc or carrot juice are not even mentioned. Nor do most physicians bother to go through the effort to learn about God's chemistry so they can teach folks to heal, since a drug prescription takes seconds and you are out the door, as well as forever dependent.

In fact, **there appears to me to be a total disconnect in medicine between non-drug research and reality**. For example, even though the researchers at Harvard showed how beta-carotene reprograms the p53 gene, this in not used in any cancer programs from there that I am aware of. Likewise, even though congestive

367

heart failure was reversed with the far infrared sauna at the Mayo Clinic, I have never seen a cardiology consult from that clinic recommend one. **Why do these pillars of medicine ignore their own researchers working in their own institutions?**

NSAIDs or non-steroidal anti-inflammatory drugs (like Motrin, Aleve, ibuprofen, etc. that are over-the-counter as well as the prescribed forms like Celebrex, Voltaren, etc.) kill over 16,000 people each year just from intestinal hemorrhage alone. And recall they also foster blood clots. Over 100,000 victims get congestive heart failure a year while who knows how many have hip and knee replacements because of the known cartilage destruction caused by these FDA-approved drugs. And this is only one category of death-producing approved drugs. Why did they ever become available without a prescription when they started out needing one?

So back to the question of which book? You can empower yourself to learn how to use food, nutrients, and detoxification to restore God's chemistry. For in the *Bible* we are warned that we "are destroyed from lack of knowledge" (*Hos* 4). And since "you yourselves are God's temple" (*I Cor* 3), why would you be like those whose "God is their stomach" (*Phi* 3) and fill that temple with junk food? For "If anyone destroys God's temple, God will destroy him; for God's temple is sacred, and you are that temple." (*I Cor* 3). Fortunately, we are "fearfully and wonderfully made" (*Ps* 139).

Or you can ignore all His chemistry and go by the book of sorcery, the *PDR* of drugs, and merely poison any ailing pathway. The unsuspecting and contentedly ignorant patient can continue to remain unencumbered by knowledge and content with the farce that absence of symptoms means the problem has been solved. "For the wisdom of this world is foolishness in God's sight" (*I Cor* 3).

As another example, all cancer drugs eventually cause cancer. "Has not God made foolish the wisdom of this world?"(*I Cor* 1). In fact "God chose the weak things of the world to shame the strong."(*I Cor* 1), for you and I have collated more knowledge about how to heal (and totally referenced from the best journals) than hundreds of highly specialized physicians. I've witnessed not only in myself the curing over 20 dead-end diagnoses, but the casting out of disease in many of you with far worse diagnoses. Sure, it's tough to be a pioneer, "For wide is the gate and broad is the road that leads to destruction and many enter through it. But small is the gate and narrow the road that leads to life, and only a few find it." (*Mat*7).

Is it not ironic "that the ancient serpent called the devil, or Satan, who leads the whole world astray" (*Rev* 12) is the symbol of drug-driven medicine? Clearly you cannot rely on someone else to cleanse your temple; you have to do it yourself. And when you chose a doctor as a partner, sure, you want one who goes by the book. But which book?

Healing the Soul

If I hadn't seen it with my own eyes, in folks I have known for decades, I wouldn't be telling you about it. But folks, including physicians specializing in nutrition and detoxification have attributed their healing to booting bitterness, resentment, anger, fear, jealousy, worry, guilt, envy, rejection, and negative emotions from their lives. This in no way means that our illnesses are all in our heads, but quite the contrary. As Dr. Art Mathias beautifully explained in his book, *In His has Own Image, We Are Wonderfully Made,* that our emotions are strong enough to not only bring on illness but also perpetuate it. This book is the best blend of psychiatry, biology, and spirituality I've ever encountered, plus it suits a "reference junkie" like myself because it's thoroughly backed by scientific citations.

It proves how undesirable emotions and stresses can bring about an actual elevation of cholesterol as well as heart disease with or without, hypercholesterolemia. **Basically if the memory still**

369

hurts, it's unresolved and not forgiven. This can perpetuate illness. Our emotions have a powerful influence over our physiology. Grief can lower the white count and set us up for infection, while **stress can elevate cholesterol levels and fibrinogen levels** (*TW* Nov 2007). I highly recommend starting with that book and then proceeding to his *Biblical Foundations of Freedom* (Wellspring Ministries of Alaska, phone 907-563-9033, web site: ak-wellspring. com).

And don't neglect simple things to de-stress your life, like just resting or having a nap. **Heart attack risk was cut 37% by taking a half-hour nap at least three times a week** according to the *Archives of Internal Medicine* (*Wall Street Journal*, A1, Feb 13, 2007).

Move Over Dr. Kevorkian, AMA Recommends Euthanasia For the Faithful

More medical articles are showing that medicine is increasingly approaching euthanasia. A few years ago a medical journal article I reviewed in *TW* stated, "Not infrequently, Christian patients and families provide religious justification for an insistence on aggressive medical care near the end of life." The article in this AMA journal ended with instructions for physicians to help patients reach "appropriate limits to life-sustaining treatment." **Translation: Doctors, don't let a patients' religious beliefs keep you from playing God and telling them how long they should live.** Can you believe an AMA journal is directing physicians to ignore Christians wanting to do everything possible to live?

I think I speak for you, too, when I say I don't want any group of physicians unknowledgeable in the molecular biochemistry of reversing disease telling me how long I can live. They want to tell you and I when it's time to stop treatments and pull the plug, when they have not a clue of what is necessary to "heal the impossible"!

I suspect you want the best form of life-saving medicine for yourself and your loved ones that I do. The new gatekeepers over your longevity (who are assuming the role of God) are the very guys who don't come to courses on nutritional, environmental and toxicological medicine nor molecular biochemistry, and never even thought of ordering bare minimum your red blood cell minerals and fatty acids, much less anything else that could save your life. They don't even know what is in a Cardio/ION Panel. They are solely into standard blood tests and the latest pharmaceutical drugs, none of which heal, but merely mask symptoms while you continue to worsen. These are definitely not the guys who should tell us when to "pull the plug".

Even more frightening is the front-page *Wall Street Journal* article I reviewed in *TW* showing that *non-physician hospital and insurance employees are now playing the most important role in the rationing of health-care by deciding who gets what.* This is downright scary. You now have low wage, "fly-by-night", poorly trained folks who do not know you and are hired by the hospital or insurance company to make the decisions of which types and how much life-sustaining therapy you can have. This is scary rationing of healthcare and promises to get worse (McQueen). You had better keep getting yourself progressively smarter and healthier, for your sake and those you love. And for Pete's sake never give up or assume something is incurable if you haven't at least had a **Cardio/ION Panel** complete with expert interpretation!

Fortunately, another article in the same journal showed that folks who request clinical services like laboratory tests, usually get them. They did state also that **folks who ask for tests**, specialist referral or particular prescriptions, but **especially specialty tests make doctors very uncomfortable.** Isn't that just too bad? The moral of the story is thousands of years old: **ask and you shall receive** (*Matt* 7:7) (Anand, Kravitz, Brett, Hiilakivi, Byrd, Denolet).

You Need Continual Vigilance

As this readies for press, a notice smack dab on the front page of *The Wall Street Journal* reads "a new *Neurology* study bolstered the growing body of evidence that cholesterol-lowering statin drugs may help stave off Alzheimer's" (*Wall St J*, A-1, August 28, 2007). This is blatantly misguided and so very scary.

If you remember back to Chapter I, I showed you the evidence right out of the *European Journal of Neuroscience* (Meske, Blockade, HMG-COA reductase activity causes changes in micro-tubules-stabilizing protein suppression of geranylgeranylpyrophosphate formation: implications for Alzheimer's disease, 17:93-102, 2003) where the biochemical evidence is detailed how statins destroy the nervous system in multiple pathways, and clearly foster Alzheimer's! And then you saw all of the other reports (Wagstaff, Jackson, Hilgendorff, Shovman, Graveline, etc.) showing how statins bring on memory loss including complete amnesia in a NASA physician/astronaut and thousands of others, as well as increased death by suicide, infection and much more.

Furthermore, you saw how statins damage the chemistry needed to process folic acid. When this happens, it can bring on elevated homocysteine. Well, half the folks who have a stroke or brain atrophy have this combination of low folate and elevated homocysteine that makes them at high risk for brain rot (Yang). There is no way you should take a statin to prevent brain atrophy when it poisons multiple pathways (not to mention cholesterol metabolism) needed to prevent it. I hope you know by now that they just don't give up trying to pull the wool over your eyes to sell more drugs. They think there is no one to stand up for you by researching the details and then explain the details to you and show you the evidence so that you can make your own decisions.

Boosting Spirituality is Healthful For the Immune System

My hat goes off to my many patients and readers who home school their children. To me this is the ultimate sacrifice. But whether you home school or not, a mounting body of evidence shows that family time spent together, as well as nurturing a belief system in a supreme being, not only improves ethics, morals and compassionate social skills in children, but is nurturing for the *neuropsychoimmunology* of the body, the brain-body-hormone connection. **In short, a healthy spirituality boosts the immune system.** That's one reason I'm excited about a few of the over hundred books I have read.

Why would I be interested in reading a book by the investigative reporter who discovered the interoffice memo proving that the Ford Motor Company knew its Pinto could burst into flames when hit from behind at only 20 mph, (which it did, killing innocent teenagers and others)? Why would I want to read a book by this same award-winning journalist and former legal editor of *The Chicago Tribune*, with a degree from Yale Law School who cracked crime cases that had stumped the police? Because Lee Strobel went far beyond Larry King, who has said of all the people in history he would have most liked to interview would have been Jesus Christ. This former agnostic legal bulldog investigative reporter par excellence didn't wait for Christ's PR agent to schedule a TV interview.

He tackled the most important question in the world by tracking down the facts and sifting through the evidence using his legal/award-winning investigative reporter skills via interviews with top world authorities. As a consequence, he became a Christian after having been assigned to interview 13 leading experts on the historical evidence for Jesus Christ. He documents this in his book, *The Case for Christ*. He then went on to write a second book interviewing even more experts, from theologians and historians to physicists, biologists, judges, law professors, and more in

The Case for Faith. And he went even further to convince the unconvinced with *A Case For A Creator.* But you have already seen enough evidence right here for a creator. **This fantastic molecular biochemistry of the human body didn't just pop out after some big bang.**

A former Hindu, Ravi Zacharias, wrote another book that was equally convincing for me. He likewise interviewed leading world experts on the evidence for Christ. He then proceeded to successfully present his evidence in spirited debates at Harvard, Oxford and other prestigious learning centers of the world. His book, *Can Man Live Without God?,* details this (all these books are available from 1-800-CHRISTIAN). If you need "convincing", these books should do it, and still several others are mentioned in Chapter VII of *Depression Cured At Last!* (1-800-846-6687 or prestigepublishing.com). For there are books written on the evidence for the resurrection by leading attorneys, historians, theologians, archeologists, mathematicians, physicists, biologists, and more.

I know that my friends, relatives, and colleagues who are Hindus, Jews, Muslims, Buddhists and agnostics, or share other belief systems will not be offended. For those who know me, know that I use Christianity as an example of the power of spirituality in general, with my examples coming from Christianity, because that's the one that I'm personally most familiar with and convinced by. The bottom line is that spirituality has proven to be healthful in a multitude of ways.

As I continually search for the molecular biochemical evidence that enables folks to heal the impossible, I'm eternally and humbly reminded of many facts. For example, as I have shown in the past, Harvard researchers have proven that high doses of beta-carotene actually cause the p53 cancer gene to revert back to a normal gene. In other words, after everything that high-tech medicine has to offer has failed, and folks were on their deathbeds, nutrients in foods were able to do expensive gene therapy that no high tech scientist or genetic engineering company is capable of. What an incredibly clever molecular biochemical system has been designed in our bodies to dovetail with the healing provisions in food! That's one of the many reasons why the protocol in *the Wellness Against All Odds* book includes hourly carrot juicing as part of a program proven to more than quadruple cancer survival (references in December 2000 *TW*).

I hope this abbreviated tome gives you a small appreciation for the magnificence of the natural, God-given healing capability that has been programmed in you. I hope it has instilled in you an appreciation for **the awesome power you have over your health. For each day you are silently called upon to exercise decisions that will lead to your getting either healthier or not**. The tough part is you are surrounded by "medical authorities" who fail to comprehend the power you have. Their solution for your every symptom is a drug.

Above all, remember that the more one studies molecular biochemistry, the more convinced he must be of the presence of a **Master Biochemist** who has absolutely and miraculously designed the human body to heal, against all odds. In that case, **shouldn't you make it a top priority to know more about this Master Biochemist**?

In closing, remember from the Bible how the serpent duped Eve into disobeying God's commands? He gave bad advice: "Now the serpent was more crafty than any of the wild animals the Lord God had made. He said to the woman, "Did God really say, you must not eat from any tree in the garden'?" (Genesis 3: 1).

Later that day, "the Lord God said to the woman,' "What is this you have done?"

"The woman said,' The serpent deceived me, and I ate." (Genesis 3: 13).

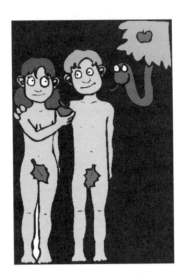

"The serpent deceived me"

Is it a coincidence that the caduceus symbol for organized, drug-oriented medicine is a winged staff with two serpents entwined? For I humbly submit to you to consider that the serpent is **still** deceiving us.

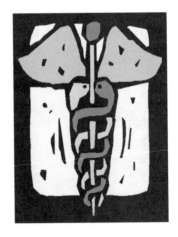

The serpent is still deceiving us.

Busy Executive Summary

The message should be loud and clear: **there is no busy executive summary**. Go back and read the details. **Many folks too busy to learn how to heal are dead.** Just as you cannot hire a clergyman to make you holy, you cannot hire a doctor to make you well. Many folks too busy to get involved with learning how to control their health have already joined the ranks of successful CEOs who were masters at delegating. They died prematurely because they never spent the time to take control of their own health. They thought they could rely on "specialists". Readers in their eighth and ninth decades write to express their gratitude at having no medications, no symptoms and great vitality. Who do you trust more than yourself to control your health?

Sources for this Chapter's Recommendations

- Health Clinic in Dallas is the American Environmental Health Foundation, aehf.com, 1-800-428-2343
- Arginine Powder, E-Gems Elite, Gamma E-Gems, carlsonlabs.com, 1-800-323-4141
- PhosChol, nutrasal.com, 1-800-777-1886
- GPLC, jarrow.com, or 1-877-VIT-AMEN
- Kyolic Liquid, wakunaga.com, 1-800-421-2998
- Corvalen Powder, corvalen.com, valenlabs.com, 1-866-CORVALEN
- Nattokinase, Lumbrokinase, allergyresearchgroup.com, 1-800-545-9960
- Wobenzyme-N, 1-877-VIT-AMEN or 1-800-669-CALM
- Magnesium Chloride Solution 200 mg/cc, (Rx needed), windhampharmacy.com, 1-518-734-3033
- Porphyrins Profile, RBC Minerals, Cardio/ION Panel, metametrix.com, 1-800-221-4640
- Book to interpret cardio/ION, *Laboratory Evaluations in Molecular Medicine,* metametrix.com, 1-800-221-4640

- Nitrostat (nitroglycerine sublingual tablets), Heparin and Magnesium Sulfate (both injectable) need Rx from your doctor
- *In He has Own Image, We Are Wonderfully Made*, and *BiblIcal* **Foundations** *of* **Freedom**, both by Art Mathias Ph.D., akwellspring.com, 1-907-563-9033

References:

Bralley JA, Lord RS, *Laboratory Evaluations in Molecular Medicine*, Institute for Advances in Molecular Medicine, 2001, Norcross GA, 1-800-221-4640

Weinhold B, Making health care healthier, *Environ Health Perspect*, 109; 8:A370-A377

Parks JS, et al, Phosphatidylcholine fluidity and structure affect lecithin: cholesterol acyltransferase activity, *J Lipid Res*, 41: 546-53, 2000

Singh RB, A randomized, double-blind, placebo-controlled trial of L-carnitine in suspected acute myocardial infarction, *Postgrad Med J*, 72:45-50, 1996

Clark RM, et al, L-carnitine increases a-tocopherol and lowers liver and plasma triglycerides in aging ovariectomized rats, *J Nutr Biochem*, 18:623-20 8, 2007

Cullen P, Evidence the triglycerides are an independent coronary heart disease risk factor, *Am J Cardiol*, 6:943-49, 2000

Yang LK, et al, Correlations between folate, B12, homocysteine levels, and radiologic markers of neuropathology in elderly post-stroke patients, *J Am Coll Nutr*, 26; 3:272-78, 2007

Lazarou J, et al, Incidence of adverse drug reactions in hospitalized patients, *J Am Med Assoc*, 279:15:1200-1205, 1998

Ebbesen J, et al, Drug-related deaths in a department of internal medicine, *Arch Intern Med*, 161:2317-23, 2001

Choudhry NK, Stelfox HT, Detsky AS, Relationships between authors of clinical practice guidelines and the pharmaceutical industry, *J Am Med Assoc*, 287;5: 612-617, Feb. 6, 2002

Levine RL, Hursting MJ, McCollum D, Argatroban therapy in heparin-induced thrombocytopenia with hepatic dysfunction, *Chest*, 129:1167-75, 2006

Levine MN, Raskob G, Beyeth RJ, et al, Hemorrhagic complications of anticoagulant therapy. The Seventh ACCP Conference on Anti-thrombotic and Thrombolytic Therapy, *Chest*, 126:287S-310 S, 2004

Jang IK, Hursting MJ, When heparins promote thrombosis: Review of heparin-induced thrombocytopenia, *Circulation*, 111:2671-83, 2002

Warkentin TE, Think of HIT when thrombosis follows heparin, *Chest*, 130:631-32, 2006

Ornish D, Scherwitz LW, Brand RJ, et al, Intensive lifestyle changes for reversal of coronary heart disease, *J Am Med Assoc*, 2: 2001-2007, 1998

Gould KL, et al, Improved stenosis geometry by quantitative coronary arteriography after vigorous risk factor modification. *Am J Cardiol,* 69: 845-853, 1992

Ornish DM, et al, Can lifestyle changes reverse coronary heart disease? *Lancet,* 336: 129-133, 1990 (and see his 1998 reference in chapter 4)

Winslow R, Study confirms better predictor of heart risk, *Wall St J,* B-1, Nov. 14, 2002

Chase M, Bacteria behind gum disease are linked to heart-attack risk, *Wall St J,* B6, September 30, 2002

Hodis HN, Mack WJ, LaBree L, et al, Serial coronary angiographic evidence that antioxidant vitamins intake reduces progression of coronary artery atherosclerosis, *J Am Med Assoc,* 273: 1849-54, 1995

Rath M, Niedzwiecki A, Nutritional supplement program halts progression of early coronary atherosclerosis documented by ultrafast computed tomography, *J Appl Nutr,* 48; 3: 67-78, 1996

Anand G, Life support. The big secret in health-care: rationing is here. With little guidance, workers on front lines decide who gets what treatment, *Wall St J,* A1, A6, Sept.12, 2003

McQueen MP, Look who's watching your health expenses, *WSJ,* D1, D4, Sept. 25, 2007

Kravitz RL, Bell RA, Thom DH, et al, Direct observation of request for clinical services in office practice. What do patients want and do they get it?, *Arch Intern Med,* 163: 1673-81, July 28, 2003

Brett AS, Jersild P, "Inappropriate" treatment near the end of life. Conflict between religious convictions and clinical judgment, *Arch Intern Med,* 163: 1645-49, July 28, 2003

Hiilakivi-Clarke L, et al, Psychosocial factors in the development and progression of breast cancer: a review, *Breast Cancer Res Treat,* 29: 141-60, 1993

Byrd RC, Positive therapeutic effects of intercessory prayer in a coronary care unit population, *South Med J,* 81: 826-29, 1988

Denollet J, et al, Personality as independent predictor of long-term mortality in patients with coronary heart disease, *Lancet,* 347: 414-21, 1996

Lagerqvist B, et al, Long-term outcomes with the drug-eluting stents versus bare-metal stents in Sweden, *New Engl J Med,* 356:1009-19, 2007

Hochman JS, et al, Coronary intervention for persistent occlusion after myocardial infarction, *New England Journal of Medicine,* 355:2395-07, 2006

CAPRIE Steering Committee, A randomized, blinded, trial of clopidogrel versus aspirin in patients at risk of ischemic events (CAPRIE), *Lancet,* 348:1329-39, 1996

Yusuf S, et al, Effects of clopidogrel in addition to aspirin in patients with acute coronary syndromes with ST-segment elevation, *New Engl J Med,* 345:494-502, 2001

Kindness G, Frackleton JP, Effect of ethylene diamine tetraacetic acid (EDTA) on platelet aggregation in human blood, *J Adv Med,* 2: 519-30, 1989

379

Corvalen references:
Ingwall JS, et al, Is the failing heart energy starved? *Circul Res*, 95:135-14 2004

Wilson R, et al, D-Ribose enhances the identification of hibernating myocardial, *Heart Drug*, 3:61-62, 2003

Perkowski D, et al, Pre-surgical loading of oral D-ribose improves cardiac index in patients undergoing "off" pump coronary artery revascularization, *FASEB J,* (part I), 19; 4:A695, 2005

Pauly DF, et al, D-Ribose as a supplement for cardiac energy metabolism, *J Cardiovasc Pharmacol Therap*, 5; 4:249-58, 2000

Omran H, et al, D-Ribose improves diastolic function and quality of life in congestive heart failure patients: a prospective feasibility study, *Eur J Heart Fail,* 5: 615-19, 2003

Seifert JG, et al, The effects of ribose ingestion on indices of free radical production during hypoxic exercise, *Free Rad Biol Med,* 33 (S1): S269, 2002

Pliml W, et al, Effects of ribose on exercise-induced ischemia in unstable coronary artery disease, *Lancet,* 340; 8818:507-10, August 1992

Sinatra S, Roberts JC, *Reverse Heart Disease Now*, J Wiley & Sons, 2007

Chapter IX

Resources

Remember NEEDS (1-800-634-1380 or needs.com) gives our readers a 25% discount on many products in this book, as does 1-877-VIT-AMEN. Check them out. Meanwhile, companies are sold, products changed, people die, etc. We have updated the information below, but it is still not immutable.

Chapter I

- Q-ODT, intensivenutrition.com, 1-800-333-7414
- Gamma E Gems, E-Gems Elite, Cod Liver Oil, Super 2 Daily, Liquid Multiple Minerals, carlsonlabs.com, 1-800-323-4141
- Phos Chol, nutrasal.com, 1-800-777-1886
- *Statin Drugs, Side Effects, and the Misguided War on Cholesterol,* and *Lipitor, Thief of Memory,* thepowerhour.com, 1-877-817-9829
- Generic statin, lef.org, 1-800-544-4440 or 1-877-877-9700

Chapter II

- Niacin-Time, carlsonlabs.com, 1-800-323-4141
- Kyolic Formula 107 Red Yeast Rice, wakunaga.com, 1-800-421-2998
- Kyolic Formula 107 Red Yeast Rice, NSC24.com, 1-800-541-3997
- Policosanol, protherainc.com, 1-888-488-2488
- Policosanol, jarrow.com or 1-877-VIT-AMEN
- Lycopene, carlsonlabs.com, 1-800-323-4141
- E-Gems Elite, Gamma E-Gems, Tocotrienols, carlsonlabs.com, 1-800-323-4141
- Sytrinol, carlsonlabs.com, 1-800-323-4141 or 1-877-VIT-AMEN

- Pantethine, carlsonlabs.com, 1-800-323-4141
- Klaire Ultrafine Pure Ascorbic Acid, protherainc.com, 1-888-488-2488
- Magnesium Chloride Solution 200 mg/cc (prescription required), windhampharmacy.com, 518-734-3033
- Magnesium Chloride Solution 85 mg/cc, painstresscenter.com, 1-800-669-CALM
- Natural Calm 200 mg/tsp, supervites.net, 1-888-800-1180
- Chelated Manganese, carlsonlabs.com, 1-800-323-4141
- Chelated Magnesium, carlsonlabs.com, 1-800-323-4141
- Super 2 Daily, carlsonlabs.com, 1-800-323-4141
- CholestSure, davincilabs.com, 1-800-325-1776

Chapter III
- Coronary calcium score (EBCT or Ultrafast Heart Scan), D.O.C. (Diagnostic Outpatient Centers), docsopenmri.com, 1-800-890-4452
- Gamma E Gems, E-Gems Elite, Niacin-Time, Tocotrienols, Cod Liver Oil, Chelated Copper, Chelated Zinc, Chelated Magnesium, B6, Vitamin B2, B12 SL, Arginine Powder Carlsonlabs.com, 1-800-323-4141
- NAC, Methylcobalamin, jarrow.com or 1-877-VIT-AMEN
- HDL Rx, integrativeinc.com, 1-800-917-3690
- Cardio/ION Panel, metametrix.com, 1-800-221-4640
- Kyolic Formula 107 Red Yeast Rice, Kyolic Liquid, wakunaga.com, 1-800-421-2998
- DMG, NAC, davincilabs.com, 1-800-325-1776
- PhosChol, nutrasal.com, 1-800-777-1886
- Folixor, Betalin 12, R-Lipoic Acid, intensivenutrition.com, 1-800-333-7414
- Wobenzyme, 1-877-VIT-AMEN or needs.com, 1-800-634-1380
- Nattokinase, allergyresearchgroup.com, 1-800-545-9960
- Macademia Nut Oil, realfoodgrocery.com, 1-877-673-2536
- Lumbrokinase, allergy researchgroup.com, 1-800-545-9960

- New York Heart Center, 1000 E Genesee St, Syracuse, NY 315-471-1044
- Ananese, intensivenutrition.com, 1-800-333-7414
- Delta-Fraction Tocotrienols, allergyresearchgroup.com, 1-800-545-9960
- Q-ODT, intensivenutrition.com, 1-800-333-7414

Chapter IV
- Organic, non-GMO grains, beans, seeds, nuts, teas, cookware, prepared foods, and so much more. There is no excuse for not eating healthfully, no matter where you live. To get catalog or place an order: natural-lifestyle.com, 1-800-752-2775
- PhosChol, nutrasal.com, 1-800-777-1886
- Far Infrared Sauna, hightechhealth.com, 1-800-794-5355
- IndolPlex and Calcium-D Glucarate, integrativeinc.com, 1-800-917-3690
- Cardio/ION, metametrix.com, 1-800-221-4640
- Cod Liver Oil, carlsonlabs.com, 1-800-323-4141
- Green tea infuser, natural-lifestyle.com, 1-800-752-2775
- Sencha Premium Organic Green tea, indigo-tea.com, 1-866-248-3516
- Books on whole foods diets, ppnf.org, 1-800-366-3748
- Dr. Ohhira's 12+ Probiotic, realfoodgrocery.com, 1-877-673-2536, or 1-877-262-7843
- GPLC, ALCA, jarrow.com or 1-877-VIT-AMEN

Chapter V
- PerioPaste, Hydro Floss, PerioScript, docharrison.com, 1-800-650-9060
- Kyolic Liquid, wakunaga.com, 1-800-421-2998
- Organic Green Barley Grass, livingfoodsusa.com, 785-856-0701
- Mastic Gum, jarrow.com or 1-877-VIT-AMEN
- Dr. Ohhira's 12 Plus, realfoodgrocery.com, 1-877-673-2536, or 1-877-262-7843, or 1-877-VIT-AMEN

- ABx Support, protherainc.com, 1-888-488-2488
- GI fx, Cardio/ION, metametrix.com, 1-800-221-4640
- Comprehensive Stool with Purged Parasites, doctorsdata.com, 1-800-323-2784
- Klaire Ultrafine Pure Ascorbic Acid Powder, protherainc.com, 1-888-488-2488
- Recancostat, integrativeinc.com, 1-800-917-3690
- R-Lipoic Acid, intensivenutrition.com, 1-800-333-7414
- Lypo-Spheric Vitamin C, livonlabs.com, 1-866-682-6193, 1-800-334-9294, or 1-877-VIT-AMEN
- Essential GSH, 1-877-VIT-AMEN
- LipoCeutical Glutathione, gshnow.com, 650-323-3238
- NSC-100 Extra Strength Formula, nsc24.com 888-541-3997
- Life Source Basics, lifesourcebasics.com, 1-877-346-6863
- Beta-1, 3-D Glucan, transferpoint.com, 1-877-407-3999

Chapter VI
- Methylcobalamin 5mg, Zinc Balance, BioSil, jarrow.com, 1-800-726-0886 or 1-877-VIT-AMEN
- Folixor 5mg, SilBoron, intensivenutrition.com, 1-800-333-7414
- NAC, DMG, davincilabs.com, 1-800-325-1776
- Liposomal GSH, 1-877-VIT-AMEN
- LipoCeutical Glutathione, gshnow.com, 650-323-3238
- Recancostat, integrativeinc.com, 1-800-917-3690
- Cardio/ION Panel, Organic Acids, ADMA, metametrix.com, 1-800-221-4640
- Kyolic Liquid Cardiovascular, Kyo-Chrome, wakunaga.com, 1-800-421-2998
- Chelated Magnesium. Nutra Support Joint, Moly B, Chelated Zinc, E Gems Elite, Chelated Chromium, Biotin, Cod Liver Oil, Vitamin D3 2000 mg, ACES with Zinc, Chelated Selenium, Chelated Manganese, Chelated Copper, Vitamin B2, Vitamin K2, Vitamin, D3, carlsonlabs.com, 1-800-323-4141

- Iodoral, optimox.com, 1-800-223-1601 or needs.com, 1-800-634-1380
- Magnesium Chloride Solution 200mg/cc, windhampharmacy.com, 518-734-3033
- Vanadium 250 Krebs, douglaslabs.com, 1-888-DOUGLAB
- IntraMin, druckerlabs.com, 1-888-881-2344
- Delta-Fraction Tocotrienols, allergyresearchgroup.com, 1-800-545-9960
- Essential Phospholipids, allergyresearchgroup.com, 1-800-545-9960
- Perfusia (Thorne), use needs.com, 1-800-634-1380

Chapter VII
- Porphyrins Profile, Cardio/ION Panel, metametrix.com, 1-800-221-4640
- Far Infrared Sauna, hightechhealth.com, 1-800-794-5355
- Detoxamin, detoxamin.com, 1-877-656-4553
- Kelatox, kelatox.com, 1-866-707-4482
- Captomer (Thorne), needs.com, 1-800-634-1380
- DMSA, vrp.com, 1-800-877-2447
- Silit fryer, sauce pans, and pressure cooker, natural-lifestyle.com, 1-800-752-2775
- Cogimax, optimox.com, 1-800-226-1601, or needs.com, 1-800-634-1380
- Lumen, lumenphoton.com, 1-828-863-4834
- SOD sublingual, intensivenutrition.com, 1-800-333-7414
- Foust Auto Air Cleaner, foustco.com, 1-800 EL FOUST

Chapter VIII
- Dr. WJ Rea, Dallas Unit, American Environmental Health Foundation, aehf.com, 214-368-4132, 1-800-428-2343
- Book to interpret Cardio/ION, *Laboratory Evaluations in Molecular Medicine,* metametrix.com, 1-800-221-4640
- Arginine Powder, E-Gems Elite, Gamma E-Gems, carlsonlabs.com, 1-800-323-4141

- GPLC, jarrow.com, or 1-877-VIT-AMEN
- Kyolic Liquid, wakunaga.com, 1-800-421-2998
- Corvalen Powder, corvalen.com or bioenergy.com, 1-866-CORVALEN
- Nattokinase, Lumbrokinase, allergyresearchgroup.com, 1-800-545-9960
- Wobenzyme-N, douglaslabs.com, 1-888-DOUGLAB
- Magnesium Chloride Solution 200 mg/cc, windhampharmacy.com, 518-734-3033
- Porphyrins Profile, RBC Minerals, metametrix.com, 1-800-221-4640
- Nitrostat, Heparin, Magnesium Sulfate, Rx needed from your doctor
- *In He has Own Image, We Are Wonderfully Made*, and *BiblIcal Foundations of Freedom,* both books by Art Mathias Ph.D., akwellspring.com, 907-563-9033

Radio Shows

Here are a few examples of where you can often hear Dr. Rogers live and call in with questions, also these shows often are available on tape, CD, or archived on the net for a month after the show.

www.kbjs.org
www.hwwshow.com
www.thepowerhour.com
www.radiomartie.com
www.tantalk1340.com
www.ksevradio.com or www.hotzehwc.com

The Cholesterol Hoax

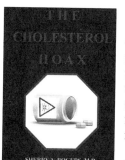

Cholesterol is not the biggest cause of heart disease nor is it predictive of heart disease. In fact, over half the folks who die of a heart attack never had high cholesterol. But they did have other warnings that could have saved their lives, had they been checked. And the cure for these is spelled out here via safe non-prescription nutrients.

Cholesterol is merely the messenger, the smoke detector, alerting you to a curable problem. Why shoot the messenger with a drug when you can find the cause and cure once and for all?

Statin drugs prescribed for high cholesterol poison cholesterol synthesis, which then leads to Alzheimer's, impotence, tooth loss, depression, sudden heart attack, fibromyalgia, chronic fatigue, polyneuropathy, tendon ruptures, insulin resistance, amnesia, suicide, heart failure and cancers, plus statins produce deficiencies of vitamin E, folic acid, and CoQ10, ushering in more diseases and shortening life. Fortunately, there are many non-prescription, cheaper, safer, and more effective agents to control cholesterol damage.

Juicy steaks, cheeses, and wine are not forbidden, but one bite of a more common food ingredient (recommended by dieticians) sends thousands of damaging molecules to every one of your body's trillions of cells and creates high cholesterol. As well, Teflon, plasticizers, PCBs, lead, arsenic, mercury and other unavoidable toxins that we all harbor can trigger coronary artery disease, with or without high cholesterol, as can hidden infections that stem from the teeth, the gut, or former "colds".

Since half the folks who have a heart attack never make it to the hospital in time, you will also learn here how to thwart death with your own home emergency box, plus crucial steps for those who have already survived one. Furthermore, complete with over 700 scientific references for evidence, you will learn more about the prevention and reversal of heart disease than most physicians know, because you need to. For no one can heal you, but you can learn how to heal yourself. Yes, having high cholesterol is one of the luckiest things that ever happened to you, because it led you to this book, which can save your life, regardless of who you are. Clearly, even if you never had high cholesterol you need this book to show you how to thwart the number one cause of death, cardiovascular disease.

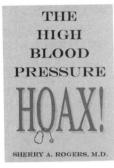

THE HIGH BLOOD PRESSURE HOAX!

SHERRY A. ROGERS, M.D.

The High Blood Pressure Hoax

Blood pressure drugs guarantee you will get worse, for they actually deplete the nutrients that cause high blood pressure, making sure you will need even more medications as your pressure goes higher and you also develop new symptoms. High blood pressure is not a deficiency of blood pressure-lowering drugs, which also shrink the brain and raise your risk of heart attack, senility, cancer and blindness. But there are dozens of ways you can permanently cure your blood pressure without drugs.

And since healthy blood vessels determine the longevity of every organ in the entire body, **you need this book even if you don't have high blood pressure, for vascular health is key to total body health and longevity.** First of all the health of every single cell of your body depends on the health of your blood vessels that supply them. For example, if you don't want to get Alzheimer's, then you need a healthy brain, but it is only as healthy as its blood supply. Likewise, if you don't want cancer (or you are trying to heal it), it starts (and spreads) in areas of poor circulation. Furthermore, obvious conditions like impotency or erectile dysfunction scream for blood vessel health to be restored.

The High Blood Pressure Hoax will show you that for every ailment, even one as simple as high blood pressure, there are multiple causes and multiple cures. You have a lot to choose from. In fact I would suggest you read the entire book before you chose your program. For by understanding how the various causes work, you (who know your body and medical history better than anyone else) have the optimum opportunity for choosing the best solution for you.

This is the ultimate plan for vascular health, but it doesn't stop there. **This book is also the sequel to the classic, *Detoxify or Die*,** for it takes off from where *DOD* left off, bringing you to even more powerful levels of detoxification. For **it is unprecedented in showing you how to detoxify heavy metals with non-prescription items that are safer, easier, and more efficacious than IV chelation.** Dr. Rogers can't wait to empower you! So let's get started.

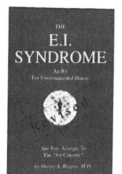

The E.I. Syndrome, Revised is a 635-page book that is necessary for people with **environmental illness.** It explains chemical, food, mold allergies, and Candida sensitivities, nutritional deficiencies, testing methods and how to do the various environmental controls and diets in order to get well.

Many docs buy this by the hundreds and make them mandatory reading for patients, as it contains many pearls about getting well that are not found anywhere else. In this way it increases the fun of practicing medicine, because patients are on a higher educational level and office time is more productive for more sophisticated levels of wellness. It covers hundreds of facts that make the difference between E.I. victims versus E.I. conquerors. It helps patients become active partners in their care and thereby get better results, while avoiding doctor burnout. It covers the gamut of the diagnosis and treatment of environmentally induced symptoms.

Because the physician author was a severe universal reactor who has recovered, this book contains mountains of clues to wellness. As a result, many have written that they healed themselves of resistant illnesses of all types by reading this book. This is in spite of the fact that no consulted physicians were able to diagnose or effectively treat them. If you are not sure what causes your symptoms, this, Dr. Rogers' very first book, is a great start.

Many veteran sufferers have written that they had read many books on aspects of allergy, chronic Candidiasis and chemical sensitivity and thought that they knew it all. Yet (they wrote that) what they learned *in **The E.I. Syndrome, Revised*** enabled them to reach that last pinnacle of wellness.

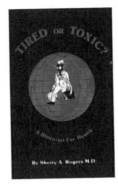

Tired or Toxic? is a 400-page book, and the first book that describes the mechanism, diagnosis and treatment of chemical sensitivity, complete with scientific references. It is written for the layman and physician alike and explains the many vitamin, mineral, essential fatty acid and amino acid analyses that help people detoxify everyday chemicals more efficiently and hence get rid of baffling symptoms, including chronic pain.

It is the first book written for laymen and physicians to describe xenobiotic detoxification, the process that allows all healing to occur. You have heard of the cardiovascular system, you have heard of the respiratory system, the gastrointestinal system, and the immune system. But most have never heard of the chemical detoxification system, which is the main determinant of whether we have chemical sensitivity, cancer, and in fact, every disease.

This program shows you how to diagnose and treat many resistant everyday symptoms and use molecular medicine techniques. It also gives the biochemical mechanisms in easily understood form, of how Candida creates such a diversity of symptoms and how the macrobiotic diet heals "incurable" end stage metastatic cancers. It is a great book for the physician you are trying to win over, and shows you how chemical sensitivity masquerades as common symptoms. It then explores the many causes and cures of chemical sensitivity, chronic Candidiasis, brain fog or toxic encephalopathy, and other "impossible to heal" medical labels.

Chemical Sensitivity

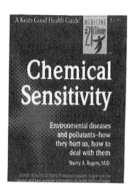

This 48-page booklet is the most concise referenced booklet on chemical sensitivity. It is for the person wanting to learn about it, but who is leery of tackling a big book. It is ideal for teaching your physician or convincing your insurance company, as it is fully referenced. And it is a good reference for the veteran who wants a quick concise review.

Most people have difficulty envisioning chemical sensitivity as a potential cause of everyday maladies. But the fact is that a lack of knowledge of the mechanisms of chemical sensitivity can be the solo reason that holds many back from ever healing completely. Some will never get truly well, simply because they do not comprehend the tremendous role chemical sensitivity plays. For failure to address the role that chemical sensitivity plays in every disease has been pivotal in failure to get well. The principles of environmental controls are of especially vital importance for cancer victims.

If you are not completely well, you need to read this booklet. If you have been sentenced to a lifetime of drugs, whether it be for high blood pressure, high cholesterol, angina, arrhythmia, asthma, eczema, sinusitis, colitis, learning disabilities, chronic pain or cancer, you need this booklet. It matters not what your label is. What matters is whether chemical sensitivity is a factor that no one has explored that is keeping you from getting well. Most probably it is, and this is an inexpensive way to start you on the path toward drug-free wellness. Then give one to your physician and friends who need to learn about pervasive everyday chemicals and their power to cause disease.

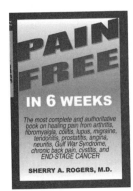

The most complete and authoritative book on healing pain from arthritis, fibromyalgia, colitis, lupus, migraine, tendonitis, prostatitis, angina, neuritis, Gulf War Syndrome, chronic back pain, cystitis, and END-STAGE CANCER

SHERRY A. ROGERS, M.D.

Pain Free in 6 Weeks

All pain has a cause, and once you know the cause, you have the cure. We don't all just look different; we have different chemistries and different underlying causes for our pain.

Old injuries, old age, autoimmune disease, chronic degeneration and even cancer are not the *reasons* for pain. They are mere *labels and excuses* for not finding the true cause and getting rid of it. In fact, the very medications prescribed for pain actually cause deterioration of bone and cartilage, guaranteeing that hip and knee replacement will be needed in the future. And total cure from pain need not be difficult, for the solution may be as simple as eliminating an unidentified food antigen, correcting a nutrient deficiency, healing the gut, or killing an unidentified stealth infection.

For others it has required getting rid of a lifetime's accumulation of everyday toxic chemicals. U.S. EPA studies of chemicals stored in the fat of humans showed that 100% of people harbor environmental chemicals that trigger mysterious back pain, hip pain, arthritis, osteoporosis, painful burning skin, migraines, prostatitis, fibromyalgia, sciatica, degenerating back discs, cystitis, neuropathies, tic doloreau, and even end-stage cancer. When folks get symptoms, they are told that they are a normal consequence of aging, and that there is no known cause or cure. This is totally wrong, as the over 500 scientific references prove. The exciting part is that the majority of folks have total power over their pain. Are you ready to reverse years of pain and become truly **pain free**?

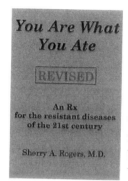

You Are What You Ate

This book is indispensable as the primer and introduction to the macrobiotic diet. The macrobiotic diet is the specialized diet with which many have healed the impossible, including end-stage metastatic cancers. This is after medicine had given up on them and they had been given only months or weeks to live. Yes, they have rallied after surgery, chemotherapy and radiation had failed. Life was seemingly, hopelessly over, yet they kicked death in the teeth.

Understandably, this diet has also enabled many chemically sensitive universal reactors, and highly allergic and even "undiagnosable people" to heal. It has also enabled those to heal who had "wastebasket" diagnostic labels such as chronic fatigue, fibromyalgia, MS (multiple sclerosis), rheumatoid arthritis, depression, chronic infections, colitis, asthma, migraines, lupus, chronic Candidiasis, and much more.

Although there are many books on macrobiotics, this is one that takes the special needs of the allergic person and those with multiple food and chemical sensitivities as well as chronic Candidiasis into account. It provides details and case histories that the person new to macrobiotics needs before he embarks on the strict healing phase, as meticulously described in the sequel, *The Cure is in the Kitchen*.

Even people who have done the macrobiotic diet for a while will find reasons why they have failed and tips to improve their success. When a diet such as this has allowed many to heal their cancers, any other condition "should be a piece of cake".

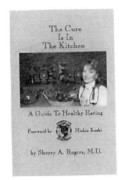

The Cure is in the Kitchen is the next book you should read after ***You Are What You Ate*** to fully understand how to successfully implement the healing macrobiotic diet. It is the first book to ever spell out in detail what all those people ate day to day who cleared their incurable diseases like MS, rheumatoid arthritis, fibromyalgia, lupus, chronic fatigue, colitis, asthma, migraines, depression, hypertension, heart disease, angina, undiagnosable symptoms, and relentless chemical, food, Candida, and electromagnetic sensitivities, as well as terminal cancers.

Dr. Rogers flew to Boston each month to work side by side with Mr. Michio Kushi, as he counseled people at the end of their medical ropes. As their remarkable case histories will show you, nothing is hopeless. Many of these people had failed to improve with surgery, chemotherapy and radiation. Instead their metastases continued to spread. It was only when they were sent home to die within a few weeks that they turned to the diet.

Medical studies confirm that this diet has more than tripled the survival from cancers. And the beauty of this diet is that you use God-given whole foods to coax the body into the healing mode. It does not rely on prescription drugs, but allows the individual to heal himself at home.

If you cannot afford a $500 consultation, and you choose not to accept your death sentence or medication sentence, why not learn first hand what these people did and how you, too, may improve your health and heal the impossible.

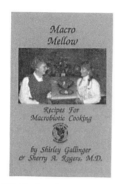

Macro Mellow is a book designed for 4 types of people: (1) For the person who doesn't know a thing about macrobiotics, but just plain wants to cook and eat better to feel better, in spite of the 21st century. (2) It solves the high cholesterol and triglycerides problem without drugs, and is the preferred diet for heart disease patients. In fact, it is the only proven diet to dissolve cholesterol deposits from arterial walls. (3) It is the perfect transition diet for those not ready for macro, but needing to get out of the chronic illness rut. (4) It spells out how to feed the rest of the family members who hate macro, while another family member must eat it in order to clear "incurable" symptoms.

It shows how to convert the "grains, greens, and beans", strict macro food, into delicious "American-looking" food that the kids will eat. This helps save the cook from making double meals while one person heals. The delicious low-fat whole food meals designed by Shirley Gallinger, a veteran nurse who has worked with Dr. Rogers for over two decades, uses macro ingredients without the rest of the family even knowing. It is the first book to dovetail creative meal planning, menus, recipes and even gardening so the cook isn't driven crazy.

Most likely your kitchen contains a plethora of cookbooks. But you owe it to yourself and your family to learn how to incorporate healing whole foods, low in fat and high in phytonutrients into their diets. **Who you have planning and cooking your meals has been proven to be as important if not more important, than who you have chosen for your doctor.** Medical research has proven time after time the power of whole food diets to heal where high tech medicines and surgery have failed.

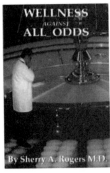

Wellness Against All Odds is the 6th and most revolutionary book by Sherry A. Rogers, M.D. It contains the ultimate healing plan that people have successfully used to beat cancer when they were given 2 weeks, some even 2 days to live by esteemed medical centers. These people had exhausted all that medicine has to offer, including surgery, chemotherapy, radiation and bone marrow transplants. Some had even been macrobiotic failures. And one of the most unbelievable things is that the plan costs practically nothing to implement and most of it can be done at home with non-prescription items.

Of course, in keeping with the other works and going far beyond, this contains the mechanisms of how these principles heal and is complete with the scientific references for physicians. In fact, this program has been proven to more than quadruple cancer survival in the most hopeless forms of cancer (Gonzales, *Nutrition & Cancer*, 33(2): 117-124, 1999).

Did you know, for example, that Harvard physicians have shown how vitamins actually cure some cancers, and over 50 papers in the best medical journals prove it? Likewise, did you know that there are non-prescription enzymes that dissolve cancer, arteriosclerotic plaque, and autoantibodies like lupus and rheumatoid? Did you know that there is a simple inexpensive, but highly effective way to detoxify the body at home to stop the toxic side effects of chemotherapy within minutes? Did you know that this procedure can also reduce chemical sensitivity reactions (from accidental chemical exposures) from 4 days to 20 minutes? Did you know that there are many hidden causes for "undiagnosable" symptoms that are never looked for, because it is easier and quicker to prescribe a pill than find (and fix) the causes?

The fact is that when you get the body healthy enough, it can heal anything. You do not have to die from labelitis. It no longer matters what your label is, from chronic Candida, fatigue, MS, or chronic pain to chemical sensitivity, an undiagnosable condition, or the worst cancer with only days to survive. If you have been told there is nothing more that can be done for you, you have the option of kicking death in the teeth and healing the impossible. Are you game? And **if you can give only one book to a friend with cancer, this is it.**

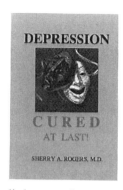

DEPRESSION CURED AT LAST! SHERRY A. ROGERS, M.D.

Depression Cured at Last!

Just when you think all has been accomplished, along comes one of the most important books of all. Unique in many ways, (1) it is written for the layperson and the physician, and is appropriate as a medical school textbook. In fact, it should be required reading for all physicians regardless of specialty. (2) It shows that it borders on malpractice to treat depression as a Prozac deficiency, to drug cardiology patients, or any other medical/psychiatric problems without first ruling out proven causes.

With over 700 pages and 1,000 complete references, it covers the **environmental, nutritional** and **metabolic** causes of all disease. It covers leaky gut syndrome, intestinal dysbiosis, hormone deficiencies, hidden sensitivities to foods, molds, and chemicals, dysfunctional detoxification, heavy metal and pesticide poisonings, toxic xenobiotic accumulations, and much, much more.

It is the best blueprint for figuring out what is wrong and how to fix it once and for all. If no one knows what is wrong with you, you need this book. If they know, but say there is no cure, you need this book. If they say you need medications to control your symptoms indefinitely, you need this book. Using depression as an example, it is the protocol for the environmental medicine work-up for all disease: how to systematically find the causes.

It is inconceivable that there is anyone who would not benefit from this book, as it surely leaves drug-oriented medicine in the dust of the 20th century. And it does so by using the only disease that by definition sports a lack of hope. We chose this disease, depression, as a prototype; to be sure to drive home the message that **just when you least expect it, there is always hope. Every symptom has a cause and a cure**. Come learn how to find the causes of yours.

The
Scientific Basis
for
Selected
Environmental
Medicine
Techniques

by

Sherry A. Rogers, M D

Scientific Basis for Selected Environmental Medicine Techniques contains the scientific evidence and references for the techniques of environmental medicine. It is designed with the patient in mind who is being denied medical payments by insurance companies that refuse to acknowledge environmental medicine.

With this guide a patient may choose to represent himself in small claims court and quote from the book showing, for example, that the *Journal of the American Medical Association* states that "titration provides a useful and effective measure of patient sensitivity". Or he may need to prove to his HMO that a U.S. Government agency stated, "an exposure history should be taken for every patient". Failure to do so can lead to an inappropriate diagnosis and treatment.

It has sections showing medical references of how finding hidden vitamin deficiencies have, for example, enabled people to heal carpal tunnel syndrome without surgery, or heal life threatening steroid-resistant vasculitis, or stop seizures, or migraines, or learning disabilities.

This book is designed for patients who choose to find the causes of their illnesses, rather than merely mask their symptoms with drugs for the rest of their lives. It is also for those who have been unfairly denied insurance coverage, or appropriate diagnosis by an HMO that is more concerned about profit than finding the cause of their patients' symptoms. And it is the ideal book with which to educate your PTA, attorney, insurance company, or physicians who still doubt your sanity.

In this era, HMO's tell people what diseases they can have, how long they can have them, and what treatments they can have. And all diseases seem to be deficiencies of drugs, for that is how they are all treated. It is as though arthritis were an Advil deficiency. This book arms you with the ammunition to defend your right to find the causes, get rid of symptoms and drugs, and get reimbursed for it by your insurance company.

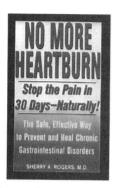

No More Heartburn

The chance of healing any condition in the body is slim to none until the gut is healthy first. Heartburn, indigestion, irritable bowel, spastic colon, colitis, gall bladder disease, gas and bloating are far from benign, for they are all signs of an ailing gastro-intestinal tract. And disease and death began in the gut.

Learn how the many prescription and over-the-counter drugs guarantee that you will not only have worse gut symptoms eventually, but that you can pile on new symptoms, seemingly unrelated to the gut, within the next few years like arthritis, heart problems or cancer.

Come learn how to find the many hidden causes of symptoms like food allergies, Candida overgrowth, Helicobacter, leaky gut, nutrient deficiencies, toxic environment and thoughts, and more. Then learn how to use non-prescription remedies to heal, not merely mask every symptom from mouth to rectum.

Since the gut houses over half the immune system and over half the detoxification system, a silently ailing gut holds back healing any condition indefinitely. This book is also full of new non-prescription Candida and other yeast fighters and protocols, since this is a common unsuspected cause of many diseases.

Learn how heartburn masked with drugs is a fast road to a heart attack or cancer, chronic fatigue, chronic pain or fibromyalgia. Explicit clear directions are given for every gut symptom, their causes and cures. For an unhealthy gut is a primary reason for many folks to be stuck at a standstill, unable to heal any further. **If your healing is stalled, chances are you need to start healing the gut first.** You need to heal from the inside out, for **the road to health is paved with good intestines.** (Over 350 references)

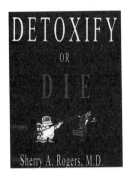

Detoxify or Die

If you don't own this book, you're missing out on the most surefire and thoroughly documented way to heal the impossible and reverse aging, regardless of how "stuck" you might feel. Environmental toxins are ubiquitous, impossible to escape. For example, the phthalates from plastic wrap of foods to Styrofoam trays and cups, plastic bottles for water, soda, juices and infant formula leach into our foods. Once inside our bodies they can create any disease and indefinitely stall the chemistry of healing. EPA studies show this pollutant is in every person and is thousands of times more plentiful than the hundreds of other environmental toxins that insidiously stockpile in the body; taking sometimes decades to produce disease seemingly overnight. Luckily there are a multitude of ways to boost your body's ability to detoxify them, starting with the *Detox Cocktail* that you can make at home every day.

Our lifetime accumulation of pesticides, volatile organic hydrocarbons, heavy metals and more contribute to every disease and symptom. The most exciting part is the proof that **getting rid of environmental toxins reverses diseases for which medicine claims there is no known cause and no known cure!** Contrast this with medicine's solution that consists of a lifetime sentencing to costly medications with a laundry list of side effects. Once you peel away the underlying causes the body is able to heal itself and disease melts away, as scientific studies in leading medical journals from the Mayo Clinic, for example, clearly prove. **Detoxification is equally crucial for the addicted individual trying to get free from alcohol or addiction to prescription or street drugs.** This is the most thorough program for medical detoxification, including detoxification for folks with infertility and parents-to-be, showing you how to do it safely at home, avoiding the pitfalls. The Resources chapter is complete with where to find everything in this book, 1-800 numbers, addresses, web sites and more, plus over 700 complete scientific references. If you buy only one book this year, make it *Detoxify or Die.*

Total Wellness Newsletter

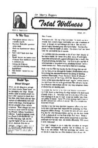

For over a decade and a half, this referenced monthly newsletter has kept folks and physicians up to date on new findings. Since Dr. Rogers is constantly researching, lecturing around the globe, maintaining a private practice of 38 years, doing television and radio shows, writing for health magazines and physicians, and has published over 20 scientific papers and over 15 books in 20 years, she is pedaling as fast as she can.

There is literally an avalanche of new information, but we don't want you to have to wait for a new book on the subject to learn about it or worse, wait decades for it to reach the media or your doctor. We want that practical and useful instruction in your hands this month.

Furthermore, the field of environmental medicine, because it is so all encompassing, can be overwhelming at times. So in addition to bringing you the new, we also focus on the overall perspective and the practical solutions you can do today.

In this era, because we cannot get the information out to you fast enough, we use the newsletter as our communication link. By sending you to the medical school of the future each month, *Total Wellness* will teach you useful facts years before they will be presented elsewhere, and it is practical and action-oriented, giving you explicit directions and sources. For pennies a day you really cannot afford to be without this life-altering unique information.

We continually receive kind letters that read, "I had to laugh last week when all the newspapers and television shows were abuzz with that hot new medical discovery. If they had been readers of your newsletter, they could have learned about it 10 years ago, as I did!"

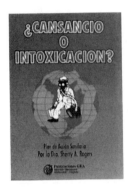

Cansancio o Intoxicacion?
(Tired or Toxic? in Spanish)

El lego informado reconoce que a medida que el mundo se vuelve más tecnológico, el hombre pierde proporcionalmente más control sobre su vida. Este libro le permitirá recuperar el control de su salud, ofreciéndole mayor capacidad para formar equipo con su medico para diagnosticar y tratar su condición.

Esta información es vitalmente importante ahora ya que a todos toca con cualquier síntoma tal como la sensibilidad química, alto colesterol, fatiga crónica, complejo relacionado a Cándida, depresion, Alzheimer, hipertensión, diabetes, enfermedad cardíaca, osteoporosis y más.

Dra. Rogers se encuentra en la avanazada de la educación pública sobre los efectos del medio ambiente en el individuo.

Otros libros escritos por Dra. Rogers que tienen que ver con prevenir enfermedades y restablecer la salud son **Eres lo que Has Comido, El Síndrome de E.A.,** y **La Cura Se Encuentra En La Cocina:** La Fase Curativa Estricta de la Dieta Macrobiotica.

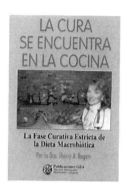

La Fase Curativa Estricta de
la Dieta Macrobiótica

Por la Dra. Sherry A. Rogers

La Cura Se Encuentra En La Cocina
(*The Cure is in the Kitchen* in Spanish)

Este libro explora la relación entre dieta, medio ambiente, salud, y enfermedad y explica como la dieta macrobiótica, basada en cereales integrales, porotos y sus productos y otros alimentos naturales integrales puede prevenir enfermedades y restablecer la salud.

Nos explica cómo una dieta muy artificial contribuye a una variedad de problemas de salud y cómo ciertos aspectos de la vida moderna también nos pueden debilitar.

Un programa macrobiótico consiste de dos fases; pasar gradualmente a una dieta macrobótica o ponerse en una fase curativa estricta de carácter temporario. El objectivo de la fase curativa de esta dieta es aclarar una condición en particular. Es necesariamente, muy estricta e individualizada, y por eso razón, la persona debe consultar un doctor entrenado en la macrobiótica.

Otros libros escritos por Dra. Rogers que tienen que ver con prevenir enfermedades y restablecer la salud son **Cansancio o Intoxicación?, Eres lo que Has Comido,** y **El Síndrome de E.A.**

Mold Plates: An Investment in Your Future Health

Mold is unavoidably ubiquitous and an unsuspected cause of many illnesses, whether common, "incurable" or mysterious. In fact one reason why many insurance companies deny coverage for mold-related damage now may be in part because it can mimic any symptoms you can name. We used to think of just mold as a cause of only typical allergic symptoms like post nasal drip, sinusitis, migraines, headaches, dizziness, ringing in the ears, recurrent soar throats, exhaustion, burning eyes, itchy eyes, bronchitis, asthma, chronic cough, eczema, hives, and more. But now colitis, arthritis, depression, schizophrenia, learning disorders, rare neurologic problems, and even behavior mimicking brain injury can be added to the list of mold mimics.

Since mold is a common, yet remedial cause of symptoms, you first need to know if you have too much. By exposing special petri dishes (or mold plates) in your bedroom, family room, and office, you have effectively assessed your 24-hour mold environment.

Each plate comes with directions for exposure and as well as instructions to enable you to assess the amount of mold contamination you have. You'll need to order one plate for each room you want to assess at home or work.

You may have an air filter that is not removing sufficient mold, or a home structural problem with hidden leaks contributing to sustained mold levels. A mold plate with a special agar that yields 30% more growth can demonstrate this. Since mold is not static, but constantly growing, you may need to periodically assess the contribution it is making to your environment, symptoms and life.

If you do not know how many molds is in your environment, you may erroneously be attributing symptoms to chemical or food sensitivities or just settling for "It's undiagnosable and untreatable". It is always best to meet the unseen enemy head on to optimally identify the cause of the problem and to be able to solve it, once and for all.

Personal Phone Consultations with Dr. Rogers

Many people are stuck. They have an undiagnosable condition. Or they have a label but have been unable to get well. Or they have a "dead-end" label that means nothing more can be done. And many are not able to find a physician who is trained in what our books explore, and need for example, help in interpreting their state-of-the art laboratory results.

These people could benefit from a personal consultation with Dr. Sherry Rogers, M.D. to explore what diagnostic and treatment options may exist that they or their physicians are not aware of. For this reason we offer prepaid, scheduled phone consultations with the doctor. Call the office, 315-488-2856 for more information.

If you wish to send copies of your medical reports and/or also have your doctor or spouse on the line, this can be helpful as well. Reports must be received at least 3 weeks prior to the consult and not be on fax paper. They should be copies and not originals as they are not returnable. Do not send records without first having secured a scheduled appointment time, for records without an appointment are discarded. Many elect to have their spouse or physician on the line with them.

Because you have not come to the office and been examined, you are not considered a patient. In spite of that, you can learn what tests your physician could order, and what plans you could follow. If he needs help in interpreting the tests, a scheduled follow-up consultation can allow you to explore treatment options with specific nutrient and other treatment suggestions. The point is, you do not have to be alone without guidance in your quest for wellness. And you owe it to yourself to explore the options that you might otherwise never even have heard of.

Price List

Books

The Cholesterol Hoax	$23.95
The High Blood Pressure Hoax	$19.95
Detoxify or Die	$22.95
Depression Cured At Last!	$24.95
The E.I. Syndrome Revised	$17.95
Tired or Toxic?	$18.95
Chemical Sensitivity (booklet)	$ 3.95
You Are What You Ate	$12.95
The Cure Is In The Kitchen	$14.95
Macro Mellow	$12.95
Wellness Against All Odds	$17.95
The Scientific Basis for Environmental Medicine Techniques	$17.95
No More Heartburn	$15.00
Pain-Free In 6 Weeks	$19.95

Spanish Translations

Cansancio o Intoxicacion?	$30.00
La Cura Se Encuentra En La Cocina .	$30.00

Total Wellness Newsletter

Monthly referenced newsletter on current wellness and healing information

Current 1 year subscription (12 issues, 8 pages, referenced)	$54.00
Back issues/1 year (12 issues)	$36.00
Individual back issues	$ 8.00

Services

Mold Plates (one room)	$25.00

Phone Consultations

Telephone consultations are available with Dr. Rogers. For scheduling information, contact Dr. Rogers' office at (315) 488-2856.

Index

Beta-glucans, 229, 230
Bile, 16, 17, 18, 51, 55, 77, 85, 93, 103, 122, 123, 126, 138, 164, 166, 167, 171, 175, 185, 261, 262, 280, 291, 307
Bile acid sequestrant, 16
Biotin, 260, 286, 385
Birth deformities, 11
Blindness, 185, 187, 218, 280, 317
Blood pressure, high, 6, 9, 11, 21, 23, 29, 106, 140, 141, 163, 182, 270, 271, 280, 302, 314, 316
Boluoke, see Lumbrokinase
BPA, 302, 303
Bufferin, 67

C

Cadmium, 116, 160, 236, 259, 267, 295, 308, 311, 318, 324, 327, 334, 363
Calcifications, arterial vascular, 253
Calcium Channel Blockers, 11, 48, 76, 104, 281, 313, 333
Calcium channels, 12, 48, 104, 164, 281, 311, 313
Calcium pumps, 11, 21
Calcium score, 96, 108, 109, 110, 151, 169, 228, 348, 382
Cancer, 1, 4, 5, 6, 7, 10, 14, 17, 18, 19, 22, 23, 24, 27, 29, 31, 33, 34, 37, 47, 49, 58, 61, 63, 64, 66, 67, 68, 70, 77, 79, 83, 90, 91, 92, 101, 102, 106, 111, 112, 116, 118, 126, 129, 133, 134, 135, 136, 155, 156, 157, 166, 170, 174, 175, 177, 179, 181, 182, 183, 189, 193, 197, 200, 211, 212, 214, 221, 229, 239, 242, 254, 255, 256, 258, 273, 274, 275, 276, 277, 280, 287, 288, 297, 298, 300, 304, 306, 309, 314, 318, 321, 322, 324,
325, 335, 337, 340, 366, 367, 368, 374
Cancer, breast, 1, 36, 87, 111, 112, 183, 198, 202, 319, 340, 379
Cancer, metastatic, 160, 171, 179, 322
Cancer, metastatic end-stage, 117
Cancer, prostate, 160, 204, 208, 309, 318, 320
Cancer, stage IV metastatic lung, 187
Cancers, 7, 11, 13, 21, 54, 57, 68, 101, 111, 117, 118, 120, 134, 146, 161, 178, 187, 188, 245, 251, 275, 284, 288, 292, 300, 304, 305, 309, 322, 335, 356, 361, 366, 367
Cancers, prostate and breast, 300, 302
Candida, 49, 145, 180, 213, 214, 224, 228, 231, 233, 234, 265, 274, 281, 283
Capillaries, 163, 165
Captomer, 327, 338, 385
Carbonic anhydrase, 258
Cardiac, sudden death, 39, 143, 203, 208, 366
Cardio/ION Panel, 29, 47, 57, 58, 64, 95, 114, 115, 122, 129, 131, 137, 148, 149, 151, 158, 169, 180, 196, 217, 219, 235, 247, 252, 259, 260, 261, 262, 266, 279, 283, 285, 286, 319, 328, 329, 334, 335, 338, 348, 356, 371, 377, 382, 383, 384, 385, 386
Cardiomyopathy, 29, 36, 163, 284, 287, 314
Carnitine, 123, 124, 162, 208, 209, 280, 283, 354, 358, 378
Catalase, 300, 313
Chelation, rectal, 341

I

J

Reactive oxygen species, 93, 167, 272, 274, 276, 277
Red Yeast Rice, 45, 46, 47, 48, 49, 50, 53, 79, 82, 83, 113
Redifferentiation, 5
Register, federal, 154
Regression, 36, 48, 64, 82, 93, 95, 96, 101, 110, 167, 278, 355
Replacements, hip or knee, 54, 106
Replacements, joint, 298
Rhabdomyolysis, 3, 14, 17, 20, 43, 48, 99, 112, 119
Rheumatoid arthritis, 237, 298
R-Lipoic Acid, 132, 151, 226, 235, 382, 384
Roberts, Dr. James, 330, 353, 358, 380
ROS, 167, 272, 274, 275, 276

S

Saccharomyces boullardii, 223
Salmon, farmed, 161, 208
Salmon, wild, 150, 161, 177, 208
SAMe, 282
Sauna, Far Infrared, 323, 338, 383, 385
Schizophrenia, 44, 77, 366
Selenium, 15, 76, 266, 273, 275, 276, 283, 284, 313, 363
Silicon, 297
Sinatra, Dr. Stephen, 162, 353, 358, 380
Smoke detector, 115, 174
SOD, super oxide dismutase, 72, 147, 175, 276, 316, 338, 385
Soy, ploy, 198
Spasm, arteial wall, 269
Spirituality, 369, 373, 374
Stage fright, 102
Stenosis (plugging), 59, 87, 110, 205, 208, 379
Stents, 39, 109, 128, 332, 333, 344, 350, 379

Stool, Comprehensive, 233, 235, 384
Strobel, Lee, 373
Stroke, hemorrhagic, 27, 89
Strokes, 12, 24, 52, 67, 127, 146, 181, 248, 312, 361
Sugar, 9, 44, 75, 131, 156, 161, 176, 182, 186, 187, 189, 263, 264, 265, 303, 304, 309, 356
Suicide, 4, 7, 15, 21, 22, 33, 38, 91, 92, 101, 102, 120, 121, 136, 258, 372
Super 2 Daily, 30, 31, 79, 81, 381, 382
Syndrome X, 9, 76, 132, 156, 264, 299, 304
Syndrome, metabolic, 9, 115, 132, 147, 156, 299, 314, 345
Sytrinol, 73, 74, 80, 88, 381

T

Taurine, 33, 123, 124, 280, 281, 282, 283, 290, 339
Tea, green, 175, 189, 201, 203
Teflon, 92, 93, 98, 116, 117, 118, 195, 295, 296, 297, 298, 299, 301, 324, 350
Tendon rupture, 13
Testosterone, 4, 114, 122, 129, 283, 299, 300, 328, 356, 364
The Power Hour, 12, 14, 386
Thyroid, 15, 68, 99, 103, 105, 128, 141, 236, 282, 299, 300, 302, 304, 311, 342, 344
TIA, transient ischemic attack, 12, 27, 32
Tingling, 9, 40, 43, 312
Tocopherols, 20, 47, 58, 61, 63, 65, 68, 72, 73
Tomography, computerized electron beam, 107
Tooth loss, 6, 29
Toprol-XL, 105, 126